AF615800

Fine Needle Aspiration Cytology and Its Clinical Applications
BREAST & LUNG

Fine Needle

and Its

Philip S. Feldman, MD
Associate Professor of Pathology and
Director of Cytology
University of Virginia Medical Center
Charlottesville, Virginia

Jamie L. Covell, BS, CT(ASCP)
Assistant Professor of Pathology (Cytology)
University of Virginia Medical Center
Charlottesville, Virginia

Aspiration Cytology

Clinical Applications

BREAST & LUNG

American Society of Clinical Pathologists Press
Chicago

Dedication
To our parents and children

Cover
Left: FNA smear showing tubular structures of tubular carcinoma in breast (see Plate 13, Figure 1). *Right*: FNA smear showing fungal hyphae that indicate the presence of mucormycosis in lung (see Plate 32, Figure 6).

Notice
Trade names for equipment and supplies described herein are included as suggestions only. In no way does their inclusion constitute an endorsement or preference by the American Society of Clinical Pathologists. The ASCP did not test the equipment, supplies, or procedures and, therefore, urges all readers to read and follow all manufacturers' instructions and package insert warnings concerning the proper and safe use of products.

Printed in the United States of America.
89 88 87 86 85 6 5 4 3 2 1

Library of Congress Cataloging in Publication Data

Feldman, Philip S., 1937-
Fine needle aspiration cytology and its clinical applications.

Includes bibliographical references and index.
1. Lungs—Biopsy, Needle. 2. Breast—Biopsy, Needle. 3. Diagnosis, Cytologic. I. Covell, Jamie L., 1946- II. Title. [DNLM: 1. Biopsy, Needle. 2. Breast Diseases—pathology. 3. Lung Diseases—pathology. WP 840 F312f]
RC734.B56F45 1985 616.07′582 84-11125
ISBN 0-89189-184-6
ISBN 0-89189-192-7 (text & slide set)

Contents

3 Technique and Interpretation *(continued)*

6 Illustrated Case Studies of Lung Diseases *(continued)*

Color Plates

Figures

Tables

Preface

In a 1934 report on needle aspiration cytology from Memorial Hospital for Cancer and Allied Diseases (Memorial Sloan-Kettering Cancer Center) in New York, Martin and Ellis stated that "knowing the source, knowing what tumors are apt to occur in the region, and being fully cognizant of the histologic criteria for the diagnosis of such tumors from ordinary sections, one may form, from the various minutiae of the smear, a sort of composite picture which permits visualization of the probable histologic process, and hence a diagnosis of the type of tumor." This principle was their basis for cytologic diagnosis by aspiration. It is interesting to note that the statement was made nine years before the publication of Papanicolaou's monograph, *The Diagnosis of Uterine Cancer,* which marked the advent of modern diagnostic cytology. Comparison of the cellular features and nuclear structure of the cells seen in smears with those seen in tissue sections has established the wealth of knowledge of diagnostic cell patterns for various benign and malignant diseases in the many body sites accessible by aspiration biopsy.

The primary objective of this atlas is to provide a wide range of illustrated diagnostic patterns for the interpretation of fine needle aspiration (FNA) cytology. The atlas also demonstrates the clinical applications and technique of FNA, and thereby, we hope, will promote more widespread understanding and use of this valuable diagnostic tool.

The material is presented in three parts. Part One contains detailed explanations and illustrations of FNA methods and processing of all cell samples. Parts Two and Three each contain an introduction to FNA of a particular body site and a description of normal cytology. This information is followed by illustrated case reports of various benign and malignant disorders selected to illustrate the expected, as well as variant, cytologic patterns of these disorders, as diagnosed by FNA. The case presentations include clinical histories, patient photographs, and roentgenograms, as well as photomicrographs of the cytologic smears and their histologic counterparts. The cases described were seen at the University of Virginia Medical Center, unless otherwise noted.

The text for each section contains detailed descriptions of the cytologic material and concludes with a list of appropriate references. The body areas to be covered are breast and lung.

Numbering System

Due to the complexity of the book, we would like to draw your attention to the numbering system used for color plates and black and white figures. The black and white figures illustrating general breast and lung fine needle aspiration technique have been numbered consecutively throughout the book with arabic numerals (Figure 1, Figure 2, etc.). The color plates corresponding to certain case reports are numbered from Plate 1 to Plate 51, each section of the color plate has its own arabic numeral, resulting in a double-numbering system for the color plates (Plate 1–1 to 1–10, etc.). There are black and white figures that correspond to certain color plates and case reports. These have been designated by letter (Figure A, Figure B, etc.), and begin with the letter "A" for each separate color plate.

An Optional Slide Set of 100 color slides (transparencies) is available. The slides correspond to selected sections of the plates. Each slide is cross-referenced to the appropriate color plate and section in the "Key to Optional Slide Set" and to the color plate alone in the "Cross-Reference for Optional Slide Set." The slides corresponding to a case study are listed immediately after it.

This visual format is designed to provide pathologists, cytotechnologists, cytotechnology students, and clinicians with a readily usable reference in the application and interpretation of FNA.

Acknowledgments

The completion of this atlas could have been accomplished only with assistance from many sources. Our first thanks must go to William J. Frable, MD, of the Medical College of Virginia (Richmond), who introduced us to fine needle aspiration (FNA) cytology. Dr. Frable, in our opinion, has contributed greatly to the revitalization of this technique in the United States during the past decade. Dr. Frable's philosophy, like that of the Swedes, is to have the same person perform the FNA as well as interpret the specimen. We followed his example and our experience has confirmed this as a sound principle. We thank him for guiding us in this direction. Throughout the years, he has shared his expertise and expanded our knowledge and interpretive ability of FNA. While in the process of completing his own textbook on FNA, he encouraged our concept of a color atlas on FNA and shared many of his interesting cases. In addition, we were able, along with Dr. Frable, and David Kaminsky, MD, of the Eisenhower Medical Center, Rancho Mirage, CA, to participate jointly in many workshop presentations and benefit greatly from these experiences.

At the University of Virginia Medical Center there are numerous individuals whose support and encouragement contributed significantly to the success of FNA in our institution. Within our Department of Pathology, we would like to acknowledge Thomas W. Tillack, MD, Department Chairman, and Robert E. Fechner, MD, Director of Surgical Pathology, for their financial backing and confidence in the FNA technique during this study; and to Dieter Gröschel, MD, for the many hours spent tracking down and translating the German-language articles for us. We express a very special thanks to Mrs. Petronella Oostingh, CT(ASCP), Mohamed Ihsan, CT(ASCP), the other cytotechnologists, the pathology residents and fellows, and the laboratory technicians in our cytology laboratory for their assistance in the performance, preparation, and screening of the FNA material. We are indebted to Ms. Tawana Drumheller for her secretarial expertise and many hours spent in preparation of this manuscript.

We are especially thankful to colleagues in the Department of Radiology for their cooperation. Most notably is Peter Armstrong, MD, who performed the lung FNAs under guidance by fluoroscopy and computerized tomography. The breast aspirates that were performed under mammographic guidance were done by Marc Read, MD. In the Department of Surgery we extend gratitude to Harold J. Wanebo, MD, Morton C. Wilhelm, MD, and George R. Minor, MD, for their faith in the efficacy of FNA and for the encouragement of its use.

The success of any atlas is dependent upon the excellence of its illustrations. We express sincere appreciation to the Department of Medical Art and Photography for their efforts and skill in the production of all artwork and black and white photographs. In particular we acknowledge Mrs. Ursula Bunch, Mr. Michael Pittard, Mrs. Patricia Pugh, and Mr. Craig Harding. The color plates were produced from Cibachrome (Ilford Inc, West 70 Century Rd, PO Box 288, Paramus, NJ 07652) prints made from Kodachrome (Eastman Kodak Co, Rochester, NY 14650) slides. All Kodachrome photomicrographs were taken by the authors and the outstanding Cibachrome prints were produced by Richmond Camera, Inc., and by Mr. John Stubblefield.

We wish to acknowledge the following contributors of FNA cases and color plates: William J. Frable, MD, Richmond, VA (Plates 13, 16, 22); William

Clark, MD, and Richard Otis, MD, Hartford, CT (Plate 28); David Kaminsky, MD, Rancho Mirage, CA (Plate 15); Richard Marshall, MD, Winston-Salem, NC (Plate 47); Marianna Masin, MD, and Francis Masin, MD, Santa Barbara, CA (Plate 24); Theodore Miller, MD, San Francisco (Plate 6); Yolanda Oertel, MD, Washington, DC (Plate 4); and J. Michael Perry, MD, Lynchburg, VA (Plate 45).

We appreciate the opportunity given us by the American Society of Clinical Pathologists to produce this atlas. Their patience and understanding throughout this endeavor has been unfailing. The quality of their reproduction of our color plates, no simple task, is superb. We found their suggestions and critique most helpful.

On a personal note (PSF), I want to thank my family. My parents, Sam and Nellie Feldman, provided me opportunities and unfailing encouragement throughout my life. To my children, Robert and Rene, I offer my apologies for the time I was unable to spend with you during the completion of this atlas. To my sister, Gloria F. Keeb, OD, many thanks for both the translations you provided and the support you gave me. To my wife, Sallie, I am grateful for your editorial assistance, your understanding, and moral support.

Two of my former teachers with whom it was a privilege and honor to study also have my deepest gratitude. Averill A. Liebow, MD, introduced me to pathology. Indeed it was the fundamentals of lung pathology acquired under his tutelage that have enabled me now to better understand lung aspirates. Lauren V. Ackerman, MD, is another individual for whom I have great respect and admiration. While training under him and later working with him at Washington University in St. Louis, I came to know a great man. Besides his valuable lessons in surgical pathology and medicine, he has enriched my life in many personal ways. It would be impossible to fully thank these two men for all they have done for me, and any expression of gratitude would be an understatement.

My personal thanks (JLC) go first to my family, especially to my parents, James and Rylma Covell. They have always given me support and encouragement through all my endeavors. On a professional level I express my gratitude to Nelson D. Holmquist, MD, and Yolande Hutson, CT(ASCP), who first introduced me to the field of cytopathology and provided my educational basis in the field.

As anyone who has ever attempted to write a book knows, it is a long, painstaking experience. We are grateful to all the people mentioned here. Our dream of publishing this atlas could not have been realized without their help and the love of our families.

PART ONE

Overview of Fine Needle Aspiration Cytology

1

Introduction

History

The technique of needle aspiration dates back to the nineteenth century.[1–4] Pravaz, in 1853, developed a metallic syringe used originally for the treatment of aneurysms and vascular diseases and subsequently for subcutaneous injections.[1] In 1882, Günther used a Pravaz syringe for a transthoracic needle aspiration to obtain organisms from a patient with a pneumonic lung.[2] Six months later, Leyden performed a lung puncture and aspirated organisms to diagnose pneumonia.[2] In 1884, Krönig was the first to diagnose lung cancer by means of a lung aspiration.[3] Ménétrier, in 1886, also diagnosed lung carcinoma by aspirating tissue through a transthoracically inserted cannula.[4] Additional reports of lung aspirations followed towards the end of the nineteenth century.[5]

In 1904, Greig and Gray performed aspirations of lymph nodes to isolate the causative agent of trypanosomiasis.[6] Ten years later, Ward noted that cells obtained by lymph node aspirations might aid in the diagnosis of lymphoblastoma.[7] In the same year, Chatard and Guthrie reported a case of trypanosomiasis diagnosed by lymph node aspiration.[8] In 1921, Guthrie reported his results with aspirations using a 21-gauge needle and syringe.[9] He successfully diagnosed cases of syphilis, tuberculosis, malignant lymphoma, leukemia, and metastatic carcinoma by needle aspirations. In 1926 Martin and Ellis, at Memorial Hospital for Cancer and Allied Diseases (Memorial Sloan-Kettering Cancer Center) in New York, began performing aspiration biopsies using an 18-gauge needle attached to a record syringe. Four years later, they reported their findings from 65 malignant tumors and are credited with introducing the needle aspiration biopsy technique.[10] By 1934, their experience with aspiration biopsies had expanded to 1,400 cases.[11] Ochsner and DeBakey stated, in 1939, that lung aspirations were "useful, relatively safe and fairly accurate."[12] The future of needle aspirations appeared most promising.

However, in 1947, Ochsner and DeBakey condemned this procedure because they had seen three patients in whom tumor implants had occurred along the site of the needle puncture.[13] They concluded that this procedure should not be used in operable patients. Their criticism was unfounded since 18-gauge needles were used in their three cases with implants, and not fine (22-gauge) needles. Although their criticism was applicable to the large bore cutting needles (18-gauge) used at that time, it has been proved invalid with the current use of the small bore needles (22-gauge). Similarly, others strongly denounced needle biopsies because of the fear of implants.[14–19] Although this resulted in a sharp decline in the use of needle aspirations in the United States, needle aspirations continued to be performed at Memorial Hospital. Godwin, in 1956, reported that about 2,500 aspirations were performed annually at that center.[20] Unfortunately, needle aspirations performed in the United States were largely confined to that hospital. An extensive discussion of the reasons for the decline of FNA in the United States is contained in an article by Cecil Fox, MD,[21] and an editorial by Leopold Koss, MD, on thin needle aspiration biopsy.[22]

Fine needle aspiration (FNA) was introduced to Sweden in 1951. This procedure was enthusiastically accepted, and the number of FNAs performed per year rose precipitously to 12,285 aspirations in 1972.[23] This figure is impressive when one considers that the Radiumhemmet, the oncologic division of the Karolinska Institute in Stockholm, at that time had 150 beds and about 60,000 outpatient visits per year.[23] The technique of needle aspirations in Sweden differed significantly from the procedure introduced by Martin and Ellis. Instead of an 18-gauge cutting needle, Franzen and Zajicek used a 22-gauge fine needle. With this smaller needle, no anesthetic was given to patients having FNA of palpable lesions. Another significant change was that the person who performed the FNA usually interpreted the smears as well. By contrast, at Memorial Hospital, surgeons performed the aspirations and pathologists interpreted the smears.

Monographs on FNA published by Lopes Cardozo,[24] Soderstrom,[25] and Dahlgren and Nordenström[5] helped establish this technique in the Netherlands and Scandinavia. During this period, reports by Franzen and Zajicek[26] from the Radiumhemmet and by Zajdela et al[27] from the Foundation-Curie Institute in France on large series of breast needle aspiration cases further documented the efficacy and accuracy of the procedure. The experiences from these centers reawakened interest in FNA. Subsequently, numerous series were reported in the United States emphasizing the merits of FNA.[28–36] The American Society of Cytology and the American Society of Clinical Pathologists sponsored numerous workshops and presentations on FNA to promote the technique and to educate pathologists and cytologists in its advantages.

Advantages

Fine needle aspiration is essentially a type of needle biopsy to sample material from palpable or roentgenographically visible lesions using a thin needle (outside diameter, 0.6 to 0.9 mm) with negative pressure supplied by an attached syringe. This type of biopsy obtains cellular material for cytologic examination, rather than a segment of tissue. The FNA technique is very different from a cutting needle (14-gauge) biopsy, which obtains a core of tissue for histologic examination. It is important not to confuse FNA with cutting needle biopsies when discussing the advantages of needle biopsy. Considerable criticism of FNA in the literature resulted from the failure to realize this difference.[13] A comparison of these two techniques for needle biopsy explains the striking contrast in results.

Because of the small diameter of the needle used for FNA, the needle can be moved in a back-and-forth motion and in different directions. This ease of movement allows material from different parts of the tumor to be sampled and greatly increases the chances of obtaining material that will accurately represent the tumor's pathology. In contrast, a cutting needle biopsy may, in its single pass, push a small, nonfixed mass aside and miss the target (Figure 1). Thus, FNA may yield the diagnosis when cutting needle biopsy fails. This was exemplified by 23 cases we observed in our hospital during a four-year period. In these cases, FNA results provided the definitive diagnosis whereas negative results were obtained by either cutting needle (15 cases) or open biopsies (eight cases). Fine needle aspiration of the breast (two), liver (two), retroperitoneum (three), lung (three), bone (five), lymph nodes (four), thyroid (two), pelvis (one), and rectum (one) were included in this series.

Results from cutting needle biopsies in the two cases involving the breast were negative and were followed by FNA findings diagnostic of carcinoma. Mastectomies confirmed the FNA findings. Results from cutting needle hepatic biopsies in two cases with suspected metastases were negative. The presence of metastatic lesions was confirmed in both cases using ultrasound-directed FNA of the liver. Retroperitoneal masses in two cases were initially approached by exploratory laparotomy with open biopsies, but no cancer was diagnosed. Results from subsequent ultrasound-directed FNA in one case showed the presence of a malignant tumor, possibly seminoma. Examination of the patient's scrotum and an orchiectomy confirmed the presence of a seminoma not suspected before the FNA. Computerized axial tomography scan-directed FNA of the right psoas muscle in another case showed a sarcoma. Exploratory laparotomy showed a retroperitoneal lesion, and biopsied tissue specimens were interpreted as retroperitoneal fibrosis. However, a repeat laparotomy six months later confirmed the FNA diagnosis of sarcoma. An example of a neck lesion "miss" was a patient with a thyroid mass, who previously had a laryngectomy due to squamous cell carcinoma. Results of thyroid FNA showed metastatic squamous cell carcinoma. An open biopsy of the thyroid was performed and on frozen section, the specimen showed no carcinoma. However, permanent sections and deeper levels did contain squamous cell carcinoma.

Shabot et al reported a prospective study on 81 patients with clinically suspicious breast masses.[37] They compared the diagnostic accuracy of physical examination, mammography, cutting needle biopsy, and FNA. Clinical diagnoses were correct in 85% (3% false-negative, 13% false-positive) and mammography was diagnostic in 53% (32% false-nega-

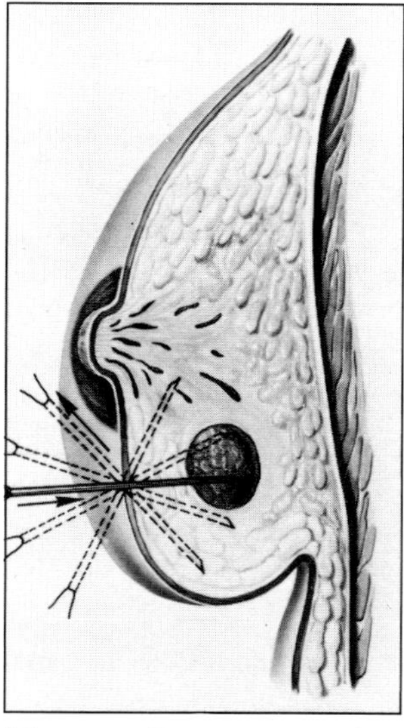
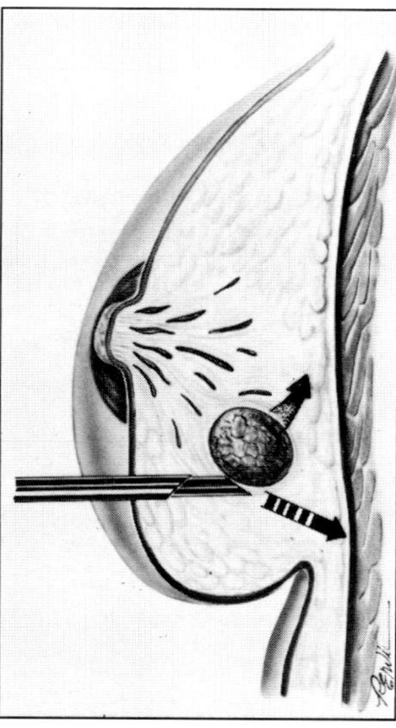

Figure 1. Comparison of FNA technique to that used for needle biopsy. *Left:* Note the small diameter of the needle used in FNA (0.6 to 0.9 mm, outside diameter). The needle can be moved in a back and forth motion and in different directions. *Right:* In contrast, biopsy needle (14-gauge, approximately 2.0 mm, outside diameter) may push small, nonfixed mass aside in its single pass, and miss target.

tive, 16% false-positive). Results of cutting needle biopsies were accurate in 79% (21% false-negative, 0% false-positive), and FNA results were diagnostic in 96% (4% false-negative, 0% false-positive) of the cases studied. They concluded that FNA was superior to cutting needle biopsies to establish the diagnosis of clinically suspicious breast masses.

Ho et al studied a group of 40 patients with suspected malignant disease of the liver by FNA.[38] They also obtained cutting needle biopsies of the liver in 24 of these patients. In this study, 16 patients had a final diagnosis of hepatic malignancy. Results of the FNAs were positive in 14 cases (87%), and those of cutting needle biopsies were positive in only four (25%). They found that radiographically guided FNA of the liver was diagnostically superior to cutting needle biopsies.

Rapidly escalating medical costs perhaps contributed to a renewed interest in FNA in the United States. A comparison of the expenses resulting from FNA versus conventional surgical biopsy disclosed a considerable cost benefit in favor of FNA.[39,40] Kaminsky investigated these differences at the Eisenhower Medical Center in California and found that FNA can be performed at 10% to 30% of the cost of a conventional biopsy procedure.[39] The cost of FNA is minimal, especially when compared with alternative procedures such as laparotomy and thoracotomy.[39,40]

The equipment for FNA is inexpensive and the technique, simple. Technical considerations of the actual aspiration procedure, slide preparation, and staining techniques are discussed in detail in chapter 2 and in the introductions for parts two and three.

A significant advantage of FNA is the rapidity of diagnostic results. The duration of FNA varies according to the site, and is longer when radiologic guidance (fluoroscopy, ultrasound, and computerized axial tomography) is used. Once the needle is in the correct position, the actual aspiration takes less than two minutes, and the aspirated material can be processed and interpreted with a definitive diagnosis within 10 to 15 minutes. If the material obtained from the FNA is insufficient, the aspiration can be repeated immediately. This contrasts strikingly with conventional cutting biopsies where the tissue sample obtained requires approximately 24 hours for processing before being available for interpretation.

Another advantage of FNA is that the patient experiences minimal discomfort during the procedure even though a local anesthetic usually is used only for radiographically guided aspirations.

The most significant advantage of FNA is the high degree of accuracy possible with the procedure. Numerous reported series have clearly documented that excellent results can be achieved with FNA of multiple body sites: breast,[26–30] lung,[29,31–36,41] lymph nodes,[28,42–44] prostate,[45–47] liver,[38,48,49] pancreas,[50–53] kidney,[54–56] thyroid,[57–59] bone,[60,61] and brain.[62] The degree of accuracy depends on the following: site of the aspiration; the size, location, and nature of the lesion; and the experience and skill of the person performing and interpreting the FNA. We observed greater accuracy in our hospital when the pathologist performed the aspiration as well as interpreted the material obtained. Others have had similar experiences.[23,26,28] For example, aspirations from the neck and oral cavity showed a statistically significant difference between the unsatisfactory (insufficient material for a diagnosis) rate achieved by the cytopathologist, 6% (10/158) and by others (noncytopathologists), 15% (11/71), ($P < .05$).[63]

During the developmental years of FNA, errors in technique and interpretation were not infrequent and contributed significantly to false-positive and false-negative diagnoses.[5,64–67] However, as experience with FNA increased, the percentage of false-positive and false-negative diagnoses decreased concomitantly. False-positive diagnoses are a rarity today in lung FNA[28,29,31–36,68] and breast FNA.[26–38,30] To clinicians, an FNA report positive for malignancy indicates that there is definitive cytologic evidence of malignancy and that they may proceed directly to therapy (surgery, radiation) without additional biopsy confirmation, for example, frozen section. This practice is not new and has been used in certain European centers for more than 10 years and more recently in the United States.[26–28,30,39,69,70]

Knowledge of the disease process before initiation of therapy, particularly surgery, is a distinct advantage to both patient and clinician. The patient can be informed of the diagnosis, can participate in the decision on methods of therapy, and can mentally prepare for any subsequent procedures, for example, mastectomy. For the surgeon, appropriate preoperative staging for metastases can be done; operating room time is shortened, as are the duration of the surgical procedure and the time that the patient is under anesthesia.

Fine needle aspiration is also very helpful in identification of the type of malignancy or benign disease. Results from reported series have shown that not only can a diagnosis of benign or malignant be made with great accuracy but usually the malignant cell type can be identified as well.[71] Recognition of the cell type is of critical importance because the histologic type of cancer plays a significant role in the choice of therapy. For example, if a patient with known extrathoracic malignancy develops a lung mass, FNA of the lung can frequently determine if the mass represents a metastasis, a new primary site, or an inflammatory process. Part three, "Fine Needle Aspiration of the Lung," includes many examples illustrating the use of FNA to identify the type of mass.

Complications

Complications resulting from FNA occur at a low rate, are frequently of a minor degree, and usually resolve spontaneously. The frequency and type of complications vary with the body site sampled (for example, breast versus lung), the procedure used for the FNA (such as guidance by fluoroscopy, ultrasound, and computerized axial tomography), the condition of the patient, and the experience of the physician performing and interpreting the FNA. The complications associated with FNA of specific organs will be discussed in detail in the appropriate parts of this atlas. For example, complications from breast FNA are rare;[26–28,36] complications of lung FNA are not.[29,31,33–35,41] However, the majority of these complications (for example, pneumothorax, hemoptysis) resolve without treatment.[33–35,41] Complications are very unusual when computerized tomography or ultrasound guidance is combined with percutaneous FNA for transabdominal aspirations.[29,72–75] Livraghi et al reviewed the literature for complications resulting from abdominal FNA in 11,700 patients and rarely found complications.[75] There was one death (0.008%) that was caused by necrotizing pancreatitis.[74] Six patients (0.05%) had major complications: one intrahepatic hematoma,[76] one peritonitis after abscess puncture,[77] two cases of bile peritonitis,[75,78] and two needle tract implants of pancreatic cancer.[72,73] In addition, 58 patients (0.49%) had less severe complications (pain, fever, hemorrhage, pancreatitis, hematuria, bacteremia).[75]

In our experience with over 200 transabdominal FNAs with computerized tomography or ultrasound guidance, no complications were encountered. In fact, when surgery was performed within days of the FNA, it was difficult and frequently impossible for the surgeon to identify the FNA puncture site. When one considers that during an FNA procedure, the needle may traverse several viscera and may even puncture major vessels, the very low rate of complications is remarkable. To study the effect of FNA on abdominal organs and the potential complications, Goldstein et al conducted an experimental study on dogs.[79] The dogs were anesthetized and several percutaneous biopsies, as well as biopsies directed into solid and hollow viscera, were performed. The FNA technique used was essentially the same as that for humans. Laparotomy at varying time intervals after the biopsies revealed no significant findings, and in most instances the needle biopsy site could not be identified.

Although the needle may traverse blood vessels, we observed no hemorrhagic complications even when major arteries were punctured (eg, carotid artery, abdominal aorta). Similarly, Lalli had needled the pulmonary artery and vein many times, the aorta, aortic aneurysm, the pericardium and the heart at least once with no resulting complications. The experience with translumbar aortograms also indicates that large vessels such as the aorta can be punctured safely with only a rare incidence of hemorrhage.[80]

Several major criticisms of FNA played a significant role in the slow acceptance of needle aspirations, particularly in the United States. Time and experience, however, have shown these criticisms to be invalid.[26–28,30,33–35,41,81–83] The foremost criticism of FNA was the fear of implanting tumor cells along the needle tract.[13–19] However, a search of the literature revealed only three cases of documented needle tract implants resulting from FNA.[72,73,84] Sinner and Zajicek noted a tumor implant at the site of a lung FNA that they had performed.[84] This was their only implant resulting from FNA of a series of 1,264 malignant lung tumors. No additional reports of implants from FNA of the lung have been reported.

Smith et al described cutaneous seeding of pancreatic cancer following FNA of the pancreas.[73] Ferrucci et al also found a subcutaneous implant after FNA of an unresectable carcinoma of the pancreas.[72] However, in their case, ten needle passes had been performed under computerized tomographic guidance. We agree with the authors who noted that "it may be prudent to restrict the number of needle passes to minimize the risk of needle tract implants." In contrast, there have been many reports of tumor implants following cutting needle biopsies. Body sites involved with cutting needle biopsy implants include the lung,[13–15,17] pleura,[85–87] liver,[88] thyroid,[19] prostate,[89–93] and parotid.[94]

Another concern was the risk of hematogenous spread of the cancer by FNA with resultant dissemination of the cancer and lower survival rates. However, studies on the survival of patients after FNA of malignancies of breast,[26,27,81,82] lung,[28,31–34,41] and kidney[56] failed to show a decrease in survival compared with control groups. Experimental studies by Engzell et al also failed to substantiate dissemination of tumor cells following FNA.[83]

Fatalities caused by needle biopsy have almost exclusively been due to cutting needles (14- and 18-gauge) and not the thin needles (22-gauge) used for FNA. We know of only one death resulting from a transthoracic FNA.[41] In this particular case the patient's death was technically preventable because he developed an unrecognized tension pneumothorax and died untreated. The only other reported fatality resulted from necrotizing pancreatitis following FNA of an enlarged normal pancreas.[74]

TABLE 1. Advantages of Fine Needle Aspiration

Accuracy
Diagnosis known to patient and surgeon/physician prior to surgery
Avoids unnecessary hospitalization, surgery, & other diagnostic procedures
Minimal complications
Minimal patient discomfort
Time
Low cost
Office/clinic/bedside procedure
Identification of benign versus malignant processes
Identification of type of malignancy
Detection of recurrence, new primary lesion, or metastasis

Summary

The effectiveness of FNA is well documented in the literature and reconfirmed in our experience. One further point should be emphasized in this discussion of FNA. For this technique to be successful, a close working relationship between the pathologist and clinician is essential. Communication between the clinician and the pathologist as to the patient's clinical history and physical findings contributes greatly to accurate interpretation of the cellular features in the FNA smear. The FNA diagnosis should be a definitive evaluation of the cytologic findings in conjunction with the clinical findings. The advantages of the technique are summarized in Table 1. These advantages explain the rebirth of FNA in this country and its extensive use throughout the world. It is fortunate that the renewed interest in FNA coincided with the advent of more sophisticated radiographic techniques, such as computerized axial tomography and ultrasound to guide placement of the needle. FNA is a diagnostic method of the present, and its uses as a routine diagnostic procedure will only increase in the future.

References

1. Pravaz C, Gabriel P: Sur un nouveau moyen d'operer la coagulation du sang dans les arteres applicable a la guerison des aneurismes. *Comptes rend. hebd. des seances de l'Acad. d. Sciences* 1853;56:88–90.

2. Leyden H: Ueber infectiose pneumonie. *Deutsch Med Wochnschr* 1883;9:52–54.

3. Krönig G: Diagnostischer Beitrag Zur Herz-und Lungen pathologie. *Berl Klin Wochnschr* 1887;24(51): 961–967.

4. Ménétrier P: Cancer primitif du Poumon. *Bull Soc Anat* (Paris) 1886;11:643.

5. Dahlgren SE, Nordenström B: *Transthoracic Needle Biopsy.* Stockholm, Almgvist & Wiltsell, 1966.

6. Greig EDW, Gray ACH: Note on the lymphatic glands in sleeping sickness. *Br Med J* 1904;1:1252.

7. Ward GR: *Bedside Hematology* Philadelphia, WB Saunders Co, 1914.

8. Chatard JA, Guthrie CG: Human trypanosomiasis. Report of a case observed in Baltimore. *Am J Trop Dis & Prev Med* 1914;1:493–503.

9. Guthrie CG: Gland puncture measure as a diagnostic puncture. *Bull Johns Hopkins Hosp* 1921;32:266–269.

10. Martin HE, Ellis, EB: Biopsy by needle puncture and aspiration. *Ann Surg* 1930;92:169–181.

11. Martin HE, Ellis EB: Aspiration biopsy. *Surg Gynecol Obstet* 1934;59:578–589.

12. Ochsner A, DeBakey M: Primary pulmonary malignancy. Treatment by total pneumonectomy. *Surg Gynecol Obstet* 1939;68:435–451.

13. Ochsner A, DeBakey M, Dixon JL: Primary cancer of the lung. *JAMA* 1947;135:321–327.

14. Allbritten FF Jr, Nealon T, Gibbon JH Jr, et al: The diagnosis of lung cancer. *S Clin North Am* 1952;32:1657.

15. Dutra R, Geraci C: Needle biopsy of the lung. *JAMA* 1954;155:21–24.

16. Aronovitch M, Chartier J, Kahana, LM, et al: Needle biopsy as an aid to the precise diagnosis of intrathoracic disease. *Can Med Assoc J* 1963;88:120–127.

17. Wolinsky H, Lischner MW: Needle track implanation of tumor after percutaneous lung biopsy. *Ann Int Med* 1969;71(2):359–362.

18. Schachter EN, Basta W: Subcutaneous metastasis of an adenocarcinoma following a percutaneous pleural biopsy. *Amer Rev Respir Dis* 1973;107:283–285.

19. Crile G, Jr, Vickery AL: Special uses of the Silverman biopsy needle in office practice and at operation. *Am J Surg* 1952;83:83–85.

20. Godwin JT: Aspiration biopsy. Technique and application. *Ann NY Acad Sci* 1956;63:1348–1373.

21. Fox CH: Innovation in medical diagnosis: The Scandinavian curiosity. *Lancet* 1979;1:1387–1388.

22. Koss LG: Thin needle aspiration biopsy, editorial. *Acta Cytol* 1980;24:1–3.

23. Zajicek J: *Aspiration Biopsy Cytology. Part 1: Cytology of Supradiaphragmatic Organs,* in Wied GL (ed): Monographs in Clinical Cytology, vol 4. New York, Karger 1974.

24. Lopes Cardozo P: *Clinical Cytology.* Leiden, Stafleu, 1954.

25. Soderstrom N: *Fine Needle Aspiration Biopsy.* Stockholm, Almgvist & Wiltsell, 1966.

26. Franzen S, Zajicek J: Aspiration biopsy in diagnosis of palpable lesions of the breast. Critical review of 3479 consecutive biopsies. *Acta Radiol* 1968;7: 241–262.

27. Zajdela A, Ghossein NA, Pilleron JP, et al: The value of aspiration cytology in the diagnosis of breast cancer: Experience at the Foundation Curie. *Cancer* 1975;35:499–506.

28. Frable WJ: *Thin Needle Aspiration Biopsy.* Philadelphia, WB Saunders Co, 1983.

29. Zornoza J (ed): *Percutaneous Needle Biopsy.* Baltimore, Williams & Wilkins Co, 1981.

30. Kern WH: The diagnosis of breast cancer by fine-needle aspiration smears. *JAMA* 1979;241:1125–1127.

31. Westcott JL: Direct percutaneous needle aspiration of localized pulmonary lesions. Results in 422 patients. *Radiology* 1980;137:31–35.

32. Jackson R, Coffin L, DeMeules J, et al: Percutaneous needle biopsy of pulmonary lesions. *Am J Surg* 1980;139:586–590.

33. Stitik F: Percutaneous lung biopsy, in Siegelman et al (eds): *Pulmonary System.* New York, Grune & Stratton, 1979, vol 1: *Multiple Imaging Procedures,* pp 181–219.

34. Sagel SS, Ferguson TB, Forrest JV, et al: Percutaneous transthoracic aspiration needle biopsy. *Ann Thorac Surg* 1978;26:399–405.

35. Lalli AF, McCormack LJ, Zelch M, et al: Aspiration biopsies of chest lesions. *Radiology* 1978;127:35–40.

36. Kline TS: *Handbook of Fine Needle Aspiration Biopsy Cytology.* St. Louis, Missouri, CV Mosby Co, 1981.

37. Shabot MM, Goldberg IM, Schick P, et al: Aspiration cytology is superior to tru-cut needle biopsy in establishing the diagnosis of clinically suspicious breast masses. *Ann Surg* 1982;196:122–126.

38. Ho CS, McLoughlin MJ, Tao LC, et al: Guided percutaneous fine-needle aspiration biopsy of the liver. *Cancer* 1981;47:1781–1785.

39. Kaminsky DB: *Aspiration Biopsy for the Community Hospital.* New York, Masson Publishing Co, 1981.

40. Frable, MA, Frable WJ: Fine-needle aspiration biopsy revisited. *Laryngoscope* 1982;92:1414–1418.

41. Sinner WN: Complications of percutaneous transthoracic needle aspiration biopsy. *Acta Radiol. Diag.* 1976;17:813–828.

42. Lopes Cardozo P: The cytologic diagnosis of lymph node punctures. *Acta Cytol* 1964;8:194–202.

43. Bloch M: Comparative study of lymph node cytology by puncture and histopathology. *Acta Cytol* 1967;11:139–144.

44. Engzell U, Jakobsson PA, Sigurdson A, et al.: Aspiration biopsy of metastatic carcinoma in lymph nodes of the neck. A review of 1101 consecutive cases. *Acta Otolaryngol.* 1971;72:138–147.

45. Franzen S, Giertz G, Zajicek J: Cytological diagnosis of prostatic tumours by transrectal aspiration biopsy. *Br J Urol* 1960;32:193–196.

46. Esposti PL: Cytologic diagnosis of prostatic tumors with the aid of transrectal aspiration biopsy. *Acta Cytol* 1966;10:182–186.

47. Kline TS, Kohler P, Kelsey DM: Aspiration biopsy cytology (ABC)—Its use in diagnosis of lesions of the prostate gland. *Arch Pathol Lab Med* 1982;106:136–139.

48. Tao L-C, Donat EE, Ho CS et al: Percutaneous fine-needle aspiration biopsy of the liver. *Acta Cytol* 1979;23:287–291.

49. Johansen P, Svendsen KN: Scan-guided fine needle aspiration biopsy in malignant hepatic disease. *Acta Cytol* 1978;22:292–296.

50. Smith EH, Bartrum RJ Chang YC, et al: Percutaneous aspiration biopsy of the pancreas under ultrasonic guidance. *N Engl J Med* 1975;292:825–828.

51. Goldstein HM, Zornoza J, Wallace S, et al: Percutaneous fine needle aspiration biopsy of pancreatic and other abdominal masses. *Gastrointest Radiol* 1978;3:295–302.

52. Tao L-C, Ho C-S, McLoughlin MJ et al: Percutaneous fine needle aspiration biopsy of the pancreas. *Acta Cytol* 1978;22:215–220.

53. Beazley RM: Percutaneous needle biopsy for the diagnosis of pancreatic carcinoma. *Semin Oncol* 1979;6:344–346.

54. Zajicek J: *Aspiration biopsy cytology. Part 2: Cytology of infradiaphragmatic organs,* in Wied G (ed): Monographs in Clinical Cytology, 7 New York, Karger 1979.

55. Lindblom K: Diagnostic kidney puncture of cysts and tumors. *Am J Roentgenol Radium Ther Nucl Med* 1952;68:209–215.

56. Von Schreeb T, Arner O, Skousted G, et al.: Renal adenocarcinoma. Is there a risk of spreading tumor cells in diagnostic puncture? *Scand J Urol Nephrol* 1967;1:270–276.

57. Lowhagen T, Granberg PO, Lundell G, et al: Aspiration biopsy cytology (ABC) in tumors of the thyroid gland suspected to be malignant. *Surg Clin North Am* 1979;59:3–18.

58. Miller J, Hamburger JI, Kini S: Diagnosis of thyroid nodules use of fine-needle aspiration and needle biopsy. *JAMA* 1979;241:481–484.

59. Frable WJ, Frable MA: Fine-needle aspiration biopsy of the thyroid. Histopathologic and clinical considerations, in Fenoglio CM, Wolff M (eds): *Progress in Surgical Pathology,* vol 1. New York, Masson Publishing Co 1980, pp 105–118.

60. Lalli AF: Roentgen guided aspiration biopsies of skeletal lesions. *J Can Assoc Radiol* 1970;21:71–73.

61. Adler O, Rosenberger A: Fine needle aspiration biopsy of osteolytic metastatic lesions. *AJR* 1979;133:15–18.

62. Maroon JC, Bank WO, Drayer BP, et al: Intracranial biopsy assisted by computerized tomography. *J Neurosurg* 1977;46:740–744.

63. Feldman PS, Kaplan MJ Johns ME, et al: Fine needle aspiration in squamous cell carcinoma of the head and neck. *Arch Otolaryngol* 1983;109:735–742.

64. Craver LF, Binkley JS: Aspiration biopsy of tumors of the lung. *J Thorac Cardiovasc Surg* 1938;8:436–463.

65. Adair FE: Surgical problems involved in breast cancer. *Ann R Coll Surg Engl* 1949;4:360–380.

66. Cornillot M, Verhaeghe M: Donnees cytologigues dans les ponctions de tumeurs du sein. *Pathol Biol* 1959;7:793–802.

67. Laumonier J, Hemet J: La cytologie des tumeurs mammaires (a partir de 1000 cytodiagnostics). *Proc Int Symp on Detection of Cancer,* Spa, Belgium, 1968, p 257–262.

68. Poe RH, Tobin RE: Sensitivity and specificity of needle biopsy in lung malignancy. *Am Rev Resp Dis* 1980;122:725–729.

69. Cornillot M, Verhaeghe M, Cappelaere P, et al.: Place de la cytologie par ponction dans le diagnostic des tumeurs du sein (2267 examens cytologignes). *Lille Med* 1971; 16:1027–1031.

70. Hajdu SI, Melamed MR: The diagnostic value of aspiration smears. *Am J Clin Pathol* 1973;59:350–356.

71. Zajdela A, Durand JC, Veith F: Cytological aspects of various particular varieties of breast epitheliomas. *Bull Cancer* 1975;62 (3):227–240.

72. Ferrucci JT, Jr, Wittenberg J, Margolies MN et al.: Malignant seeding of the tract after thin needle aspiration biopsy. *Radiology* 1979;130:345–346.

73. Smith FP, MacDonald JS, Schein S, et al: Cutaneous seeding of pancreatic cancer by skinny needle aspiration biopsy. *Arch Intern Med* 1980; 140:855.

74. Evans WK, Ho C-S, McLoughlin MJ Tao L-C: Fatal necrotizing pancreatitis following fine-needle aspiration biopsy of the pancreas. *Diag Radiol* 1981;141:61–62.

75. Livraghi T, Damascelli B, Zombardi C, et al: Risk in fine-needle abdominal biopsy. *J Clin Ultrasound* 1983;11:77–81.

76. Lundguist A: Fine needle aspiration biopsy of the liver. *Acta Med Scand* 1971;520:1–25.

77. Schnyder PA, Candardjis G, Anderegg A: Peritonitis after thin needle aspiration biopsy of an abscess. *AJR* 1981;137:1271–1272.

78. Schulz TB: Fine needle biopsy of the liver complicated with bile peritonitis. *Acta Med Scand* 1976;199:141–142.

79. Goldstein HM, Zornoza J, Wallace S, et al: Percutaneous fine needle aspiration biopsy of pancreatic and other abdominal masses. *Radiology* 1977;123:319–322.

80. Lalli AF: Roentgen-guided aspiration biopsies of thoracic, renal and skeletal lesions, in Meaney TF, Lalli AF, Altidi RJ (eds): *Complications and Legal Implications of Radiologic Special Procedures.* St. Louis, CV Mosby Co., 1973; pp 83–91.

81. Robbins GF, Brothers JH, Eberhart WF, et al: Is aspiration biopsy of breast cancer dangerous to the patient? *Cancer* 1954;7:774–778.

82. Berg JW, Robbins G: A late look at the safety of aspiration biopsy. *Cancer* 1962;15:826–827.

83. Engzell U, Esposti PL, Rubio C, et al: Investigation on tumour spread in connection with aspiration biopsy. *Acta Radiol* 1971;10:385–398.

84. Sinner WN, Zajicek J: Implantation metastasis after percutaneous transthoracic needle aspiration biopsy. *Acta Radiol Diag* 1976;17:473–480.

85. Mestitz P, Purves MJ, Pollard AC: Pleural biopsy in the diagnosis of pleural effusion. A report of 200 cases. *Lancet* 1958;275:1349–1353.

86. Schachter EN, Basta W: Subcutaneous metastasis of an adenocarcinoma following a percutaneous pleural biopsy. *Am Rev Resp Dis* 1973;107:283–285.

87. Jones FL, Jr: Subcutaneous implantation of cancer. A rare complication of pleural biopsy. *Chest.* 1970;57:189–190.

88. Sakurai M, Seki K, Okamura J, et al: Needle implantation of hepatocellular carcinoma after percutaneous liver biopsy. *Am J Surg Pathol* 1983;7:191–195.

89. Clarke BG, Leadbetter WF, Campbell JS: Implantation of cancer of the prostate in site of perineal needle biopsy. Report of a Case. *J Urol* 1953;70:937–939.

90. Goldman EJ, Samellas W: Local extension of carcinoma of the prostate following needle biopsy. *J Urol* 1960;84:575–576.

91. Burkholder GV, Kaufman JJ: Local implantation of carcinoma of the prostate with percutaneous needle biopsy. *J Urol* 1966;95:801–804.

92. Labardini MM, Nesbit RM: Perineal extension of adenocarcinoma of the prostate gland after punch biopsy. *J Urol* 1967;97:891–893.

93. Desai SG, Woodruff LM: Carcinoma of prostate. Local extension following perineal needle biopsy. *Urology* 1974;3:87–88.

94. Yamaguchi KT, Strong MS, Shapshay SM, et al: Seeding of parotid carcinoma along Vim-Silverman needle tract. *J Otolaryngol* 1979;8:49–56.

2

Technique for Palpable Lesions

Proper technique is essential to the maintenance of a high level of accuracy in fine needle aspiration (FNA). A procedure protocol for the performance of FNA should be established by the laboratory (Figure 2), and distributed to all clinicians interested in the procedure. All cytopathologists, clinicians, radiologists, nurses, and technologists involved in the performance of FNA must be instructed in the correct technique for sampling the lesion and preparing the cytologic smears. They must be well versed in the indications, contraindications, and complications of the procedure.

The patient's complete clinical history must be obtained before the aspiration; it is imperative for accurate FNA interpretation. The end result of the procedure should be an adequate sample of well-fixed and correctly stained cellular material for microscopic evaluation. Improper technique in either the performance of FNA or in the preparation of the smear will directly contribute to inconclusive or incorrect cytologic diagnoses.

The methods described here are used primarily to sample palpable masses. Specialized procedures for particular organs and those procedures using ra-

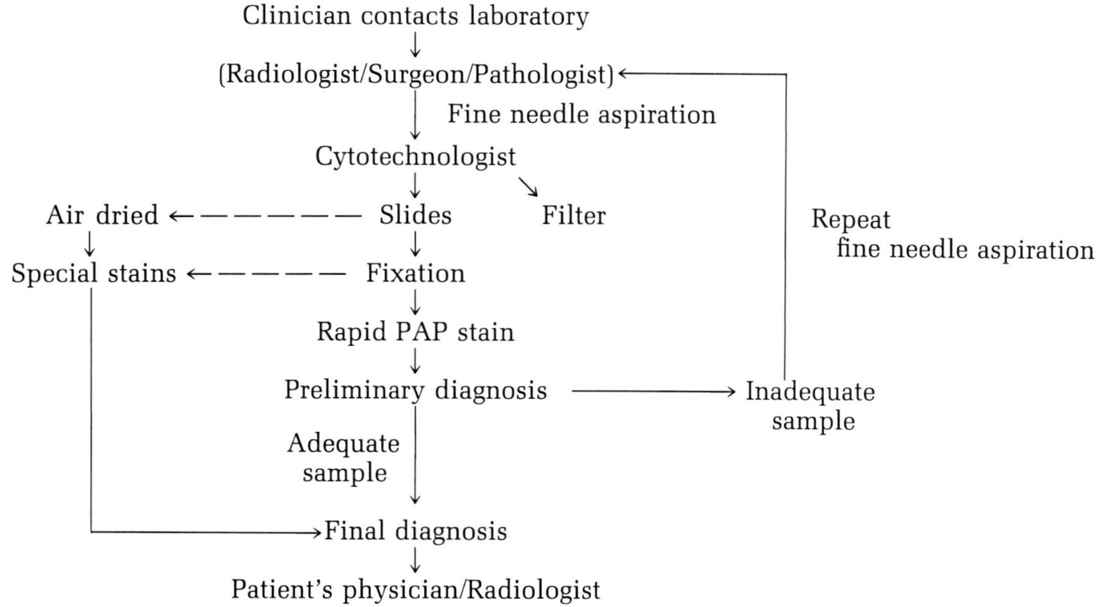

Figure 2. Procedure protocol for FNA used at University of Virginia.

diographic or ultrasound guidance for FNA of deep visceral lesions will be discussed in the appropriate chapters.

Who Performs Fine Needle Aspiration

The question of who should perform the aspiration—the internist, the surgeon, the radiologist, or the pathologist—has caused considerable debate in the literature.[1–5] There are many interconnected factors that influence the decision, including the number of aspirations the physician has performed and the experience and attitudes of clinicians and pathologists involved.

In 1966, Soderstrom stated that "the simple answer is that the aspirate should be performed by the person who is to examine the smears."[2] His answer reflects the Swedish experience since the early 1950s. The advantage of this position is that the person who will interpret the cytologic smears has a complete clinical picture of the patient and the lesion to be aspirated. This includes a physical examination of the mass, the clinical history of the patient, and the gross appearance of the aspirated material. Detailed clinical information complements the interpretation of the cytologic material when making a definitive diagnosis. This reasoning favors the opinion that FNA should be performed by the pathologist. Unfortunately, in hospitals where numerous aspirations are done on a daily basis, such an organizational structure may not be feasible.

In 1978, when FNA was introduced as a routine diagnostic procedure at the University of Virginia Medical Center, all aspirations were performed by pathologists. An initial apprehension that surgeons would be reluctant to allow pathologists to perform what can be considered a surgical procedure was unfounded. Once the technique was firmly established, the number of aspirations performed greatly increased, and a decision was made to train clinicians and radiologists in this procedure. This training was accomplished by allowing clinicians to do needle passes under the direction of pathologists. After clinicians had obtained sufficient experience in the correct technique, they routinely performed one needle pass with the pathologist doing a second aspiration.

The major consideration in the decision of who does the aspiration is that whoever is designated to perform this procedure is adequately trained in all aspects of sampling the lesion and preparing the cell smears. A high degree of accuracy can be maintained regardless of who performs the FNA if that person has the necessary training and experience. If the aspirations are done by clinicians, close communication with pathologists concerning the clinical aspects of the case is essential.

Articles by Koss and by Fox provide excellent discussions of the Swedish and American experiences with the FNA technique in regard to this basic organizational question.[3,4]

Procedure

Equipment and Materials

1. Cameco Syringe Pistol (Precision Dynamics Corp, Burbank, CA) or Aspir-Gun (Everst Co, Linden, NJ)
2. 20-mL Disposable plastic syringe with Leur Loc tip (McKenna Medical Products, Richmond, VA)
3. Needles: 22-gauge, 1½-in. disposable needles and 22-gauge, 3½-in. disposable spinal needles (McKenna Medical Products)
4. Alcohol swabs
5. Sterile gauze pads
6. Glass slides
7. 95% Ethyl alcohol in Coplin jars
8. Modified Carnoy's fixative in Coplin jars

At the University of Virginia Medical Center, a cytotechnologist is present at every aspiration to assist the physician and prepare the cytologic smears. All necessary equipment (Figure 3) is easily transported to the patient's side in a compartmentalized basket or tray (Figure 4).

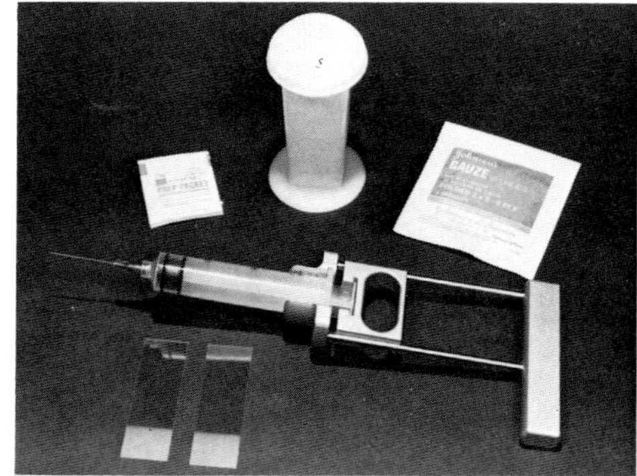

Figure 3. Equipment needed for FNA.

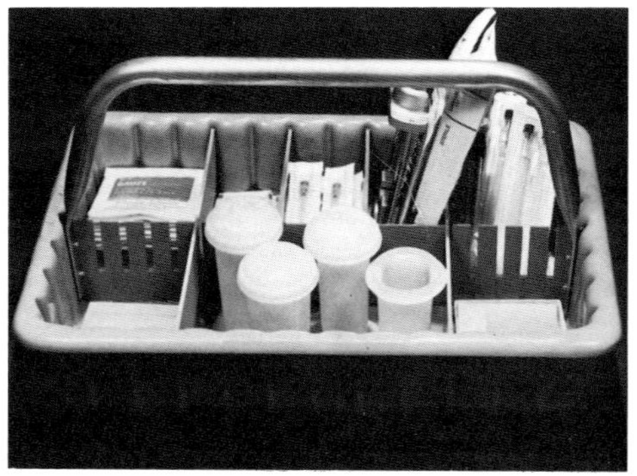

Figure 4. Equipment is transported to patient's side in compartmentalized basket.

Patient Preparation

When preparing the patient for FNA, carefully explain the safety and simplicity of the procedure, and answer all questions. Since no anesthesia is used for FNA of palpable lesions, most patients are anxious; therefore, make all efforts to calm and reassure them. A consent form is then signed by the patient or guardian and witnessed. Pediatric patients are often given a "cocktail" consisting of meperidine hydrochloride (Demerol), 1 mg/lb (2 mg/kg); promethazine hydrochloride (Phenergan), 0.5 mg/lb (1 mg/kg); and chlorpromazine (Thorazine), 0.5 mg/lb (1 mg/kg), which helps them relax and overcome their fear of the procedure. The maximum dose of meperidine hydrochloride in children is 50 mg, administered intramuscularly (IM).

Palpation

Place the patient in a comfortable lying or sitting position that allows the lesion to be easily aspirated. Before performing the aspiration, palpate the mass to identify the depth of the target and its relation to surrounding structures.

Aspiration*

1. Clean the skin overlying the region to be aspirated with an alcohol swab and immobilize the area with the thumb and index finger of one hand (Figure 5).

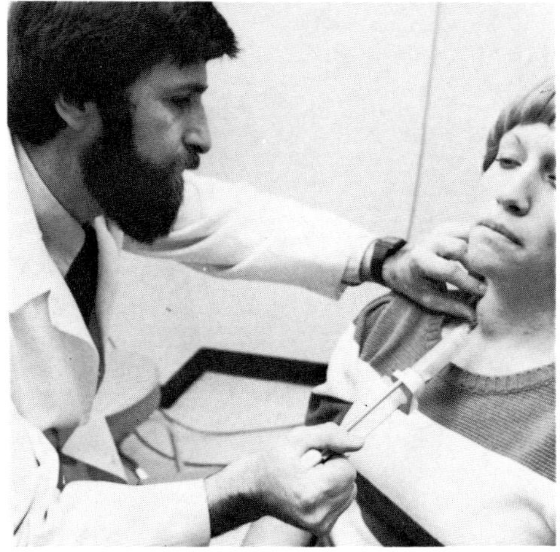

Figure 5. Immobilize area to be aspirated with thumb and index finger of one hand.

2. Attach a 20-mL disposable plastic syringe with Leur Loc tip to a 22-gauge needle (1½ to 3½ in.) and fit it into a syringe holder that is held with the other hand (see Figure 3). The syringe holder enables one-handed withdrawal and release of the syringe plunger.

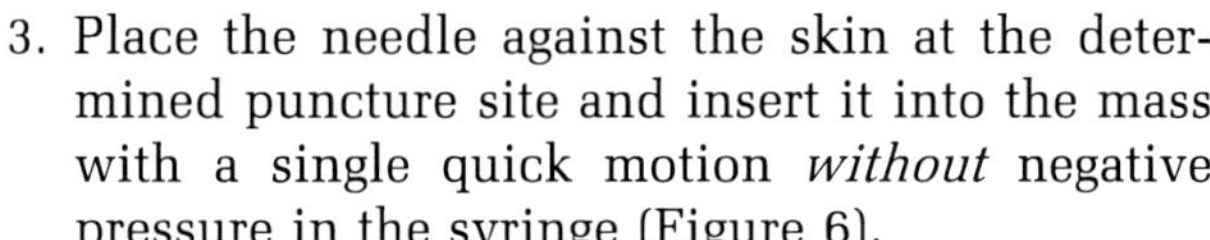

3. Place the needle against the skin at the determined puncture site and insert it into the mass with a single quick motion *without* negative pressure in the syringe (Figure 6).

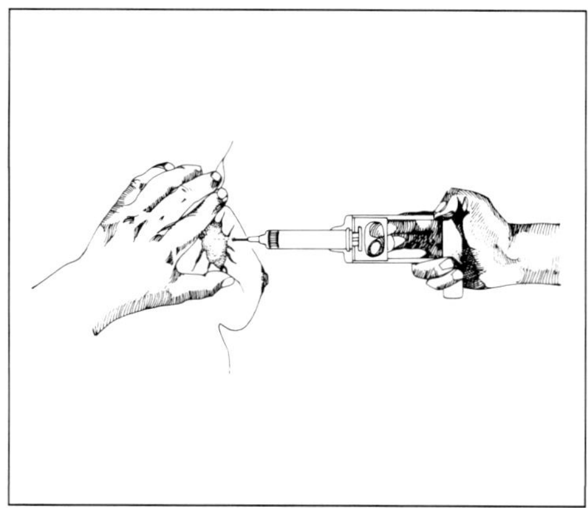

Figure 6. Technique for FNA of palpable lesions. Attach needle to syringe and insert into lesion without negative pressure in syringe.

4. Once the needle is in the mass, retract the plunger of the syringe (Figure 7) to create negative pressure in the syringe and needle lumen. This draws material into the needle.

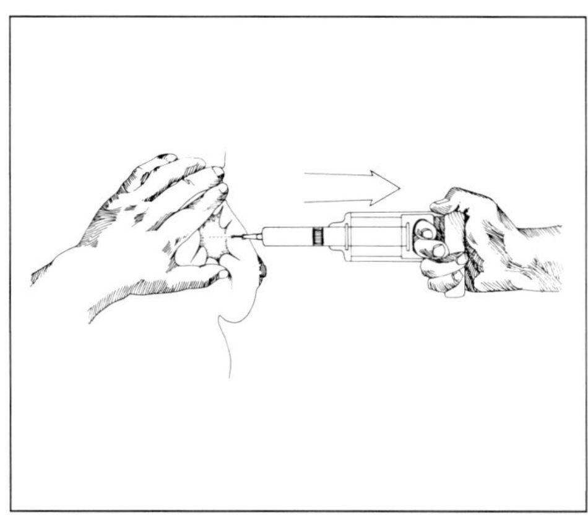

Figure 7. Retract plunger of syringe to produce negative pressure in syringe.

* These techniques are adapted from the FNA procedures established by William J. Frable, MD, at the Medical College of Virginia (Richmond).[6]

5. Move the needle back and forth several times and direct it into different areas of the mass (Figure 8). This fanning motion allows for sampling a wide area of the lesion.

6. Maintain constant negative pressure in the syringe throughout this manipulation by keeping the plunger of the syringe retracted (see Figure 8).

7. Closely observe the junction of the needle and syringe. At the first sight of material, the aspiration is completed.

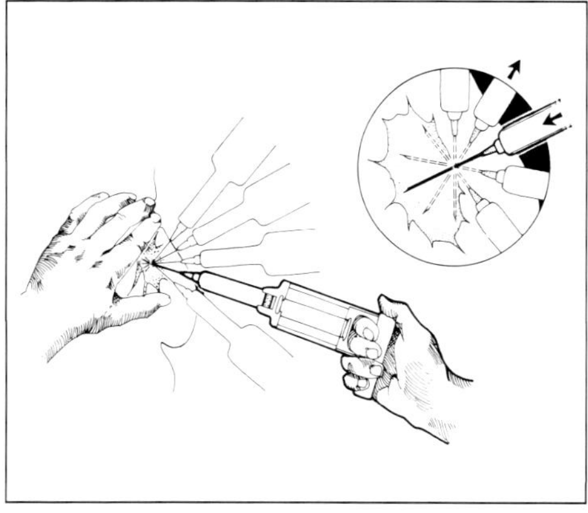

Figure 8. Move needle in back and forth motion in different directions under constant negative pressure.

8. Allow the pressure in the syringe to return to atmospheric pressure by gently releasing the plunger (Figure 9). The aspirated material should remain within the needle.

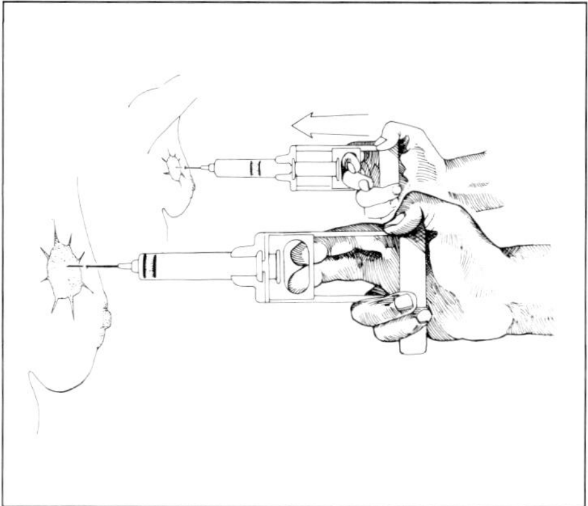

Figure 9. Release plunger to allow pressure in syringe to return to atmospheric pressure.

9. Withdraw the needle from the lesion and apply pressure to the puncture site with a sterile gauze pad. *The needle should never be removed while any negative pressure is applied to the syringe.* Such pressure would force aspirated material out of the needle and into the syringe making the preparation of smears difficult. The possibility of drawing tumor cells along the needle tract, increasing the risk of implantations must also be considered. This risk is more theoretical than real, although rare cases of implantation have occurred with FNA. At our institution, two passes are generally performed on all palpable masses.

   It is important not to dilute the cellular material with fluid or blood. If a cyst is encountered during the aspiration, evacuate all fluid from the cyst (Figure 10). Perform a second aspiration on any residual mass using a new syringe and needle.

   If blood is aspirated into the syringe, stop the procedure immediately and choose another aspiration site. Use a new syringe and needle for the repeat aspiration.

   If pus is encountered, withdraw as much of the material as possible and perform a repeat aspiration in an adjacent area.

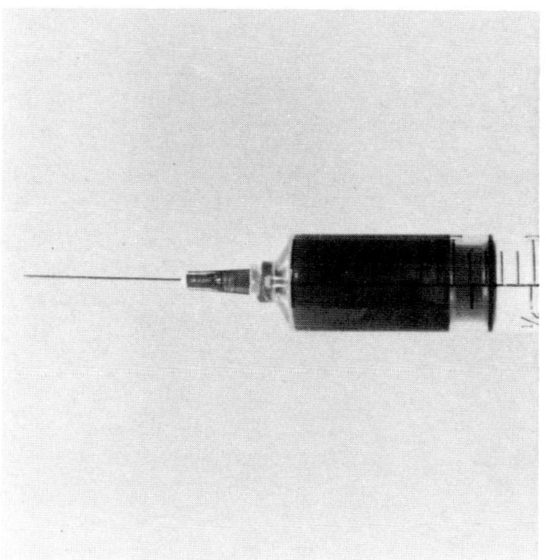

Figure 10. Fluid evacuated from a cyst.

10. When an infectious process is included in the differential diagnosis, culture of the aspirated material is often desirable. Perform a separate aspiration and eject the collected material into the appropriate culture tube. The needle should remain sterile and not be allowed to touch any contaminated surface.

Smear Preparation

1. After the needle is removed from the mass, detach it from the syringe, fill the syringe with air (Figure 11), and reattach the needle (Figure 12).

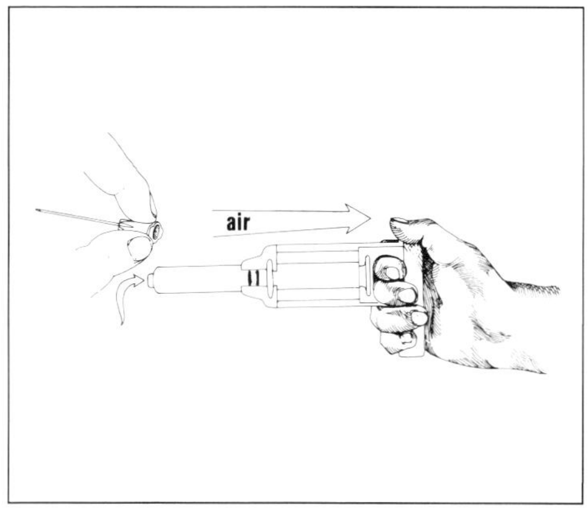

Figure 11. Withdraw needle from lesion, disconnect syringe from needle, and fill with air by retracting plunger.

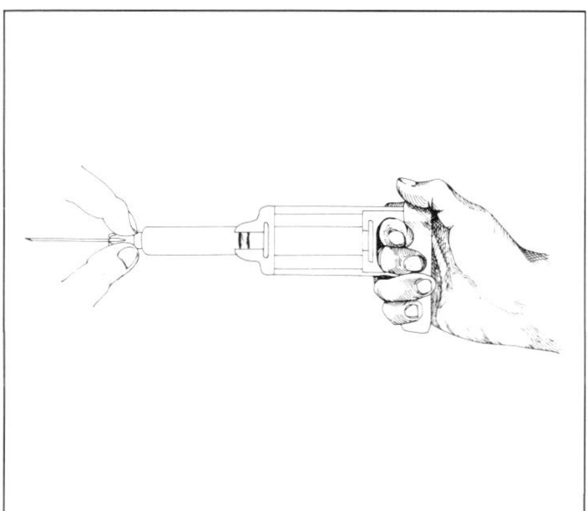

Figure 12. Reattach needle to syringe.

2. Place the bevel of the needle against a glass slide with no intervening air space and express a small drop of aspirated material onto the center of the slide (Figure 13). This needle position helps to prevent drying artifacts in alcohol-fixed smears. If too much material is expressed onto the slide, withdraw the syringe plunger slightly and reaspirate a portion of the material.

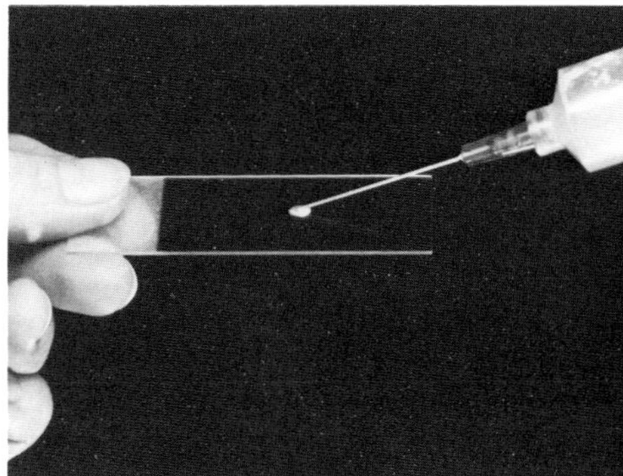

Figure 13. Place bevel of needle against a glass slide leaving no intervening air space. Express a small drop of aspirated material onto slide.

3. If the cellular material is semisolid in nature, place another slide on top of the drop (Figure 14) and pull them gently and quickly apart as the drop spreads from the weight of the slide (Figure 15).

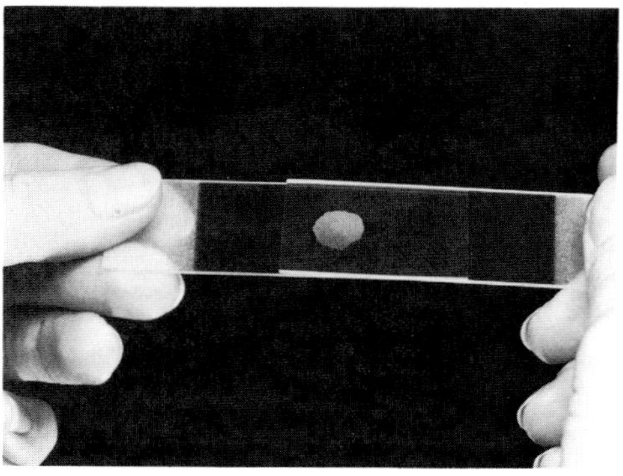

Figure 14. Place another slide on top of drop.

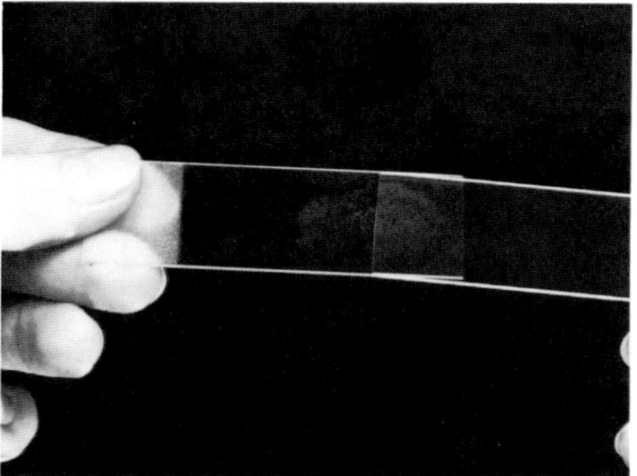

Figure 15. Pull slides gently and quickly apart.

4. Aspirated material diluted by fluid or blood is smeared using the technique for differential blood smears. Back the edge of a slide or cover glass into the drop (Figure 16). As the material spreads along the edge, move the slide forward pulling the cellular material away from the fluid or blood (Figure 17). In this type of preparation, cells tend to collect around the outer rim of the smear (Figure 18). Be careful not to exert too much pressure when preparing these smears to avoid cell distortion or crush artifacts.

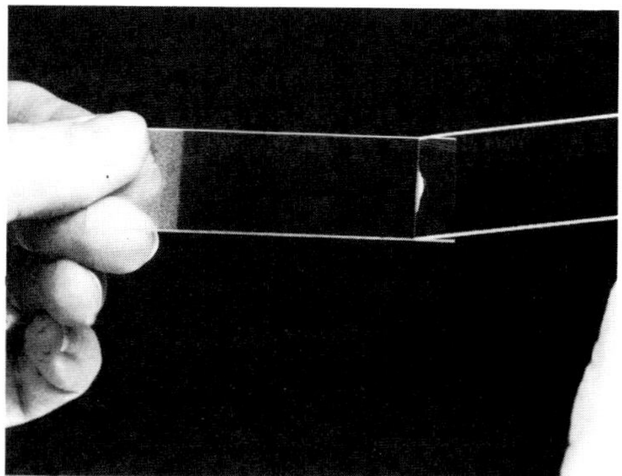

Figure 16. Back edge of slide into drop.

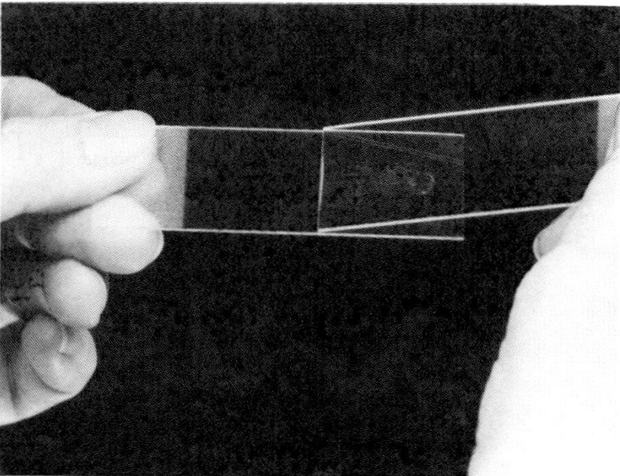

Figure 17. Move slide forward pulling cellular material away from fluid or blood.

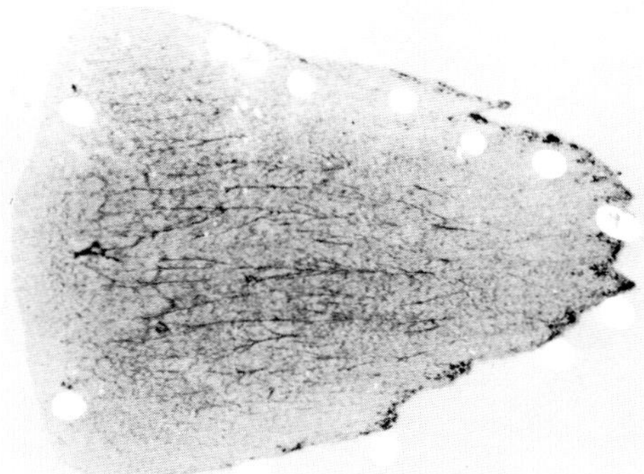

Figure 18. An FNA smear showing tendency of cells to collect around outer rim of smear.

5. Immediately wet-fix smears in 95% ethyl alcohol for the Papanicolaou and hematoxylin and eosin (H & E) stains (Figure 19). Place bloody slides in modified Carnoy's fixative for approximately 30 seconds to lyse the red blood cells. Then transfer these slides to 95% ethyl alcohol for final fixation.

6. Allow smears for hematology stains and certain special stains to air-dry.

7. Request that the patient remain in the clinic or treatment room until the adequacy of the aspiration is determined.

8. Stain a few of the fixed slides with a rapid Papanicolaou stain or frozen section, H & E method for an immediate preliminary diagnosis. The Diff-Quik (Scientific Products, Newark, NJ) stain set, modified Wright-Giemsa stain, or modified May-Grünwald-Giemsa stain may be used on air-dried slides for this preliminary diagnosis.

9. If the material obtained is inadequate or nondiagnostic, repeat the aspiration without further delay (See Figure 2).

10. Stain the remaining slides by the routine Papanicolaou method or using any desired special stains.

11. In cases of scant cellularity, a filter preparation of needle washings is often desirable. Draw 5 to 10 mL of saline or another balanced electrolyte solution into the syringe and then force the liquid back through the needle into the filtration apparatus (Figure 20).

12. Prepare and stain the filters in the routine manner. Gelman Metricel filters (Gelman Sciences, Inc, Ann Arbor, MI) are used in our laboratory.

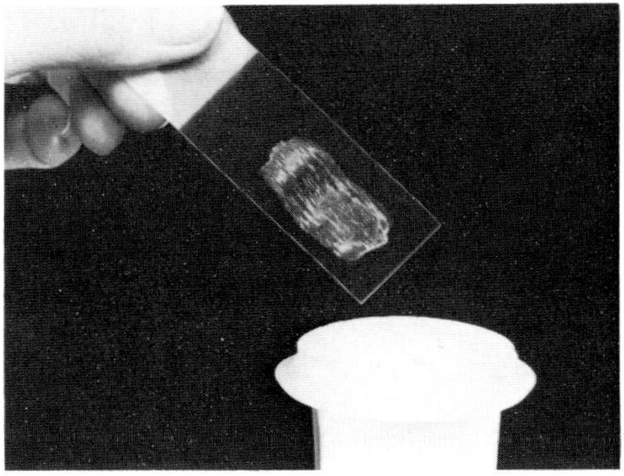

Figure 19. Immediately wet-fix smears in 95% ethyl alcohol.

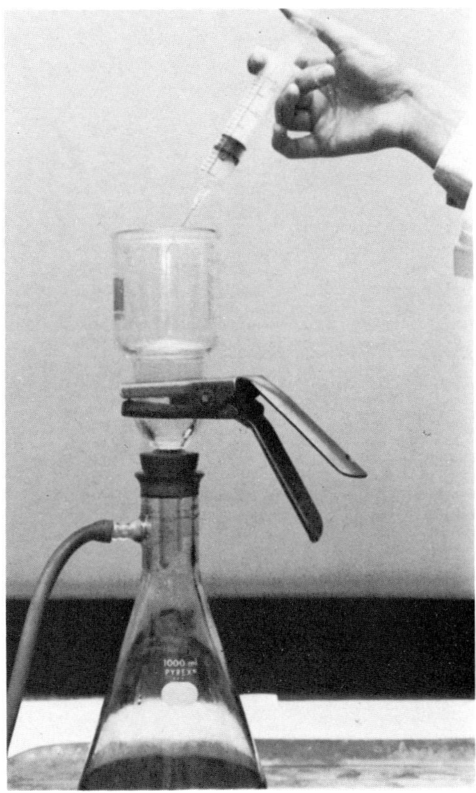

Figure 20. Filter preparation of needle washings is often desirable.

Stains

As mentioned previously, aspiration smears may be stained with routine Papanicolaou, modified Wright-Giemsa, H & E, or modified May-Grünwald-Giemsa stains. Any formula for these stains in standard laboratory use is satisfactory. The Diff-Quik stain set is a commercial stain kit that yields rapid results with good cellular detail on air-dried smears. The results are comparable to those obtained with the modified Wright-Giemsa.

Rapid Papanicolaou Stain

The rapid Papanicolaou staining procedure described in this chapter was developed in our laboratory and provides a fast staining method (about three minutes) for immediate FNA diagnosis. The nuclear stain is a standard alum hematoxylin which is used in its undiluted form. The cytoplasmic counterstain recipes were modified from the formulas developed in the Cytopathology Laboratory of the Johns Hopkins Hospital in Baltimore, Maryland. This staining procedure provides the same excellent definition of cellular morphology as the routine Papanicolaou methods.

Alum Hematoxylin (as prepared by Lillie-Mayer)

For 2,000 mL of stain, mix as follows:
Hematoxylin powder . . . . 10 g
Ammonium alum . . . . 100 g
Glycerin . . . . 600 mL
Distilled water . . . . 1,400 mL
Then add the following:
Sodium iodate . . . . 0.4 to 8 mL
Normal acetic acid. . . . . 40 mL
(6 mL glacial acetic acid in 100 mL distilled water)
Filter before use.

Counterstains

To assure constant reproducible results, the counterstains are prepared as volumetric solutions, taking into account the percentage content of actual dye in each batch of dyestuff.

Orange G

Stock solution. Prepare a 0.2 M orange G (CI [color index] No. 16230) aqueous stock solution by dissolving 9.05 g orange G dye in distilled water up to the 100 mL volumetric flask.

Working solution. To prepare a working orange G solution, combine the following ingredients:
Orange G stock solution . . . . 10 mL
Phosphotungstic acid . . . . 1 g
95% Ethyl alcohol. . . . . 395 mL
Glacial acetic acid . . . . 2 mL

The staining solution may be used immediately and should be filtered before use.

Eosin Polychrome

Stock solution. Prepare the following stock solutions individually by dissolving the indicated amounts of dye in 100 mL of distilled water.
0.05 M Light green SF yellowish (CI No. 42095). . . . . 3.96 g
0.30 M Eosin Y (CI No. 45380) . . . . . . 20.8 g

Working solution. To prepare a working eosin polychrome solution, combine the following:
Light green stock solution . . . . 10 mL
Eosin stock solution . . . . 20 mL
Phosphotungstic acid . . . . 2 g
95% Ethyl alcohol. . . . . 280 mL
Absolute methyl alcohol . . . . 100 mL
Glacial acetic acid. . . . . 8 mL

The staining solution may be used immediately and should be filtered before use.

Staining Procedure

Use this staining procedure on wet-fixed smears. Staining time is less than five minutes.

1. Tap water. . . . . Rinse thoroughly
2. Alum hematoxylin. . . . . 10 to 15 seconds
3. Tap water. . . . . Rinse thoroughly
4. Tap water. . . . . Rinse thoroughly
5. 95% Ethyl alcohol (ETOH) . . . . . . 15 dips
6. 95% ETOH . . . . 15 dips
7. Orange G . . . . 15 dips
8. 95% ETOH . . . . 15 dips
9. 95% ETOH . . . . 15 dips
10. Eosin polychrome . . . . . . 15 to 20 seconds
11. 95% ETOH . . . . 15 dips
12. Absolute ETOH . . . . 15 dips
13. Absolute ETOH . . . . 15 dips
14. Absolute ETOH . . . . 15 dips
15. Absolute ETOH . . . . 15 dips
16. Xylene . . . . 15 dips
17. Xylene . . . . 30 seconds

After staining, mount with mounting resin.

Water rinses should be changed after each use. Alcohol rinses should be changed frequently. Hematoxylin is filtered daily. Counterstains should be filtered weekly and replenished as necessary.

Immunoperoxidase Method

The standard morphologic criteria used in evaluating H & E- or Papanicolaou-stained sections often prove inadequate to identify the origin of neoplastic cells. This fact provided incentive for the development of ancillary diagnostic techniques. Special histochemical stains are helpful in some cases, but lack tissue or organ specificity. For example, a mucin stain may confirm a diagnosis of metastatic adenocarcinoma but does not aid in determining the primary site.

With the introduction of immunofluorescent methods by Coons et al in 1941,[7] a specific technique became available for identifying cells according to their antigenic constitution or products. Although immunofluorescence methods have been very successful in some areas of pathology (for example, renal biopsy), they have not achieved widespread application because of several disadvantages: (1) fresh tissue is required; (2) morphologic detail is poor; (3) the stain is not permanent; and (4) specialized microscopy is required.[8] These technical problems stimulated the development of an alternative antibody-labeled method that avoids these disadvantages. The immunoperoxidase technique has the following advantages: (1) it may be used on formalin- or alcohol-fixed tissue; (2) morphologic detail is equivalent to H & E-stained sections; (3) the stain is permanent; (4) slides are visualized directly with standard light microscopy; and (5) the sensitivity greatly exceeds that of immunofluorescence.[8]

Although the immunoperoxidase technique was initially used on histologic sections, Nadji has recently reported the application of these methods to cytologic material as well.[8–12] For example, FNA of a cervical lymph node may show a metastatic adenocarcinoma from an unknown primary site. Using the immunoperoxidase technique, the prostatic origin of the carcinoma may be indicated by the presence of prostatic acid phosphatase.[13]

Cell smears from FNAs and touch imprints are suitable for evaluation of immunoperoxidase reactions. Filter specimens are not used because the nonspecific background stain of the filter masks the underlying cellular reaction.[8] In our laboratory, the smear preparations are fixed in 95% ethyl alcohol. Frequently, the decision to use the immunoperoxidase technique is made after the Papanicolaou-stained material is examined. If no unstained slides are available in these cases, a selected slide is destained in acid alcohol and then carried through the steps of the immunologic reaction.

Peroxidase Antiperoxidase Method

Our laboratory currently uses an adaptation of the unlabeled antibody, peroxidase antiperoxidase (PAP) procedure pioneered by Sternberger.[10] This adaptation of the PAP method for cytologic material was described by Nadji and is currently the method of choice for our cytologic specimens.[8]

It is beyond the scope of this atlas to present detailed information on the theoretical and technical aspects of the immunoperoxidase method. Recent articles by Sternberger,[10] Taylor,[11] and Nadji et al[13] provide excellent discussions of this invaluable technique.

Procedure

1. Circle the specimen on the glass slide with a diamond tipped marker.
2. Hydrate in decreasing grades of ethyl alcohol.
3. Block endogenous peroxidase by placing slide in 0.3% hydrogen peroxide in methyl alcohol for 30 minutes.
4. Rinse in tap water for five minutes then wash in phosphate-buffered saline (PBS) for five minutes.
5. Cover the circle with normal swine serum (1:20) to reduce nonspecific background staining. Leave swine serum on for 30 minutes.
6. Decant excess normal swine serum and add drops of rabbit antiserum to the antigen under study. Proper dilution of primary rabbit antiserum should be determined by checkerboard study.
7. Wash with three changes of PBS, ten minutes each.
8. Add drops of swine antirabbit immunoglobulin (1:20). Leave immunoglobulin on for 30 minutes.
9. Wash with three changes of PBS, ten minutes each.
10. Add drops of rabbit peroxidase antiperoxidase; proper dilution should be determined from checkerboard study.[8] Leave PAP on for 30 minutes.
11. Wash with three changes of PBS, ten minutes each.
12. Add drops of 3,3′-diaminobenzidine tetrahydrochloride (DAB) solution containing hydrogen peroxide (6 mg DAB + 10 mL PBS + 4 drops 3% hydrogen peroxide). Leave solution on for three to eight minutes. This solution should be prepared fresh before administration. While working with DAB, use caution and wear a mask and gloves. The DAB reaction should preferably be carried out under a ventilated hood.
13. Wash with running tap water for five minutes.

14. Counterstain with hematoxylin or other nuclear stains.
15. Dehydrate with increasing grades of ethanol.
16. Clear in xylene and mount.

General Interpretation

For many organ systems, the diagnostic criteria used in the evaluation of routine cytologic material can be applied to FNA specimens with excellent results. However, FNA may sample lesions in body sites not ordinarily accessible to conventional cytologic techniques (eg, lymph nodes, salivary gland, bone, pancreas). Because FNA yields a direct sample of a lesion rather than exfoliated cells, the cellular artifacts present may differ from those familiar to the cytologist. Additional or different diagnostic criteria are sometimes necessary for the accurate interpretation of FNA. Cytologists will often require additional study to gain the experience and confidence necessary to feel comfortable with the widely varied material obtained by FNA.

The specific diagnostic features for the various body sites will be discussed in the appropriate chapters. However, there are several factors that must always be kept in mind when evaluating FNA cytology:

1. Be sure to obtain cellular samples that are adequate and of good quality.
2. Be aware of the limitations of the technique for the body site sampled.
3. Maintain good lines of communication with the clinicians in charge of the patient's care.
4. Have adequate knowledge of the patient's clinical history and physical findings.
5. Be realistic as to the cytologic expertise of the physician who initially interprets the smears.
6. Be aware of the diagnostic pitfalls for each body site sampled as a source of false-positive and false-negative results.
7. Correlate tissue results and patient follow-up with the FNA diagnoses for continuing education and quality assurance.

Reporting Results

Cellular evaluations of FNA are reported in four general categories: unsatisfactory, negative for malignancy, suspicious, or positive for malignancy. Aspirations with insufficient cellular material are reported unsatisfactory and no cellular evaluation is given. Repeat aspiration or biopsy is recommended to evaluate the lesion. Therefore, the unsatisfactory FNAs are not included in our statistical analyses of false-negative diagnoses. (See chapters 3 and 5.)

Smears containing adequate, well-preserved benign cells are reported as negative for malignancy. Frequently, a distinctive pattern of cells allows a definitive diagnosis of the benign disease, such as inflammatory disease, benign tumor, regenerative process. In those cases, a comment on the cell pattern is added to the negative findings. The presence of microorganisms and the results of any special stains are also included in the written report. If the clinical findings are compatible with the benign cytologic interpretation, the mass is either excised or its progress monitored. A clinical impression of malignancy requires further investigation (ie, repeat aspiration or biopsy) regardless of the negative cytologic results.

Aspirations that show cells with significant cytologic atypia but not conclusive evidence of malignancy are reported as suspicious. This category necessitates repeat FNA or tissue biopsy for a conclusive diagnosis before therapy.

An FNA report positive for malignancy indicates to the clinician that there is definitive cytologic evidence of malignancy and that therapeutic procedures may be instituted without additional biopsy confirmation. Under these circumstances it is absolutely essential that the pathologist evaluate the case (aspiration slides and clinical findings) carefully and be totally convinced of the malignant nature of the aspirate. If there is any doubt as to the diagnosis, the positive category should not be used. As previously described, false-positive diagnoses may have catastrophic results, such as unnecessary surgery. The tumor type is also indicated whenever the cell pattern is sufficiently distinctive to allow typing.

Summary

Although the interpretation of FNA is dependent on many factors, technical expertise plays a major role in the accuracy of the cytologic diagnosis. The smears should contain an adequate amount of well-fixed, properly stained cellular material showing good nuclear detail and cytoplasmic definition. Each step in the FNA procedure has been described in detail in this chapter because of its important effect on the overall quality of the microscopic preparations. Careful adherence to an established protocol and practical experience with the technique will contribute greatly to the diagnostic accuracy achieved by FNA.

References

1. Zajicek J: *Aspiration Biopsy Cytology.* part I: *Cytology of Supradiaphragmatic Organs,* in Wied GL (ed): Monographs in Clinical Cytology. New York, Karger, 1974, vol 4.

2. Soderstrom N: *Fine Needle Aspiration Biopsy.* Stockholm, Almqvist & Wiksell, 1966.

3. Koss LG: Thin needle aspiration biopsy. *Acta Cytol* 1980;24:1–3.

4. Fox C: *Innovation in medical diagnosis; the Scandinavian curiosity. Lancet* 1979;1:1387–1388.

5. Soderstrom N, Pfitzer P, Fox C, et al: Thin needle aspiration biopsy. *Acta Cytol* 1980;24:468–470.

6. Frable W, Schwinn C: Fine needle aspiration biopsy. (workshop handout), *Fall Meeting of Virginia Society for Pathology, Inc,* Richmond, VA, 1977.

7. Coons AH, Creech JH, Jones RN: Immunologic properties of an antibody containing a fluorescent group. *Proc Soc Esp Biol* 1941;47:200–202.

8. Nadji M: The potential value of immunoperoxidase techniques in diagnostic cytology. *Acta Cytol* 1980;24:422–447.

9. DeLellis RA, Sternberger LA, Mann RB, et al: Immunoperoxidase technics in diagnostic pathology: Report of a workshop sponsored by the National Cancer Institute. *Am J Clin Pathol* 1979;71:483–488.

10. Sternberger LA: *Immunocytochemistry,* ed 2. New York, John Wiley & Sons Inc, 1979, pp 1–354.

11. Taylor CR: Immunohistological approach to tumor diagnosis. *Oncology* 1978;35:189–197.

12. Taylor CR: *Immunoperoxidase techniques: Practical and theoretical aspects. Arch Pathol Lab Med* 1978;102:113–121.

13. Nadji M, Tabei SZ, Castro A, et al: Prostatic origin of tumors: An immunohistochemical study. *Am J Clin Pathol* 1980;73:735–739.

PART
TWO

Fine Needle Aspiration of the Breast

3

Technique and Interpretation

Introduction

In 1930, Martin and Ellis at the Memorial Hospital for Cancer and Allied Diseases (Memorial Sloan-Kettering Cancer Center) in New York reported 65 malignant tumors diagnosed by aspiration biopsy, six of which were from the breast.[1] In 1933, Stewart, at the same hospital, reported that they had aspirated nearly 500 breast lesions.[2] By 1934, Martin and Ellis had expanded their experience and obtained positive diagnoses of cancer by needle aspiration biopsies in more than 1,400 cases.[3] In this series, 280 breast cancers were diagnosed by aspiration. Needle aspirates of the breast continued to be used extensively at Memorial Hospital; and in 1949, Adair reported a five-year experience using needle aspirations in 1,579 cases of breast cancer.[4] Despite the pioneering work of Martin and Ellis, the medical world largely ignored needle aspirates for the next 20 years.

In the early 1950s in the United States, Saphir[5] and Godwin[6] recommended fine needle aspiration (FNA) of breast lesions. A very significant impetus for breast FNA was the introduction of this procedure at the Radiumhemmet in Sweden in 1955; and by 1968, 4,700 consecutive mammary aspiration biopsies were reported by Franzen and Zajicek.[7] Similarly in France, Zajdela et al, in 1954, began aspirating all palpable lesions of the breast and, by 1975, had obtained 2,772 aspirations.[8] The experience from these centers resulted in a reawakened interest in needle aspirations. Numerous series have since been reported documenting the results of breast FNA. Tables 2 and 3 summarize the results of many of the larger series of breast FNAs. Table 2 includes only series with results from FNA with histologic confirmation.[4,7,9–31]

Despite these reports showing the efficacy of FNA, many clinicians and pathologists remained skeptical. Pathologists were reluctant to diagnose breast carcinoma based on the cytologic appearance of individual cells for several reasons. Material obtained from an FNA consists of a smear preparation of cells and not a tissue fragment; thus, tissue architecture is not available for interpretation. This represented a major change in criteria for pathologists. Until recently, pathologists were trained to diagnose breast cancer from histologic sections and not from the cytologic specimens obtained by aspiration. In the past, pathology residents in the United States received little or no training in aspiration cytology and then only in a few centers. Only recently has resident training in this technique expanded. Because of this insufficient training, pathologists were apprehensive about interpreting aspiration specimens. The major fear was making a false-positive diagnosis with catastrophic results (eg, a mastectomy in the absence of carcinoma). Pathologists were also fearful of making a false-negative diagnosis causing a delay in therapy. They were thus apprehensive of medicolegal implications resulting from an erroneous FNA diagnosis.

Pathologists needed evidence showing the merits of FNA versus tissue biopsy. Studies from New York,[19,20] Sweden[7,13,16] and France[8,12,17] furnished such conclusive data on the accuracy and safety of FNA (see Tables 2 and 3) that today its diagnostic value is recognized by most pathologists as a definitive technique for establishing the diagnosis of breast masses.

Surgeons were also apprehensive of FNA for several reasons. As mentioned, a false-positive diagnosis could result in unwarranted surgery, eg, a mastectomy. It was, therefore, understandable that surgeons would mistrust this newer technique until

TABLE 2. Accuracy of Diagnosis Based on Results of Fine Needle Aspiration: Malignant Breast Lesions

Author	Year	Total Breast FNA	Dx Based on FNA with Histology	Histologic Dx: Malignant	FNA Diagnoses: Positive	Suspicious	Atypia	Negative	Unsatisfactory	False-Negative*
Adair[4]	1949	ND	1,579	1,579	1,343 (85)	ND	ND	236 (15)	ND	236 (15)
Cornillot & Verhaeghe[10]	1959	500	500	276	231 (84)	ND	ND	25 (9)	20 (7)	25 (9)
Schiller-Volkova & Agamova[11]	1960	576	263	165	98 (60)	22 (13)	7 (4)	4 (2)	34 (21)	9 (5)
Klimanova[12]	1961	160	71	49	38 (78)	8 (16)	ND	3 (6)	ND	3 (6)
Zajicek et al[13]	1967	2,200	1,220	651	485 (75)	94 (14)	13 (2)	←———	59 (9) ———→	ID
Franzen & Zajicek[7]	1968	3,479	1,686	873	662 (76)	117 (13)	17 (2)	←———	77 (9) ———→	ID
Laumonier & Hemet[14]	1968	1,000	1,000	456	335 (73)	21 (5)	ND	51 (11)	49 (11)	51 (11)
Winship[15]	1969	ND	487	469	436 (93)	33 (7)	ND	ND	ND	ND
Zajicek et al[16]	1970	4,700	2,111	1,068	823 (77)	139 (13)	17 (2)	←———	89 (8) ———→	ID
Cornillot et al[17]	1971	2,267	2,267	1,335	1,173 (88)	ND	ND	62 (5)	100 (7)	62 (5)
Rajcic[18]	1971	2,890	1,759	582	551 (95)	31 (5)	ND	ND	ND	0
Rosen et al[19]	1972	208	206	179	147 (82)	"32 (18) needle aspirates were nondiagnostic and included clearly Benign and Atypia below which cancer could be diagnosed"				ID
Hajdu & Melamed[20]	1973	456	tissue and/ or follow up, 456	379	315 (83)	"64 (17) needle aspirates reclassified as negative & included Suspicious/Atypia/Unsatisfactory"				ID
Stavric et al[21]	1973	400	250	108	103 (95)	0	ND	5 (5)	ND	5 (5)
Geier et al[22]	1975	974	ND	72	57 (79)	10 (14)	ND	5 (7)	ND	5 (7)
Zajdela et al[9]	1975	2,772	2,772	1,745	1,539 (88)	54 (3)	ND	63 (4)	89 (5)	63 (4)
Rimstein et al[23]	1975	984	381	107	76 (71)	14 (13)	13 (12)	4 (4)	ND	17 (16)
Koivuniemi[24]	1976	1,270	503	192	138 (72)	19 (10)	24 (13)	7 (4)	4 (2)	31 (16)
Kreuzer & Boquoi[25]	1976	602	602	247	185 (75)	29 (12)	ND	33 (13)	ND	33 (13)
Manheimer & Rywlin[26]	1977	221	127	90	69 (77)	10 (11)	ND	11 (12)	ND	11 (12)
Deschenes et al[27]	1978	2,050	405	118	92 (78)	13 (11)	ND	9 (8)	4 (3)	9 (8)
Schöndorf[28]	1978	2,778	519	307	283 (92)	18 (6)	ND	6 (2)	ND	6 (2)
Kern[29]	1979	161	161	93	45 (48)	29 (31)	ND	19 (20)	0	19 (20)
Kline et al[30]	1979	3,545	1,076	341	213 (62)	89 (26)	ND	35 (10)	4 (1)	35 (10)
Frable[31]	1983	600	ND	233	191 (82)	20 (9)	ND	22 (9)	ND	22 (9)
Feldman & Covell	1983	300	190	100	80 (80)	15 (15)	ND	0	5 (5)	0

Note: Numbers in parentheses are percentages of the cases in the "Histologic Dx: Malignant" column that were also diagnosed using the results of fine needle aspiration.

Abbreviations: Dx = diagnoses; ID = insufficient data; ND = no data.

*"False-Negative" statistics include cases in "Atypia" and "Negative" columns. "Unsatisfactory" cases are not included in the "False-Negative" statistics.

TABLE 3. Accuracy of Diagnosis Based on Results of Fine Needle Aspiration: Benign Breast Lesions

Author	Year	Total Breast FNA Procedures	Dx Based on FNA with Histology	Histologic or Follow-up Dx: Benign	FNA Diagnoses					
					Positive	Suspicious	Atypia	Negative	Unsatisfactory	False-Positive*
Cornillot & Verhaeghe[10]	1959	500	500	200	4 (2.0)	ND	ND	171 (86)	25 (13)	4 (2.0)
Zajicek et al[13]	1967	2,200	1,220	542	0	19 (4)	55 (10)	← 468 (86) →		0
Franzen & Zajicek[7]	1968	3,479	1,686	807	1	23 (3)	35 (4)	← 748 (93) →		1†
Laumonier & Hemet[14]	1968	1,000	1,000	544	13 (2.0)	23 (4)	← 424 (78) →		84 (15)	13 (2.0)
Zajicek et al[16]	1970	4,700	2,111	1,009	1	28 (3)	41 (4)	← 939 (93) →		1†
Cornillot et al[17]	1971	2,267	2,267	932	15 (2.0)	ND	ND	831 (89)	86 (9)	15 (2.0)
Stavric et al[21]	1973	400	250	142	2 (1.0)	7 (5)	ND	133 (94)	ND	2 (1.0)
Zajdela et al[9]	1975	2,772	2,772	1,027	3 (0.3)	42 (4)	ND	916 (89)	66 (6)	3 (0.3)
Rimstein et al[23]	1975	984	381	274	0	2 (1)	46 (17)	← 226 (82) →		0
Koivuniemi[24]	1976	1,270	503	311	0	27 (9)	ND	242 (78)	42 (14)	0
Kreuzer & Boquoi[25]	1976	602	602	355	4 (1.0)	46 (13)	ND	305 (86)	ND	4 (1.0)
Kern[29]	1979	161	161	68	0	8 (12)	ND	60 (88)	0	0
Kline et al[30]	1979	3,545	1,076	3,177	0	59 (2)	← 3,118 (98) →		ND	0
Feldman & Covell	1983	300	190	200	0	5 (3)	← 160 (80) →		35 (18)	0

NOTE: Numbers in parentheses are percentages of the cases "Histologic or Follow-up Dx: Benign" that were also diagnosed using the results of fine needle aspiration.

ABBREVIATIONS: Dx = diagnoses; ID = insufficient data; ND = no data.

*"False-Positive" statistics include only the cases in the "Positive" column. "Suspicious" cases are not included in the "False-Positive" statistics.

†The same case was reported in both series. The specimen from the mastectomy performed at another hospital showed no evidence of cancer in routine sectioning. Review of the FNA reaffirmed the cytologic interpretation of malignancy. Unfortunately, the mastectomy specimen had been discarded and was unavailable for further study. The breast mass was less than 1 cm in diameter.

convinced otherwise. The experiences found in the literature, especially in certain centers, clearly documented the accuracy of FNA.[7,9,13,15–20,28,31,32]

Another problem for surgeons was the fear of implanting tumor cells along the FNA needle tract. This criticism of FNA has been proved invalid.[33,34] Those rare reports of tumor implants have resulted from larger cutting needles (14-gauge) and not the 22-gauge needles used for FNA.[35] In a review of 3,479 consecutive breast aspirations, Franzen and Zajicek found no evidence of tumor-cell seeding along the needle tract.[7] A review of the literature on breast aspirations failed to disclose a single instance of tumor implant resulting from FNA.[9,13,16,17,19,31] This is not surprising since following an FNA diagnosis of malignancy, the needle tract is eradicated by either surgery or irradiation.

Another concern for surgeons was the possibility that the manipulation of the cancer during FNA might increase systemic dissemination of the cancer.[12,33,34,36] In 1954, Robbins et al investigated whether aspiration biopsy of breast cancer was dangerous to the patient.[33] From their findings, they concluded that aspiration biopsy had no effect on long-term survival rates. In 1962, Berg and Robbins reexamined their earlier series (1954) and compared 370 patients with breast carcinoma diagnosed by FNA and 370 patients with breast carcinoma diagnosed by other means.[34] They found no statistical differences in morbidity or mortality in these patients for the ten-year period.[34] Thus, FNA did not seem to compromise the patients' later course.

Advantages

There are numerous advantages of breast FNA not only for the patient but also for the surgeon, hospital and pathologist. One of the more significant advantages of breast FNA is the provision of a rapid diagnosis to the patient and surgeon, enabling the patient to play a more active role in selecting the mode of therapy. The procedure is accomplished in only two to five minutes, and the material obtained from the aspiration can be processed and interpreted within ten minutes. This results in an immediate diagnosis during the patient's initial clinic or office visit. The patient's anxiety as to the nature of the "lump" can be greatly reduced; and in many cases, fears are totally alleviated with the diagnosis of a benign process.

This procedure contrasts strikingly with the common management in some centers of patients with a breast lump. For instance, the patient comes in with a breast lump that may or may not be palpable, and the surgeon feels further investigation is warranted. The patient is apprised of the surgeon's impressions and a cutting needle biopsy or open biopsy is performed. If necessary, admission to the hospital, operating room time, and anesthesia time are all arranged. This, in itself, is time-consuming and costly. The patient is admitted most often in a frightened, unknowing state of mind. She is put to sleep in the operating room and the open biopsy is performed. If a frozen section is done, a thirty-minute delay for diagnosis is standard (in the case of a cutting needle biopsy, a definite diagnosis may come as much as 24 hours later). If a positive diagnosis is rendered, the patient may very well awaken with the breast having been removed.

Performing the FNA procedure in the office more often than not can give the patient and surgeon an immediate diagnosis. Treatment options (breast removal or radiation therapy, or both) can be discussed, and the patient can make a well-informed decision in advance about therapy. In patients with malignant breast lesions requiring mastectomy, the surgeon can more efficiently plan operating room time. As it is now, a biopsy is scheduled in the operating room with possible mastectomy. With FNA, more accurate operating room scheduling and reduced anesthesia time can be accomplished. Breast FNA also greatly benefits the surgeon when a benign diagnosis is given, eg, fibrocystic disease. FNA may also be used for follow-up in patients with a history of benign or malignant disease. Surgeons at our hospital strongly support FNA for many of the aforementioned reasons and feel that the decrease in patient anxiety is one of the greater benefits.

The simplicity of the procedure and its accuracy support the enthusiastic reception FNA has had at our institution. The breast aspiration can be performed virtually anywhere: a hospital bed, physician's office, or clinic. At our institution, no special equipment, and therefore no extra cost, is required of the surgeon because the pathologist can provide all necessary instruments. Occasionally, patients are apprehensive about the procedure, but with careful preparation, most experience little discomfort during the aspiration. We advise patients that the pain experienced from injecting a local anesthetic surpasses the pain of the FNA itself. Local anesthesia is, of course, an available option to those who feel they would be unable to tolerate the FNA without it. Another advantage is that there are only occasional and minimal complications resulting from breast FNA. Small hematomas may occur adjacent to the puncture site. This may be prevented by providing adequate compression of the skin immediately after the needle is withdrawn. It is interesting to note that frequently no bleeding occurs when the needle is withdrawn.

Estrogen Receptor Levels

If the breast FNA is diagnostic of malignancy, no frozen section is usually obtained before mastectomy in our hospital. A major concern for surgeons and pathologists was the possibility that steroid receptor activity would deteriorate during the mastectomy with its attendant devascularization and the delay in cooling the specimen. However, several studies have shown that the estrogen receptor levels measured in mastectomy specimens were not significantly different from estrogen receptor levels in biopsy specimens.[37–40] They also noted estrogen receptor content of the mastectomy specimens was actually slightly higher than that of the biopsy specimens.[40] When conditions of specimen acquisition are well controlled and prolonged storage at room temperature is avoided, estrogen receptor assay of tumor tissue from mastectomy specimens gives valid results. Based on these findings, the performance of an incisional biopsy or frozen section solely for the performance of estrogen receptor analysis is unnecessary.[38]

Although we have not attempted estrogen receptor analysis from FNA, Silfverswärd et al in Sweden have reported excellent results with estrogen receptor determination from FNA.[41,42] In 20 of 22 cases of inoperable carcinoma successful estrogen receptor assays were obtained from the FNAs. There are several advantages for using FNA rather than surgical biopsy for estrogen receptor determination in patients with inoperable conditions, recurrent cancer, and those selected for preoperative irradiation treatment.

Gunduz and Fisher investigated estrogen receptor values from FNA by means of fluoresceinated estrone binding. Findings from the aspirated cells were compared with results from aliquots of the same tumors following surgical excision. They observed no consistent differences between estrogen receptor values obtained by FNA and those from the resected specimen.[43]

Indications

The indications for breast FNA vary in different medical centers. In some hospitals, FNA is performed on all palpable breast lesions.[7,9,13,23,25,30,31,44] In other hospitals, FNA is recommended only in cases that clinically appear to be malignant.[19,20] Other hospitals do not specifically list their indications for breast FNA. At the University of Virginia Medical Center, palpable lesions of the breast are aspirated on request and nonpalpable breast masses are aspirated in conjunction with mammographic guidance. A survey of the literature and our own experiences have shown no contraindications for FNA of the breast.[7,9,28–31]

Procedure

Palpable Masses

The technique for FNA of palpable masses has been described in detail in chapter 2 and, therefore, will not be repeated here. However, there are several aspects of this technique when used for palpable breast masses that warrant further discussion.

If a cyst is encountered during the aspiration, it should be evacuated as completely as possible. Following this, the breast should be reexamined for any residual mass; and if one is found, a second aspiration should be performed.

A 22-gauge, 1½-in. needle is the standard size used for breast FNA in our hospital. However, 22-gauge, 3 in. needles are used for deep-seated lesions in large breasts. Breast masses are sometimes deceptively deeper than initially appreciated and this results in sampling error.

If the initial attempt at aspiration yields scant material because of the presence of dense fibrous tissue, a larger (18- to 20-gauge) needle is required and should be used for the repeat aspiration. An example of a tumor containing dense fibrous tissue is scirrhous carcinoma. We have not found it necessary or advantageous to use a screw-type needle for breast FNA.

Nonpalpable Masses

Mammography is used extensively for screening patients with a family history of breast carcinoma and in patients with symptoms of breast disease. This has resulted in the detection of increasing numbers of small nonpalpable tumors by mammography in asymptomatic patients.[45,46] The diagnostic accuracy of mammography reported in the literature varies between 68% to 97% with significant numbers of false-positive and false-negative diagnoses (6% to 20%).[45,47] For a precise evaluation of a radiographically suspicious, nonpalpable lesion, a microscopic examination is required. This may be obtained either with an excisional biopsy or FNA under mammographic guidance using the following technique.

Aspiration for Nonpalpable Masses

1. Take initial mammograms to localize the breast lesion (Figure 21). Once the lesion is localized, use a localizing compression cone (Figure 22) to obtain a film. The localizing compression cone is used in conjunction with a film cassette holder that enables the film to be developed without releasing compression of the breast. The cone is made of acrylic plastic and has a matrix of holes with identifying numbers and letters. The holes, in conjunction with the film, are used to guide the needle to the lesions.

   Approach the lesions from different angles according to where they are located: lesions in the upper half of the breast, from a craniocaudad position; lesions in the lower inner quadrant, from a mediolateral position; and lesions in the lower outer quadrant, from a lateromedial position.

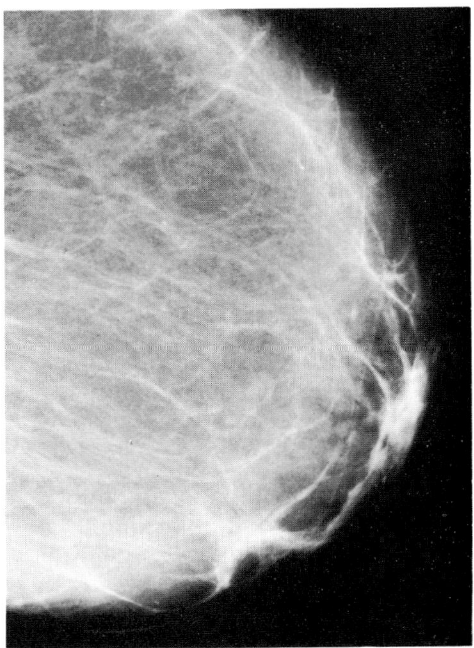

Figure 21. Mammogram taken initially to localize breast lesion.

2. Use the initial film made with the localizing compression cone to determine the hole closest to the lesion (Figure 22). Insert the needle through the chosen hole into the skin and push it at least halfway through the breast (Figure 23). With the needle in place, take another film to confirm the position of the needle with respect to the lesion (Figure 24).

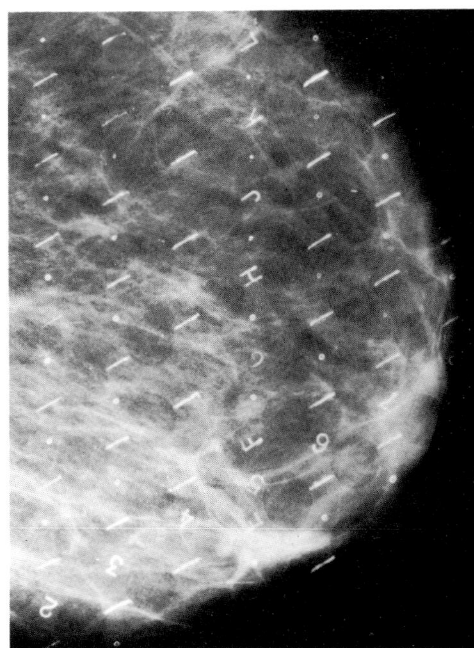

Figure 22. Mammogram using localizing compression cone.

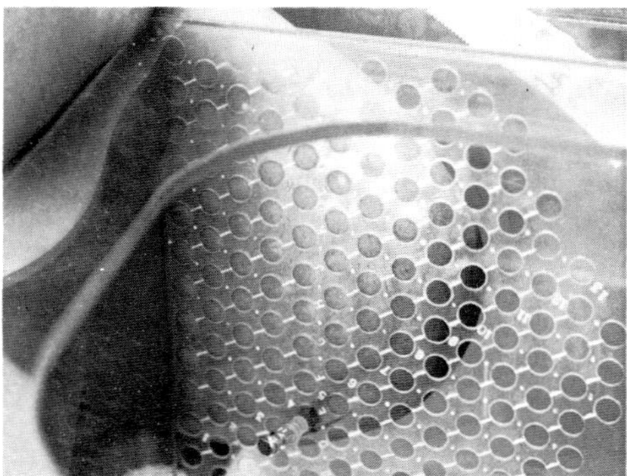

Figure 23. Needle is then inserted through hole located nearest the tumor.

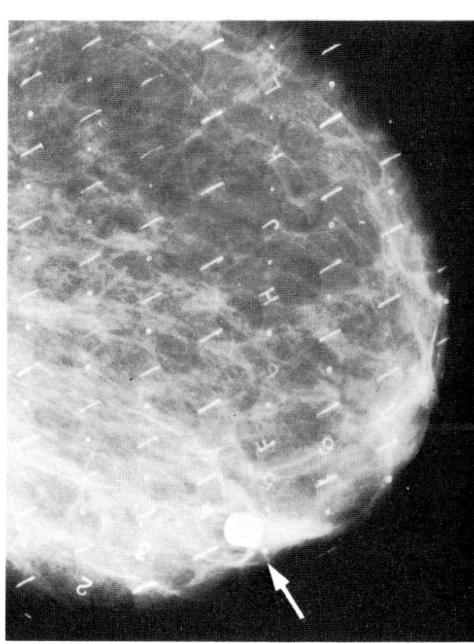

Figure 24. Mammogram confirming needle placement within lesion.

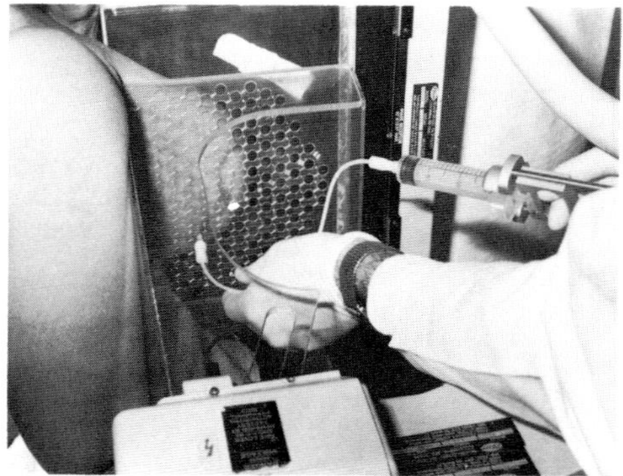

Figure 25. Needle is attached by plastic tube to aspiration syringe, then same procedure as that used for palpable breast lesions is used.

3. Release the breast compression by lifting the compression cone over the needle hub. While holding the needle, carefully reposition the breast for another film at right angles to the first (that is, mediolateral for lesions in the upper half of the breast or craniocaudad for lesions in the lower half of the breast). Compress the breast and take the film. The purpose of the second film is to show whether the needle tip is beyond the lesion. If the needle is beyond the lesion, withdraw the needle the appropriate distance while the breast is still compressed. Repeat the film and withdrawal of the needle until the needle tip is adjacent to the lesion. Connect the syringe to the aspirating needle by a plastic tube and use the same procedure as that used for palpable breast lesions given in chapter 2 (Figure 25). Prepare and stain the smears in the same manner as previously described for palpable masses (chapter 2).

If the FNA results are questionable, an open biopsy should be performed on the breast mass. A wire guide as provided with the Kopans breast localizer needle (Cook, Inc., Bloomington, IN), can be left in the breast as the needle is withdrawn, thus facilitating localization of the lesion for surgery. A final film with the wire guide in place is usually obtained to confirm the FNA needle's final position with respect to the lesion.

Accuracy

The clinical diagnosis of palpable breast lesions is imprecise. False-positive and false-negative diagnoses of breast cancer are common with palpation.[23,25,45,47,48] Kreuzer and Boquoi found an 8% incidence of false-positive clinical diagnoses and a 3% incidence of false-negative clinical diagnoses in their series.[25] Other studies have observed even a higher discrepancy between the clinical and histologic diagnosis. Ackerman and del Regato noted that "even the most experienced examiner can diagnose accurately only some 70% of [breast] carcinomas at clinical examination."[48] Even one of the most experienced diagnosticians, Dr. Haagensen, reported in his material a certain frequency of wrong diagnoses by palpation.[36] With this degree of accuracy, the surgeon cannot rely solely on the patient's clinical history and physical examination for a definitive diagnosis.

The surgeon requires an unequivocal diagnosis upon which he or she can formulate an opinion regarding the appropriate therapy. In the past, histology was the universally accepted means of establishing such a diagnosis, whereas the use of needle aspiration cytology for diagnosing breast cancer was considered controversial.[12,36,44] This criticism largely stemmed from the high incidence of false-negative diagnoses and occasional false-positive diagnoses in the earlier reports on FNA.[4,7,10,11,17] However, a review of the literature (see Tables 2 and 3) shows that the incidence of false-positive and false-negative readings has significantly decreased as experience with FNA has increased.

For example, during the period 1955 to 1964 at the Radiumhemmet in Sweden, there were 1,068 histologically proved carcinomas of the breast that were studied by FNA.[16] The FNA diagnoses were negative for malignancy in 9.9% of the total series.[16] However, in the FNA results reported from the Radiumhemmet in 1964, the false-negative reports had been reduced to 6.1%.

Similarly, others have reported a reduction in false-negative diagnoses with increased FNA experience.[24] Of the first 300 breast FNA cases at the University of Virginia Medical Center, 105 patients had diagnoses of malignancy; however, only 100 had histologically confirmed diagnoses of malignancy. Five patients were considered inoperable but had obvious clinical evidence of malignant disease. Eighty-five of these 105 patients (81%) had FNA results positive for malignancy. Fifteen cases (14%) were classed as suspicious for malignancy and biopsy was recommended. Five of the aspirations (5%) had insufficient material for adequate evaluation. There were no cases with false-positive or false-negative diagnoses in our series (Tables 2 through 4).

False-Negative Diagnoses

Failure to diagnose breast carcinomas by FNA may be due to either failure to aspirate representative material from the tumor (sampling error) or failure to recognize the malignant nature of the aspirated cells.[7]

Sampling Error

Factors related to the failure to obtain representative material from the tumor are many and may be divided into two categories: (1) *characteristics of the tumor* (size, location in the breast, degree of fibrosis, cellularity, differentiation, and location in relation to benign cysts); and (2) *technical factors.*

Characteristics of the Tumor. Kreuzer and Zajicek reviewed cytologic smears and tissue sections from 100 breast carcinomas that had false-negative diagnoses.[49] There were 46 tumors less than 1 cm in diameter; and of these, 23 (50%) had false-negative FNA results, 15 (33%) were suspicious for malignancy, and only 8 (17%) were correctly diagnosed as malignant by FNA. Their experience thus indicated that tumor size was related to the frequency of false-negative diagnoses. Zajdela et al and Smith et al also noted that smaller lesions were associated with more false-negative diagnoses.[9,50]

In Zajdela's series, false-negative diagnoses were

TABLE 4. Correlation of Cytologic and Histologic Findings

FNA Diagnoses		Histologic Findings		
Type	No. of Procedures	Malignant	Benign	Clinical Follow-up
Positive	85	80	0	5*
Suspicious	20	15	5	
Negative	160	0	55	105†
Unsatisfactory	35	5	30	
Total	300	100	90	110

Note: The data used in this table are from the first 300 breast fine needle aspiration procedures performed at the University of Virginia Medical Center.

*Inoperable cases.

†Benign follow-up.

encountered in 6% of T1 tumors (tumor-node-metastases staging system developed by the American Joint Committee for Cancer Staging and End Results Reporting) as compared with 3% for T2 to T3 lesions.[9] Kline also noted that the size of the tumor is a limiting factor; for example, 0.8 cm was the maximum diameter in 12 of her 40 false-negative diagnoses.[51] However, Schöndorf was not able to confirm that the smaller the tumor, the greater the risk for false-negative diagnosis.[28] He noted 19 malignant lesions measuring less than 1 cm in diameter and 23 between 1.0 and 1.5 cm. There was only one false-negative diagnosis and two suspicious diagnoses in these small tumors.

Kreuzer and Zajicek noted that larger sized masses in the breast may also be missed with FNA.[49] This was exemplified by six cases in which a carcinoma was located adjacent to a cyst that was evacuated by FNA. In five of these six cases, the mass measured 2 cm or more. These cases were observed in the early part of their experience with FNA, and the fluid, which in three cases was hemorrhagic, was discarded without being microscopically analyzed. Because a palpable mass persisted in these cases, a surgical biopsy specimen was obtained and carcinoma diagnosed. These cases illustrate that if a mass persists after FNA, the aspiration should be repeated or a biopsy of the mass performed, or both.

Schöndorf felt that the location of the tumor and consistency of the tissue were more important than size since proper palpation, essential for location and aspiration, is dependent mainly on these two factors.

We agree that undoubtedly the location of the tumor is an important factor in the accuracy of FNA. The deeper the tumor is located in the breast, the more difficulty one encounters in performing the FNA. Breast tumors frequently are deeper than initially appreciated, and longer needles may be required to aspirate the lesion. In large breasts, masses may be very difficult to aspirate, especially if the lesion is small. In these circumstances, we have found that mammographic guidance for FNA has been most helpful.

The degree of fibrosis in tumors is another factor considered in explaining the failure to obtain representative material in FNA. Fibrotic tissue usually yields few cells, and this may be attributed to difficulty in detaching cells from their surrounding stroma by means of negative pressure.[49] When Kreuzer and Zajicek reviewed a series of 300 breast carcinoma cases, they noted that fibrosis was more common in tumors that received a false-negative diagnosis (72%) than in cytologically diagnosed carcinomas (35%).[49] Others have also noted that aspiration may fail to yield sufficient cellular material from malignant neoplasms with a severe desmoplastic reaction, eg, scirrhous carcinoma.[7,9,24,29,51]

There is universal agreement on the therapeutic and diagnostic value of aspirations of breast cysts. However, many researchers in the past have disagreed on what to do with the aspirated fluid. Saphir, in 1952, felt that fluid aspirated from a cyst should aways be examined cytologically.[5] The opposite view was expressed by Haagensen, who noted that "if I withdraw characteristic cyst fluid and no definite palpable evidence of disease remains, the cystic fluid is not examined microscopically because I have learned it is a waste of time."[37] Similarly, numerous others have agreed with Haagensen that routine submission of breast cyst fluid is not necessarily indicated.[7,29,31,51–53] At the University of Virginia Medical Center, fluid samples aspirated from breast cysts are not examined microscopically and are discarded only if the fluid is transparent and no residual mass can be palpated. If the fluid aspirated is turbid or hemorrhagic, it is routinely analyzed cytologically. In the past when FNA samples were first being studied, fluid was frequently discarded without being analyzed.[49] This resulted in false-negative diagnoses. Kreuzer and Zajicek noted three cases where hemorrhagic fluid was aspirated and discarded without microscopic analysis, and these patients were eventually shown to have cancer.[49]

When a palpable mass remains after evacuating the cyst, the fluid from the FNA is analyzed microscopically and a repeat aspiration of the mass is obtained.[7,9,31,51,52] If results from the repeat FNA are suspicious, a biopsy of the mass should be performed.[7] The persistence of a palpable mass may be due to a cystic carcinoma or a carcinoma coincidental with the cyst. The latter condition is much more frequent. Zajdela et al noted three false-negative cases where a carcinoma was present adjoining a cyst and not detected by FNA.[9]

The histologic type of carcinoma and degree of differentiation are other factors related to tumor characteristics and false-negative diagnoses. Schöndorf noted that small-cell carcinomas of the breast and carcinomas with a monomorphic appearance contribute to false-negative diagnoses.[28] Zajdela and associates observed that the lack of cytologic abnormalities in malignant cells such as in well-differentiated carcinoma was related to false-negative diagnoses.[9] For example, of 63 malignant tumors with false-negative diagnoses, 37 (59%) were histologically classified as well-differentiated carcinomas and only 8 (13%) were poorly differentiated carcinomas.[9] When Kline reviewed her false-negative diagnoses, 43% of the aspirations from infiltrating lobular carcinoma were diagnosed as negative in contrast to 7% from infiltrating duct carcinomas.[51] Similarly, aspirations from small-cell duct carcinomas, comprising only 15% of the series reported by Zajicek et al, accounted for 70% of their total false-negative results.[16]

Technical Factors. Technical factors are also related to failures of the FNA. The skill and experience of the physician performing the FNA is of paramount importance. Diagnostic accuracy is known to increase as the person performing the FNA gains experience with the technique of FNA.[4,7,50] Our experience has shown that the two most important factors related to accuracy and directly related to false-positive and false-negative diagnoses are the experience of the physician who performs the FNA and the experience of the cytopathologist who analyzes and interprets the FNA smears. Ideally, the physician who performs the FNA is also the one who interprets the FNA smears. Such optimal conditions are present in only certain centers, such as the Radiumhemmet in Stockholm,[7,13] Foundation-Curie in Paris,[9] and Center Oscar-Lambert in Lille, France.[17] More recently in the United States, FNAs are performed and interpreted by pathologists in several centers.[31,52,54] In initial studies at the Memorial Sloan-Kettering Hospital in New York, surgeons and not pathologists performed the FNA and that procedure is still followed today.[2,3,19,20] Kline also interprets but does not perform the FNAs.[51]

Why should the person performing the FNA be the one who interprets the FNA? Surely the surgeon who has more experience with palpation could obtain better results with FNA. Our results negate this theory. There are multiple reasons why the person performing the FNA should also be the one who analyzes and interprets the material. The cytologic diagnosis from the FNA should not be based only on the microscopic evaluation of slides, but also on a summation of the clinical assessment made before the FNA and observations made during and after needling the breast mass.[7]

For the initial 1,000-plus FNAs performed at our hospital, the cytopathologists performed all the FNAs. Surgeons and radiologists began performing some of the aspirations after the FNA technique was carefully explained and illustrated. Although faculty surgeons obtained good results, the results obtained from FNA performed by surgical residents were far from ideal because of their inexperience with this technique. Similarly, Adair at Memorial Sloan Kettering Hospital noted a 10% failure rate with breast aspirations by surgeons experienced with this technique versus a 20% failure rate when the aspirations were performed by doctors new to the technique of aspiration biopsy.[4]

The pathologist performing the FNA can see the patient and his or her chart, obtain the clinical history, and discuss the case with the patient's clinician. When performing the FNA, the size, consistency (solid, cystic, soft, hard), and location of the mass can be ascertained. These findings may have considerable bearing on the results of the FNA. A key factor is assessing the adequacy of the sample from the FNA. An inexperienced operator tends not to appreciate whether sufficient material for diagnosis has been obtained. However, a physician experienced with FNA can usually evaluate the adequacy of the material by macroscopic inspection of the aspiration.

At our center, a cytotechnologist always accompanies whoever performs the aspiration and quickly processes and stains the slides. The patient remains in the clinic until the pathologist microscopically reviews the material from the FNA. If the material is inadequate, the aspiration is repeated. Unfortunately, because of the rapidly escalating numbers of FNAs performed in our hospital, it is not practical for the pathologist to do all the FNAs. However, when others performed the aspirations, the incidence of unsatisfactory aspirations increased. The results are simply not the same when the pathologist has not both seen the patient and performed the FNA.

Rapid processing of the material yields a preliminary diagnosis within 10 to 15 minutes. In this way, even with inexperienced physicians performing the FNA, failures of this technique are minimized. When the cytopathologist performs FNA, he or she does the initial FNA and then allows the surgical or pathology resident to do a second aspiration while the cytopathologist observes and instructs the resident on the correct technique. This has resulted in more successful aspirations by residents, and when they leave the university, they can correctly perform FNA. Residents are eager to learn this technique and are more inclined to request FNA as a diagnostic procedure if they are allowed to perform some of the aspirations.

We frequently receive FNA slides from other

hospitals for consultation. Although the clinical information is usually good, slides are sometimes poorly prepared (that is, staining or fixation) or contain insufficient aspirated material. These slides are not optimal for obtaining accurate diagnostic results. Fortunately, when material is sent to us for consultation from former residents who are well acquainted with the FNA technique, better results are obtained.

Failure to Recognize Malignant Cells. Failure to recognize the malignant nature of the aspirated cells is another important factor contributing to false-negative diagnoses and is related to the experience of the pathologist analyzing the FNA. When Kreuzer and Zajicek reviewed 100 cases of carcinoma of the breast that had received a false-negative cytologic report, they found that in 58 cases, malignant cells were absent in the aspiration.[49] However, in the other 42 cases, malignant cells were present in the aspirated material but not recognized at the time of diagnosis. They felt that increased experience in FNA interpretation reduced the false-negative rate by about 20%.

In the other 22%, the monomorphic pattern and lack of significant atypia would have prevented recognition of malignancy. Similarly, Koivuniemi reviewed the cytologic findings in 192 histologically verified breast cancers.[24] There were 8.8% false-negative diagnoses, but on reviewing the aspirated material, only 5.1% still had a negative diagnosis.[24] Thus, experience and correct interpretation of the aspirated material would have reduced the number of false-negative diagnoses.

False-Positive Diagnoses

In the early reported series, false-positive diagnoses were more frequent (see Table 3)[10,14,27,25] and resulted in severe criticism of breast FNA.[12,36] The medical philosophy of the not too distant past (1960) is exemplified by an article by Klimanova extolling the virtues of breast FNA and the comments of the editorial board that followed the paper.

> Puncture biopsy in breast carcinomas has become undeservedly popular and cannot under any conditions be substituted for the more reliable method of excision biopsy. It is not possible to conclude reliably whether the tumor is malignant or benign. Injury to the tumor even with a fine needle may cause dissemination of the tumor cells and thus puncture biopsy of the breast cannot be recommended for widespread use.[11]

False-positive diagnoses in breast FNA have usually been the result of the inexperience of the physician interpreting the smears. The major sources of error appear to have been the incorrect interpretation of atypical smears from benign breast disease or the rendering of diagnoses on inadequate or poorly prepared material.[7,21,25] Microscopic experience and careful application of diagnostic criteria are necessary to avoid these pitfalls.

Fortunately, breast FNA has advanced sufficiently that false-positive diagnoses are a rarity (see Table 3).[19,20,23,24,29,31,52] Today the diagnostic accuracy of breast FNA has reached the point that mastectomies are performed without confirmation by frozen section in cases with positive cytologic diagnoses.[7,9,19,20,29,31,52] This practice is not experimental and has been used in certain European centers for more than ten years,[7,9,17] and more recently in the United States.[29,31,52,54] To believe that one would have enough confidence to diagnose carcinoma from cells alone and not from a tissue biopsy would have been sacrilegious a few years ago. However, pathologists with experience in FNA technique are now sufficiently confident of their FNA diagnoses to diagnose malignancy, being fully aware of the consequences. There is no room for error because a mistake would be disastrous resulting in, eg, unnecessary mastectomy. The acceptance of FNA as an equivalent to tissue biopsy represents a major advance in diagnostic cytopathology. Of the first 80 patients with breast cancer who were diagnosed by FNA at our hospital, 48 had a mastectomy without frozen section. The mastectomy sections confirmed the presence of malignancy in every patient; there were no false-positive diagnoses. Thirty-two patients had a frozen section before mastectomy. These cases occurred early in the series before surgeons had developed confidence in the accuracy of FNA. Surgeons at our hospital now routinely perform mastectomies without frozen section when the FNA results give a definitive diagnosis of malignancy.

Interpretation of Breast Fine Needle Aspirations

Our experience at the University of Virginia Medical Center has shown that the differential diagnosis between benign and malignant lesions is clear from most breast FNAs with the careful application of the cytologic criteria for malignancy. The malignant features include cellular and nuclear variation in size and shape, hyperchromatism, irregular chromatin clumping, abnormal chromatin distribution, nuclear molding, prominent or macronucleoli, abnormal mitotic figures, increased nuclear:cytoplasmic (N:C) ratio, and overlapping and crowding of nuclei. When present, these features are excellent indicators of malignancy. Unfortunately, there are a small but significant number of malignant lesions in which these criteria are less well defined, and the differentiation of these lesions from benign proliferations of duct epithelium (eg, ductal hyperplasia, gynecomastia, and fibroadenoma) may be difficult.

Since duct carcinomas comprise approximately 90% of all breast cancers, their differentiation from benign lesions is of the greatest diagnostic significance. A report by Dziura and Bonfiglio in 1979 analyzed the various cytologic features of mammary ductal lesions seen in FNA.[55] They concluded that large nuclei, large variation in nuclear size, and the presence of macronucleoli were specific features of malignant lesions. Chromatin clumping was a useful indicator, if present. However, their most notable conclusion was that nuclear overlap was the most consistently useful feature in the diagnosis of ductal breast lesions and was the only criterion that could be applied reliably in every case studied. They noted that a continuum of overlap existed such that hyperplasia could be distinguished from malignancy.

A similar analysis of diagnostic cytologic criteria in breast FNA for benign and malignant diseases was conducted in our laboratory. The features evaluated included slide background, cellular arrangement, cell configuration, cytoplasmic features, nuclear configuration, nuclear:cytoplasmic ratio, chromatin pattern, and nucleoli. Our results from the first 300 breast FNAs conducted at the University of Virginia Medical Center are summarized in Table 4 and our general findings for the various types of breast carcinoma are summarized in Table 5. However, there are certain points that should be discussed in more detail.

Slide Background

Most breast FNAs had a similar background of scattered red blood cells as a result of the sampling procedure. The necrotic debris of tumor diathesis was seen only occasionally in cases of malignancy. However, necrosis was also noted in certain cases of benign disease such as abscess and fat necrosis.

The presence of bare nuclei in the smear background is a frequently reported indication of benign disease. Our studies have supported this theory in general; however, we have noted similar bare nuclei in two cases of duct carcinoma. The presence of large pools of mucin was noted only in cases of colloid carcinoma and, therefore, has only limited application as a criterion for malignancy.

The cellularity of the aspiration varied with each particular lesion and had limited application in differentiating benign and malignant processes. In general, malignant and atypical hyperplastic lesions were hypercellular, and benign lesions yielded less-cellular aspirates.

Cellular Arrangement

This category yielded perhaps the most consistent criteria for distinguishing benign from malignant samples in breast aspiration smears. In general, the benign lesions showed good cellular cohesion and well-organized cell sheets with distinct cell borders. Single cells were not numerous, and there was little or no nuclear overlapping within the cell groups. The exceptions to these features were some ductal hyperplasias that may mimic carcinoma.

The malignant lesions were usually arranged in aggregates with indistinct cell borders and frequent nuclear overlapping and crowding. Single, abnormal cells were seen in almost every case. These features were noted regardless of the presence or absence of nuclear criteria of malignancy. An excellent example of this is the cytologic presentation of lobular carcinoma. These cells show a distinct absence of obvious nuclear abnormality; however, the cell pattern of monomorphic, mostly dissociated cells, is unique to this tumor type.

Cell Configuration

Obvious cellular pleomorphism was often a good criterion for diagnosing malignancy; however, its absence does not exclude malignancy. This feature is noticeably absent in lobular carcinomas, papillary carcinomas, cystic carcinomas, and some duct carcinomas. Bizarre forms may occasionally be seen in benign lesions. We have noted two cases of fibrocystic disease that yielded bizarre, pleomorphic cells from the cyst wall. These cells lacked the nuclear criteria of malignancy, which aided in the diagnosis of benign disease.

Cytoplasmic Features

We found no cytoplasmic features that were reliable in differentiating benign and malignant lesions.

Nuclear Configuration

Round or oval nuclei were common to all breast lesions and, therefore, nuclear shape was of little di-

TABLE 5. Cytologic Features of Primary Breast Carcinomas

	Carcinoma Type				
Feature	Infiltrating Duct	Apocrine Cell	Medullary	Colloid (Mucinous)	Infiltrating Lobular
Slide Background	Bloody, occasional necrotic debris	Bloody, occasional necrotic debris	Bloody, inflammation (primarily lymphocytes), occasional necrotic debris	Bloody, pools of mucin	Bloody, occasional necrotic debris
Cellular Arrangement	Abundant cells, isolated and in clusters; may mimic duct structure; occasional syncytial arrangements and sheets	Numerous cells, isolated and in syncytial arrangements	Numerous cells, isolated, in syncytial arrangements or clusters	Numerous cells, isolated, in clusters or sheets	Innumerable cells, mainly isolated and in small aggregates, occasional "Indian file" arrangement and clusters mimicking the structure of the terminal ducts; signet-ring forms may be seen
Cytoplasm	Basophilic staining; granular or finely vacuolated; occasional larger vacuoles; scant	Basophilic or eosinophilic staining; finely granular; moderate to abundant	Basophilic staining; finely vacuolated; scant to abundant	Basophilic staining; finely vacuolated with occasional larger discreet vacuoles; scant to abundant	Basophilic staining; finely granular; scant
Nuclear Configuration	Small and uniform or larger and pleomorphic; round, oval, and irregular	Enlarged, round or oval; size varied	Enlarged with pronounced variation in size and shape	Enlarged with pronounced variation in size and shape; occasionally eccentrically placed	Small with some mild variation in size; round or oval
Nuclear:Cytoplasmic Ratio	Increased	Normal or increased	Increased	Increased	Slightly increased
Chromatin Pattern	Predominately finely granular; evenly, irregularly distributed; mild or moderate hyperchromatism	Finely granular or granular; evenly distributed	Finely granular or granular, evenly or irregularly distributed; normal or mild hyperchromatism	Finely granular, evenly distributed, mild or moderate hyperchromatism	Finely granular; evenly distributed, normal or mild hyperchromatism
Nucleolus	Usually prominent or macronucleoli, occasional micronucleoli, uniform or irregularly shaped	Prominent or macronucleoli, sometimes multiple	Usually multiple macronucleoli, some irregular shapes	Multiple, prominent or macronucleoli, occasionally irregularly shaped	Usually single, uniform, micronucleoli or prominent nucleoli

agnostic value. Irregular shapes usually indicated malignancy, although they were occasionally seen in benign lesions. Nuclear enlargement was noted in most breast diseases, but it was more noticeable in cases of malignancy. Variation in nuclear size was seen in cases of gynecomastia, ductal hyperplasia, and carcinoma; however, it was more pronounced in the malignant lesions.

When present, nuclear molding and nuclear membrane irregularities were also useful malignant criteria. The membrane irregularities were often subtle and required high-power magnification for distinction. Extreme nuclear molding (ie, "Indian-file" arrangement) was noted only in cases of infiltrating carcinoma, generally of either ductal or lobular type.

Nuclear: Cytoplasmic Ratio

Relative nuclear area varied widely between benign and malignant diseases, as well as among the various histologic patterns of carcinoma. The nuclear: cytoplasmic ratio was generally increased in most malignancies and in some benign lesions. It was found to have minimal definitive diagnostic value.

Chromatin Pattern

The vast majority of breast lesions, both benign and malignant, showed a finely granular chromatin pattern. Irregularities of chromatin distribution were usually confined to the malignancies; however, these irregularities were often subtle and difficult to discern without careful high-power examination. Mild to moderate hyperchromatism was noted in carcinomas, some hyperplasias, and gynecomastia. Intense hyperchromatism was rarely seen.

Nucleoli

Micronucleoli or prominent nucleoli were common in cells from many breast diseases, including carcinoma. Macronucleoli were usually confined to malignant lesions; however, large nucleoli were seen in some cases of gynecomastia. Nucleolar number varied from case to case and was therefore of little value in making differential diagnoses.

It is clear from this discussion that there was no one feature or pattern of the cells that was universally applicable in the differentiation between benign and malignant diseases. We strongly emphasize that the evaluation of nuclear features and cell patterns in combination with the clinical history and physical findings is essential for making accurate diagnoses from breast FNA smears.

Differential Diagnosis of Breast Malignancies

Schöndorf noted that "the interpretation of breast fine needle aspiration is limited to recognition of the benign or malignant potential of the cells."[28] He felt that "in order to specify the type of lesion, examination of tissue sections was necessary." Similarly, others have considered it impossible to differentiate among the various histologic types of breast cancer with aspiration biopsies.[22,56] Geier et al observed that "a histologic classification of mammary carcinoma solely based on cytologic studies is not possible."[22] On the other hand, Wallgren and Zajicek reported that after reviewing 542 histologically verified mammary cancers, most of the histologic variants of invasive carcinoma could be recognized cytologically.[57] Similarly, others have been able to recognize from FNA smears the patterns corresponding to histologic types of breast cancer.[19,31,51,52,58] For the first 100 histologically confirmed breast cancers diagnosed by FNA at the University of Virginia Medical Center, our accuracy in typing the malignancy was 96% (Table 6). The remaining 4% of the cases were interpreted as malignant but typed incorrectly.

When evaluating an FNA, the first step is to differentiate the benign from the malignant breast mass. If the mass is malignant, the second step is to

TABLE 6. Typing of Breast Malignancies by Fine Needle Aspiration

MALIGNANCY	HISTOLOGY	FNA
Duct carcinoma	80	78
Lobular carcinoma	6	5
Medullary carcinoma	2	2
Papillary carcinoma	3	3
Mucinous carcinoma	3	2
Comedocarcinoma	2	2
Sarcoma	2	2
Metastatic carcinoma	2	2
Total	100	96 (96%)*

NOTE: Data in this table are from 100 histologically confirmed breast malignancies diagnosed using results of fine needle aspiration performed at the University of Virginia Medical Center.

*Although four cases were not typed correctly by FNA, they were correctly diagnosed as malignant.

try typing the breast cancer from the FNA.

When we initially began interpreting breast FNAs, we were content to separate a benign from a malignant process. However, through examination of numerous aspiration preparations and by comparative study of smears and tissue sections, we were able to distinguish among the various histologic types of breast cancer, based on FNA. The cases presented in this atlas were intentionally selected to illustrate the various cytologic patterns seen in breast cancer. From the FNA, one should be able to recognize the pattern of infiltrating duct carcinoma, medullary carcinoma, mucinous (colloid) carcinoma, signet-ring carcinoma, apocrine carcinoma, tubular carcinoma, lobular carcinoma, and sarcomas.

The interpretation of infiltrating lobular carcinoma and small cell duct carcinoma presents problems for several reasons.[1,31] First, lobular carcinoma is not clearly distinguishable from the small-cell form of infiltrating duct carcinoma. Second, smears from these carcinomas may be either highly cellular or rather sparse in cells. The tumor cells are bland, only slightly variable in size and shape, and may be arranged in a single-file pattern. Obvious malignant nuclear criteria are usually absent. Caution is thus indicated before reporting an FNA diagnosis of these carcinomas. This conservative diagnostic approach is warranted because of the aforementioned reasons and especially since a mastectomy without frozen section would be performed for a positive diagnosis of malignancy. A frozen section or other tissue biopsy is requested before mastectomy to confirm the diagnosis in these types of carcinoma.

Reporting Results

The results for breast FNA are reported using the four categories (unsatisfactory, suspicious, negative for malignancy, or positive for malignancy) as described in chapter 2. The type of malignant lesion should also be included in the report whenever possible. Because of their significance to patient management, further discussion of the suspicious and positive categories is necessary when applied to breast FNA.

The incidence of suspicious diagnoses in the literature varies widely: Franzen and Zajicek, 14%; Zajdela et al, 3%; and Kern, 23%.[7,9,29] This incidence tends to reflect not only the experience of the pathologist interpreting the smears, but also the consequence of malignant diagnoses for the surgeon. In centers where a positive FNA results in mastectomy without frozen section, the incidence of suspicious diagnoses is higher to avoid unnecessary surgery.[9,19,20,28] At the University of Virginia Medical Center, mastectomy is performed without frozen section diagnosis when the breast FNA before surgery is positive for malignancy. Therefore, if there is any question or doubt as to the cytologic interpretation, the suspicious category is used.

In our first 300 breast FNAs, there were 20 suspicious diagnoses (7%). The majority of these cases occurred during the first year of performing breast FNA. With experience, the number of cases in this category has been greatly reduced. An open biopsy or repeat FNA was done on all these 20 cases. Results showed carcinoma in 15 of the 20 suspicious cases (75%).

A report of positive for malignancy indicates to the surgeons that there is conclusive evidence of malignancy and that they may proceed to mastectomy or radiation therapy, or both, without further tissue confirmation. After careful evaluation of the case, pathologists must be totally convinced of the malignant diagnosis. If they are not, another diagnostic category should be used because a false-positive diagnosis could result in unnecessary mastectomy. As previously discussed, the exceptions to this general rule are small-cell duct carcinomas and lobular carcinomas for which frozen section or biopsy is routinely recommended before mastectomy despite a positive cytology report.

Normal Cytology

Normal duct epithelial cells from the breast have distinct cell borders and are seen lying singly or in sheets, clusters, and aggregates. They have a monomorphic appearance with uniform, vesicular nuclei and micronucleoli as seen in Color Plate 1, chapter 4. Occasional fragments of adipose tissue may also be aspirated. In alcohol-fixed preparations, the cells are recognized as sheets of large spherical- to polyhedral-shaped cells with a large empty space occupying most of the volume of the cytoplasm of each cell. The cell nuclei are displaced to the periphery, and the basophilic-staining cytoplasm is reduced to a thin rim that gives the sheet a netlike appearance.

Summary

In summary, FNA is a highly accurate, safe, inexpensive, and rapid procedure to distinguish between benign and malignant breast diseases. For the FNA to be successful, the following are essential: (1) there is close communication between the surgeon and the cytopathologist; (2) correct technique is employed; and (3) cytologic criteria are carefully applied for interpretation of the cellular material. It is imperative for the surgeon to understand what FNA diagnoses mean: unsatisfactory FNA results require repeat FNA or biopsy; negative FNA results do not exclude malignancy; suspicious FNA results necessitate repeat FNA or open biopsy; and positive FNA results enable the surgeon to proceed to mastectomy without frozen section or radiation therapy if clinically indicated.

References

1. Martin HE, Ellis EB: Biopsy by needle puncture and aspiration. *Ann Surg* 1930;92:169–181.
2. Stewart FW: The diagnosis of tumors by aspiration. *Am J Pathol* 1933;9:801–812.
3. Martin HE, Ellis EB: Aspiration biopsy. *Surg Gynecol Obstet* 1934;59:578–589.
4. Adair FE: Surgical problems involved in breast cancer. *Ann R Coll Surg Engl* 1949;4:360–380.
5. Saphir O: Early diagnosis of breast lesions. *JAMA* 1952;150:859–861.
6. Godwin, JT: Aspiration biopsy: Technique and application. *Ann NY Acad Sci* 1956;63:1348–1373.
7. Franzen S, Zajicek J: Aspiration biopsy in diagnosis of palpable lesions of the breast. *Acta Radiol Therapy Physics Biology* 1968;7:241–262.
8. Zajdela A: Valeur et intérêt de diagnostic cytologique dans les tumeurs du sein par ponction—Etude de 600 cas confrontés cytologiguement et histologiquement. *Arch Anat Pathol* 1963;11:85–87.
9. Zajdela A, Ghossein NA, Pilleron JP, et al: The value of aspiration cytology in the diagnosis of breast cancer: Experience at the Fondation Curie. *Cancer* 1975;35(2):499–506.
10. Cornillot M, Verhaeghe M: Donnees cytologiqũes dans les ponctions de tumeurs du sein. *Pathol Biol* 1959;7:793.
11. Shiller–Volkova NN, Agamova KA: Cytological investigation of punctates as a method for the diagnosis of mammary tumours. *Vopr Onkol* 1960;65–71.
12. Klimanova ZF: Cytological examination of breast tumor punctates. *Prob Oncol* 1961;7:7–11.
13. Zajicek J, Frazen S, Jakobsson P, et al.: Aspiration biopsy of mammary tumors in diagnosis and research—a critical review of 2,200 cases. *Acta Cytol* 1967;11:169–175.
14. Laumonier J, Hemet J: La cytologie des tumeurs mammaires (a partir de 1000 cytodiagnostics). *Proc Int Symp on Detection of Cancer,* 1968, pp 257–262.
15. Winship T: Aspiration biopsy of breast cancers by the pathologist. *Am J Clin Pathol* 1969;52:438–440.
16. Zajicek J, Caspersson T, Jakobsson P, et al: Cytologic diagnosis of mammary tumors from aspiration biopsy smears. Comparison of cytologic and histologic findings in 2111 lesions and diagnostic use of cytophotometric. *Acta Cytol* 1970;14:370–376.
17. Cornillot M, Verhaeghe M, Cappelaere P, et al.: Place de la cytologie par ponction dans le diagnostic des tumeurs du sein (2267 examens cytologigues). *Lille Med* 1971;16:1027–1031.
18. Rajcic, V: Cytologic studies of aspiration biopsy of the breast: Critical review of 2,890 consecutive biopsies. *Minerva Ginecol* 1971;23:417–419.
19. Rosen P, Hajdu SI, Foote FW: Diagnosis of carcinoma of the breast by aspiration biopsy. *Surg Gynecol Obstet* 1972;134:837–838.
20. Hajdu S, Melamed MR: The diagnostic value of aspiration smears. *Am J Clin Pathol* 1973;59:350–356.
21. Stavric G, Tevcev D, Kaftandjiev D, et al: Aspiration biopsy cytologic method in diagnosis of breast lesions—A critical review of 250 cases. *Acta Cytol* 1973;17:188–190.
22. Geier G, Schuttmann R, Kraus H: Mammapunktionszytologie. Aspiration cytology of the breast. *Beitr Path Bd* 1975;156:223–240.
23. Rimstein A, Stenkuist B, Johanson H, et al: The diagnostic accuracy of palpation and fine needle biopsy and an evaluation of their combined use in the diagnosis of breast lesions: Report on a prospective study in 1,244 women with symptoms. *Ann Surg* 1975;182(1):1–8.
24. Koivuniemi AP: Fine-needle aspiration biopsy of the breast. *Ann Clin Res* 1976;8(4):272–283.
25. Kreuzer G, Boquoi E: Aspiration biopsy cytology, mammography and clinical exploration: A modern set up in diagnosis of tumors of the breast. *Acta Cytol* 1976;20:319–323.
26. Manheimer LH, Rywlin AM: Fine needle aspiration cytology. *South Med J* 1977;70(8):923–925.
27. Deschenes L, Fabia J, Meisels A, et al: Fine needle aspiration biopsy in the management of palpable breast lesions. *Can J Surg* 1978;21:417–419.
28. Schöndorf H: *Aspiration Cytology of the Breast.* Philadelphia, WB Saunders Co, 1978.
29. Kern WH: The diagnosis of breast cancer by fine-needle aspiration smears. *JAMA* 1979;241(11):1125–1127.
30. Kline TS, Joshi LP, Neal HS: Fine-needle aspiration of the breast: Diagnoses and pitfalls. *Cancer* 1979;44:1458–1464.
31. Frable WJ: *Thin Needle Aspiration Biopsy.* Philadelphia, WB Saunders Co, 1983.
32. Vilaplana EV, Ayala MJ: The cytologic diagnosis of breast lesions. *Acta Cytol* 1975;19:519–526.
33. Robbins GF, Brothers JH, Eberhart WF, et al.: Is aspiration biopsy of breast cancer dangerous to the patient? *Cancer* 1954;7:774–778.
34. Berg JW, Robbins GF: A late look at the safety of aspiration biopsy. *Cancer* 1962;15:826–827.
35. Ochsner A, DeBakey M, Dixon, JL: Primary cancer of the lung. *JAMA* 1947;135:321–327.

36. Haagensen CD: *Diseases of the Breast,* ed 2. Philadelphia, WB Saunders Co, 1971, chap 5.

37. Haason J, Luhan PA, Kohn MW: Comparison of estrogen receptor levels in breast cancer samples from mastectomy and frozen section specimens. *Cancer* 1981;47:138–139.

38. Jakowatz JB, Cullen ML, Anderson KM, et al: The stability of estrogen and progesterone receptors as an operative advantage in breast cancer. *Breast* 1981;7:2–5.

39. Meyer JS, Stevens SC, White WL, et al: Estrogen receptor assay of carcinomas of the breast by a simplified dextran-charcoal method. *Am J Clin Pathol* 1978;70: 655–664.

40. Meyer JS: Estrogen receptor assays on tumor removed from mastectomy specimens, letter to the editor. *Cancer* 1982;50:606.

41. Silfverswärd C, Humla S: Estrogen receptor analysis on needle aspirates from human mammary carcinoma. *Acta Cytol* 1980;24:54–57.

42. Silverswärd C, Gustafsson JA, Gustafsson SW, et al: Estrogen receptor analysis on fine needle aspirates and on histologic biopsies from human breast cancer. *Eur J Cancer* 1980;16:1351–1357.

43. Gunduz N, Fisher B.: Fluoresceinated estrone binding by cells from human breast cancers obtained by needle aspiration. *Cancer* 1983;52:1251–1256.

44. Webb AJ: The diagnostic cytology of breast carcinoma. *Brit J Surg* 1970;57:259–264.

45. Shephard D, Soder P, Cooper D, et al: Mammography: an aid in the treatment of carcinoma of the breast. *Ann Surg* 1974;179:749–756.

46. Hennig K, Johansson H, Rimsten A, et al: X-ray and fine needle biopsy in diagnosis of non-palpable breast lesions. *Acta Cytol* 1975;19:7–10.

47. Shabot MM, Goldberg IM, Schick P, et al: Aspiration cytology is superior to tru-cut needle biopsy in establishing the diagnosis of clinically suspicious breast masses. *Ann Surg* 1982;196:122–126.

48. Ackerman LV, del Regato JA: *Cancer,* ed 4, St. Louis, CV Mosby Co, 1970, p 851.

49. Kreuzer G, Zajicek J: Cytologic diagnosis of mammary tumors from aspiration biopsy smears. III: Studies on 200 carcinomas with false negative or doubtful cytologic reports. *Acta Cytol* 1972;16:249–252.

50. Smith IH, Fisher JH, Lott JS, et al: The cytological diagnosis of solid tumors by small needle aspiration and its influence on cancer clinic practice. *Can Med Assoc J* 1959;80:855–861.

51. Kline TS: *Handbook of Fine Needle Aspiration Biopsy Cytology.* St. Louis, CV Mosby Co, 1981.

52. Kaminsky DB: *Aspiration Biopsy for the Community Hospital.* New York, Masson Publishing Co, 1981.

53. Cowen PN, Benson EA: Cytological study of fluid from breast cysts. *Br J Surg* 1979;66(3):209–211.

54. Oertel YC: Fine needle aspiration cytology—A diagnostic tool. Read before the 1983 Spring Meeting of the American Society of Clinical Pathologists and the College of American Pathologists; Chicago, April 19, 1982.

55. Dziura BR, Bonfiglio TA: Needle cytology of the breast. A quantitative and qualitative study of the cells of benign and malignant ductal neoplasia. *Acta Cytol* 1979;23(4):332–340.

56. Bauermeister DE: The role and limitations of frozen section and needle aspiration biopsy in breast cancer diagnosis. *Cancer* 1980;46:947–949.

57. Wallgren A, Zajicek J: Cytologic presentation of mammary carcinoma on aspiration biopsy smears. *Acta Cytol* 1976;20:469–478.

58. Zajicek J: *Aspiration biopsy cytology. Part I: Cytology of Supradiaphragmatic Organs,* in Wied GL (ed): Monographs in Clinical Cytology. New York, Karger, 1974, vol 4.

4

Illustrated Case Studies of Breast Diseases

PLATE 1

Breast Abscess

Note: Most of the patients whose conditions are described in chapter 4 were seen at the University of Virginia Medical Center.

Clinical History. A 31-year-old woman was seen in the surgery clinic because of a lump in her right breast that she first noticed about six months previously. The mass had been increasing in size, and she recently noticed tenderness over this area. The patient denied any breast discharge or trauma. The physical examination showed a firm, tender, mobile 2-cm mass located in the lower inner quadrant of the right breast. The skin overlying this region was erythematous.

Cytologic Findings. The smears from the FNA of the breast mass were characterized by innumerable acute and chronic inflammatory cells (primarily polymorphonuclear leukocytes, lymphocytes, and plasma cells) in varying stages of preservation, and scattered lipid-laden macrophages, which were indicative of tissue breakdown (Plate 1–1). The dense smear background consisted of proteinaceous material and cellular debris (Plate 1–2). A few clusters and sheets of benign ductal cells were also present (Plate 1–2, 1–3). These ductal cells had uniform, round or oval, vesicular nuclei with single, small nucleoli. Their cytoplasm was scanty and basophilic. All groups showed good cohesion and uniform arrangement, although cell borders were sometimes indistinct. This cytologic pattern was interpreted as consistent with an abscess.

Follow-up. Culture of the material from the aspiration grew *Staphylococcus aureus.* She was treated with cephalexin (Keflex) and the mass resolved.

Refer to Slide 1 in Optional Slide Set.

PLATE 1

Fat Necrosis

Clinical History. A 44-year-old woman experienced trauma to her left breast and subsequently noticed tenderness and a lump in this area. A tender, firm 3-cm mass adjacent to the areola of the left breast was found during the physical examination.

Cytologic Findings. Smears from the breast FNA contained a mixture of lymphocytes, numerous macrophages, and occasional multinucleated giant cells in a background of amorphous basophilic material. The macrophages had abundant, basophilic, finely vacuolated cytoplasm (Plate 1–4). Some macrophages showed discrete larger vacuoles (Plate 1–5). Their nuclei were round or oval and vesicular with distinct nucleoli. The multinucleated giant cells contained five to ten mirror-image vesicular nuclei with prominent nucleoli (Plate 1–6, 1–7). Their basophilic cytoplasm was abundant and had a dense granular texture. A Sudan IV-stained slide showed abundant lipid material within the vacuoles of the macrophages and in the smear background (Plate 1–8). This cellular pattern was indicative of fat necrosis in the breast.

Pathologic Findings. An open biopsy of the breast excised a well-circumscribed, firm, yellow-grey, 2-cm mass. Microscopic sections confirmed the diagnosis of fat necrosis with lipid-laden macrophages and chronic inflammation (Plate 1–9). Other areas of the tissue showed scattered multinucleated giant cells.

Refer to Slide 2 in Optional Slide Set.

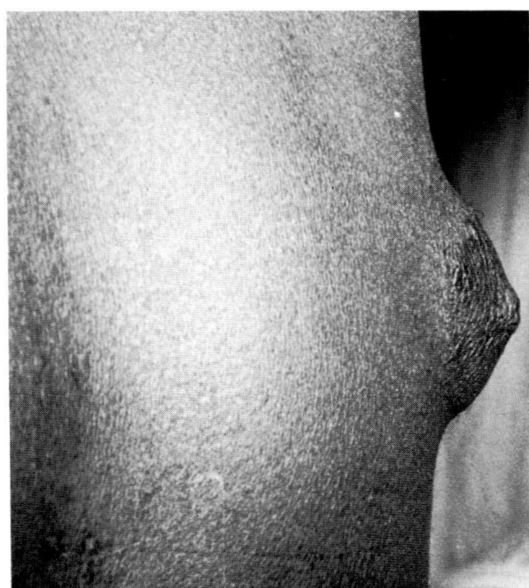

Figure A. Enlargement of breast beneath left areola.

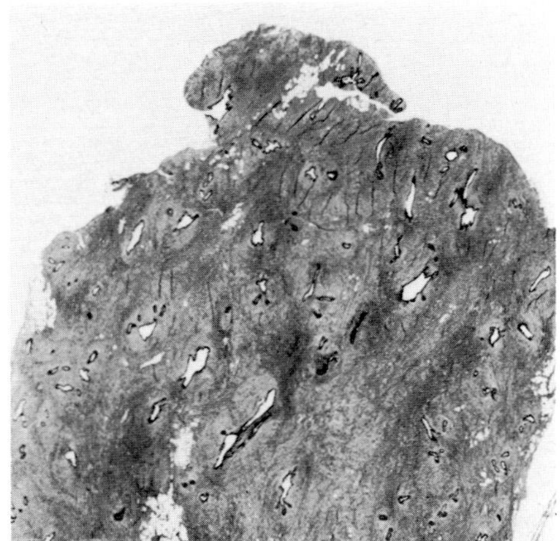

Figure B. Microscopic section of gynecomastia (×10).

PLATE 1

Gynecomastia

Clinical History. A 53-year-old man was referred to the University of Virginia Medical Center by his family physician because of a breast mass noticed by the patient about one month previously. The patient noticed that his left breast became slightly tender and a "little bit puffy" (Figure A). He was receiving spironolactone (Aldactone) for essential hypertension. The physical examination showed a freely movable area beneath his left areola. There was no discharge from the nipple. The left axilla and the right breast were normal. The clinical diagnosis was gynecomastia.

Cytologic Findings. The FNA smears of the breast contained numerous cohesive sheets of duct cells (Plate 1–10, 1–11). Single cells were only occasionally seen. The duct cells had scant or moderate basophilic cytoplasm. Their nuclei were round or oval but variable in size. Overlapping of nuclei was frequently seen within the sheets but cell polarity was preserved. The nuclear membranes were smooth and even. The chromatin pattern was finely granular and evenly distributed with occasional chromocenters present. Prominent nucleoli were noted in many cells. These cells were interpreted as atypical but benign, and together with the clinical history were consistent with a diagnosis of gynecomastia.

Pathologic Findings. For cosmetic reasons, an excisional biopsy of the breast lesion was performed, and the specimen consisted of a 2.0 × 1.8 × 0.7-cm, pink-tan, rubbery mass. Sectioning revealed a fairly well-circumscribed tan lesion. Microscopic sections showed an increased number of budding ducts with ductal hyperplasia (Figure B) and periductal stromal fibrosis. The ductal hyperplasia was characterized by the "piling up" of cells with variations in nuclear size and prominent nucleoli (Plate 1–12, 1–13).

Refer to Slide 3 in Optional Slide Set.

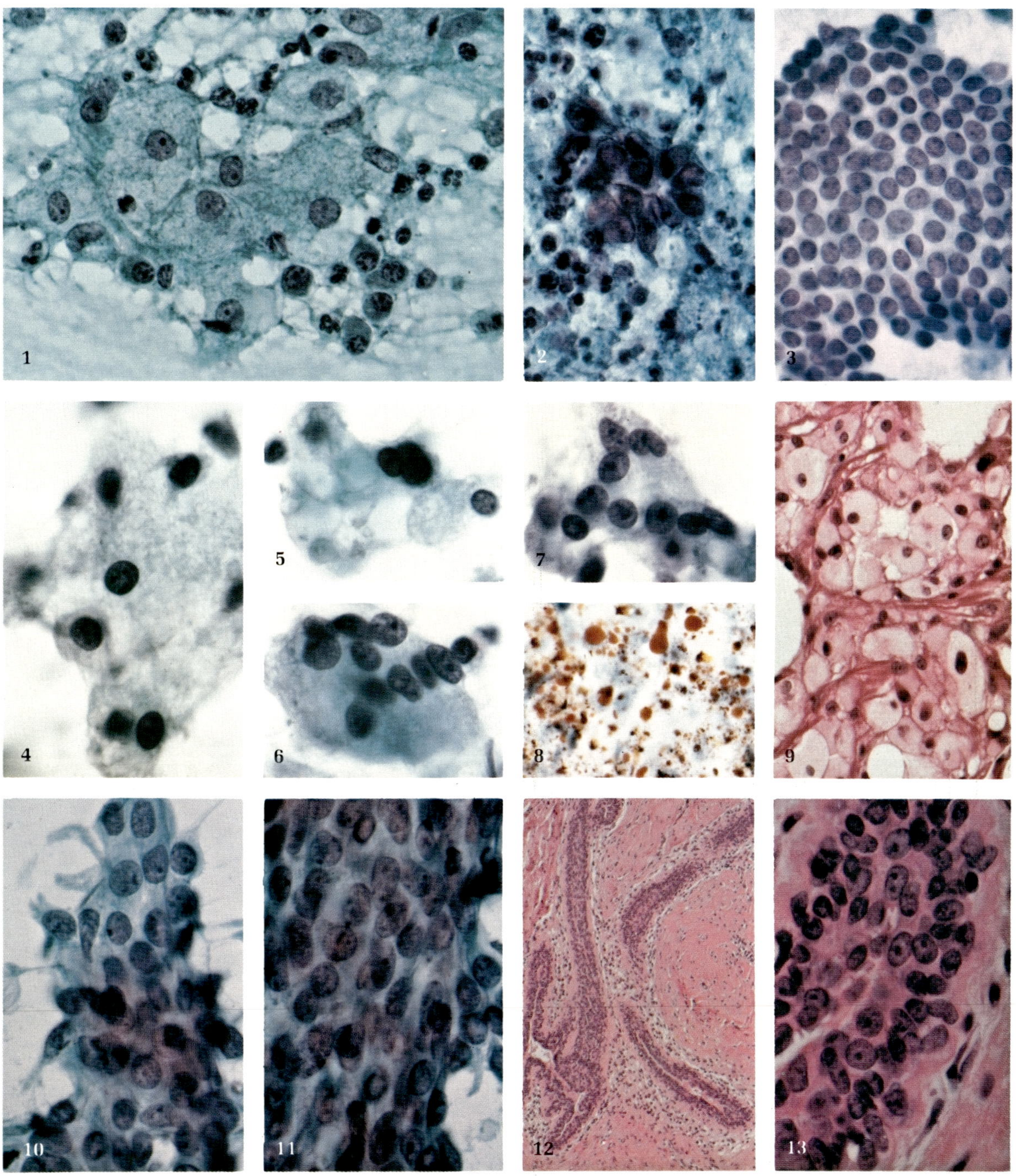

PLATE 1

Breast Abscess

Plate 1–1 to 1–3. Inflammatory cells, necrosis, and benign duct cells from breast abscess in FNA smear (Papanicolaou stain, × 400).

Fat Necrosis

Plate 1–4 to 1–7. Lipid-laden macrophages from fat necrosis of the breast in FNA smear (Papanicolaou stain, × 400).

Plate 1–8. Lipid material demonstrated by Sudan IV in FNA smear of the breast (× 100).

Plate 1–9. Microscopic section of fat necrosis of the breast. (H & E, × 200).

Gynecomastia

Plate 1–10, 1–11. Atypical ductal cells from gynecomastia in FNA smear of the breast (Papanicolaou stain, × 400).

Plate 1–12, 1–13. Microscopic section of gynecomastia of the breast (H & E; 1–12, × 40; 1–13, × 400).

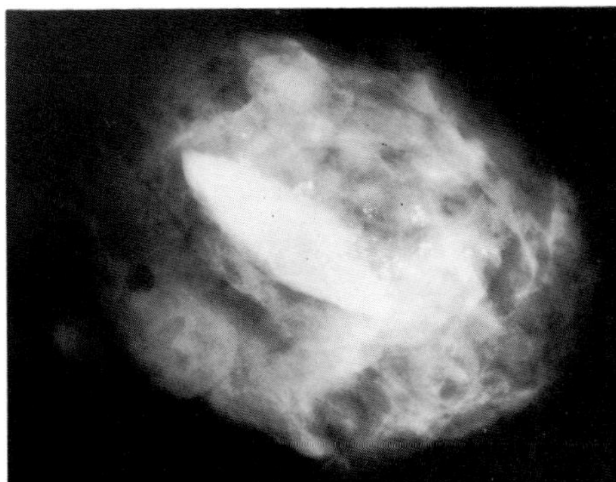

Figure A. Mammogram showing microcalcifications.

PLATE 2

Fibrocystic Disease

Clinical History. A 43-year-old woman with a history of fibrocystic disease noticed a new lump in her left breast and was referred by her physician to the University of Virginia Medical Center. The physical examination showed a firm, approximately 1.5-cm mass in the upper outer quadrant of the left breast. There was no axillary adenopathy. A mammogram showed microcalcifications (Figure A) and biopsy of this region was suggested.

Cytologic Findings. The FNA smears from the breast mass contained two distinct cell populations. In some areas, the cells were arranged in sheets or clusters of round or oval cells with well-defined cell borders (Plate 2–1 to 2–3). Some elongated forms were also seen, giving the cells a somewhat plump, columnar appearance. The cytoplasm was abundant, dense, granular, and showed either eosinophilic or basophilic staining. The nuclei were round to oval and sometimes eccentrically placed. The nuclear membranes were smooth and even. The chromatin pattern was finely granular and evenly distributed with occasional chromocenters. Nucleoli were prominent and present in almost every cell. These cells were interpreted as apocrine metaplasia, which was confirmed by tissue section (Plate 2–4, 2–5).

There were also numerous papillary fragments of benign ductal epithelium (Plate 2–6) and areas of calcification (Plate 2–7). The epithelial cells showed good cohesion and generally uniform size and shape (Plate 2–8). Their nuclei were round to oval with finely granular, evenly distributed chromatin. Chromocenters and single, round nucleoli were often seen. The calcified material was recognized by its refractile, pale-staining, crystalline appearance (Plate 2–7). This material was frequently associated with the benign duct cells. This cytologic pattern was interpreted as sclerosing adenosis, which was confirmed by tissue section (Plate 2–9, 2–10). These combined cellular features were consistent with a diagnosis of fibrocystic disease.

Pathologic Findings. The patient had a needle localization of the right breast mass by mammography and then had an open biopsy. The biopsy specimen consisted of a 4 × 4 × 3–cm segment of tissue, and the specimen radiograph showed microcalcifications. No definite mass was detected. Microscopic sections showed extensive fibrocystic disease with apocrine metaplasia (Plate 2–4, 2–5), numerous small calcifications, and sclerosing adenosis (Plate 2–9, 2–10), but no carcinoma.

Refer to Slide 4 in Optional Slide Set.

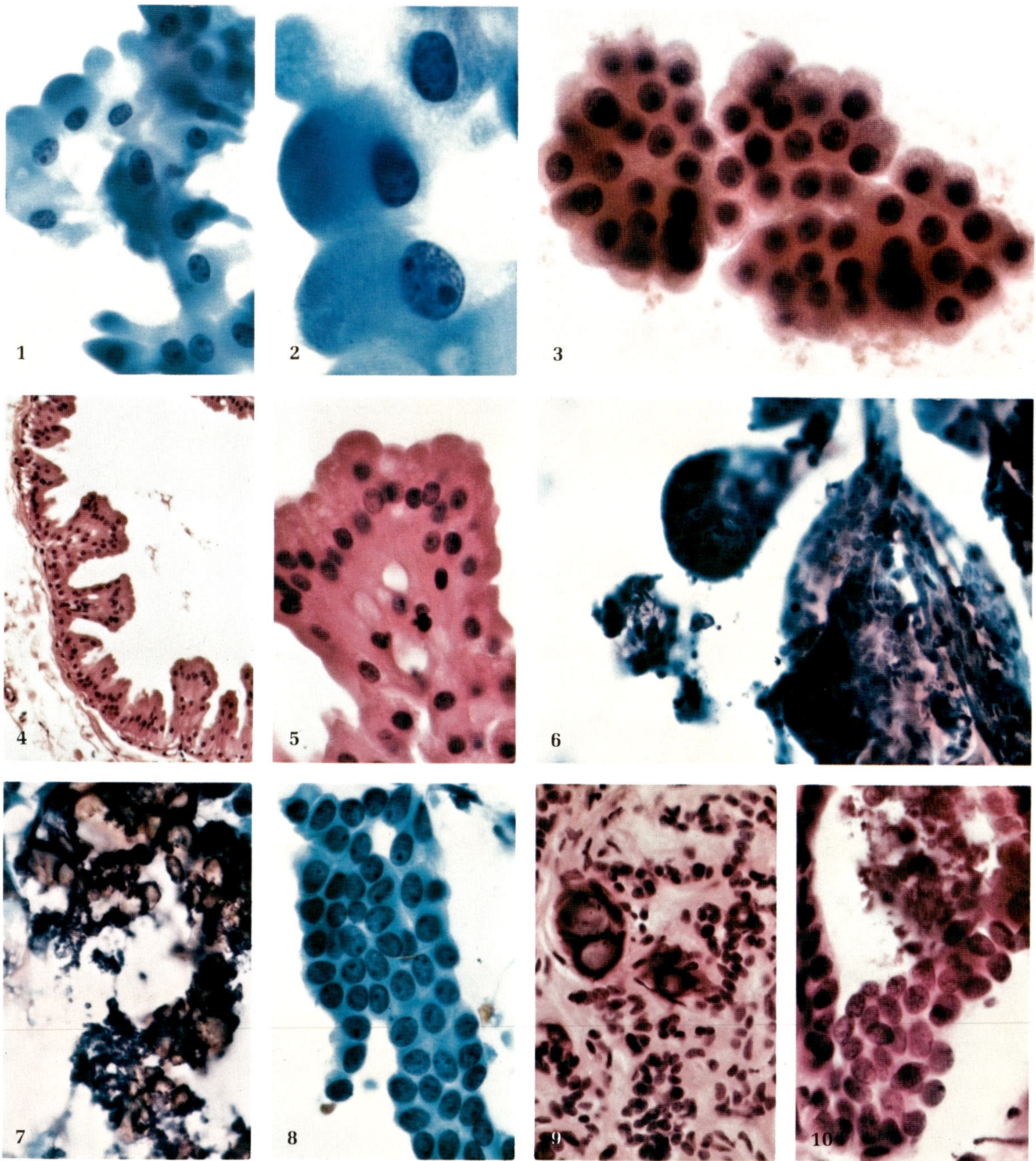

PLATE 2

Fibrocystic Disease

Plate 2–1 to 2–3. Apocrine metaplasia in FNA smear of the breast (Papanicolaou stain; 2–1, 2–2, × 400; 2–3, × 1,000).

Plate 2–4, 2–5. Microscopic tissue section of the breast showing apocrine metaplasia (H & E; 2–4, × 100; 2–5, × 400).

Plate 2–6 to 2–8. Benign ductal cells and calcified material consistent with sclerosing adenosis in FNA smear of the breast (Papanicolaou stain; 2–6, × 200; 2–7, 2–8, × 400).

Plate 2–9, 2–10. Microscopic tissue sections of the breast showing sclerosing adenosis (H & E; 2–9, × 200; 2–10, × 400).

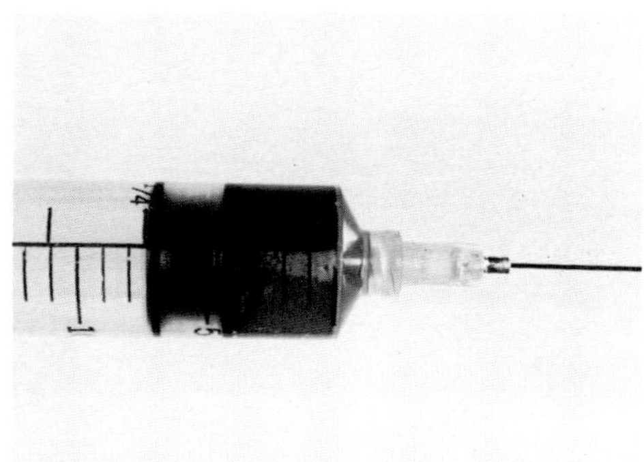

Figure A. Cystic fluid obtained by breast FNA.

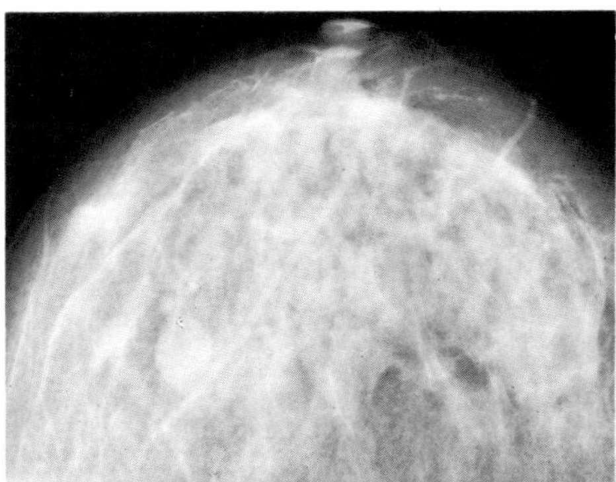

Figure B. Mammogram showing suspicious area of microcalcifications and cystic lesion.

PLATE 3

Fibrocystic Disease with Cellular Atypia

Clinical History. A 39-year-old woman with a history of fibrocystic disease noticed a mass in her left breast while bathing. She was seen the following week in the surgery clinic where a firm, nontender, movable, 4 × 3–cm mass was seen above the nipple of the left breast. Several small, left axillary lymph nodes were palpable.

Cytologic Findings. The FNA smears of the breast yielded approximately 4 mL of cloudy, green-brown fluid, and the mass resolved with the removal of the fluid (Figure A). Filter preparations of the aspirated material contained numerous inflammatory cells, foam cells, and scattered atypical cells lying singly and in sheets (Plate 3–1 to 3–6). The atypical cells had moderate or abundant, basophilic, finely granular cytoplasm. Cell borders were distinct, and the cells were arranged uniformly within the groups (Plate 3–1 to 3–4). Occasional, irregularly shaped, elongated, single cells were seen (Plate 3–3, 3–4). The nuclei of these cells showed enlargement and variation in size, but otherwise appeared vesicular. The chromatin pattern was finely granular and evenly distributed. Chromatin staining was normal. The small or prominent nucleoli were rounded and present in almost every cell. The foam cells had abundant, vacuolated basophilic cytoplasm and uniform, vesicular nuclei with occasional prominent nucleoli (Plate 3–5, 3–6). This cellular pattern was interpreted as benign atypical cells consistent with fibrocystic disease.

Pathologic Findings. The following day, mammograms showed a suspicious asymmetric area of increased density and microcalcifications in the region of palpable abnormality. There was also a rounded lesion with smooth borders having the appearance of a cyst (Figure B). She had a needle localization of the mass under fluoroscopy, and a biopsy of this area was performed. The x-ray films of the biopsy specimen showed that the suspicious area was included in the specimen. The biopsy consisted of a 34-g segment of breast tissue that contained multiple cysts but no gross evidence of carcinoma (Plate 3–7). Microscopic sections showed fibrocystic disease with no evidence of malignancy (Plate 3–8). In the wall of several of the cysts, there were plump, atypical, elongated cells that most likely represented benign mesenchymal cells (Plate 3–9). Two years later, the patient was alive and well with no evidence of disease.

Refer to Slides 5 and 6 in Optional Slide Set.

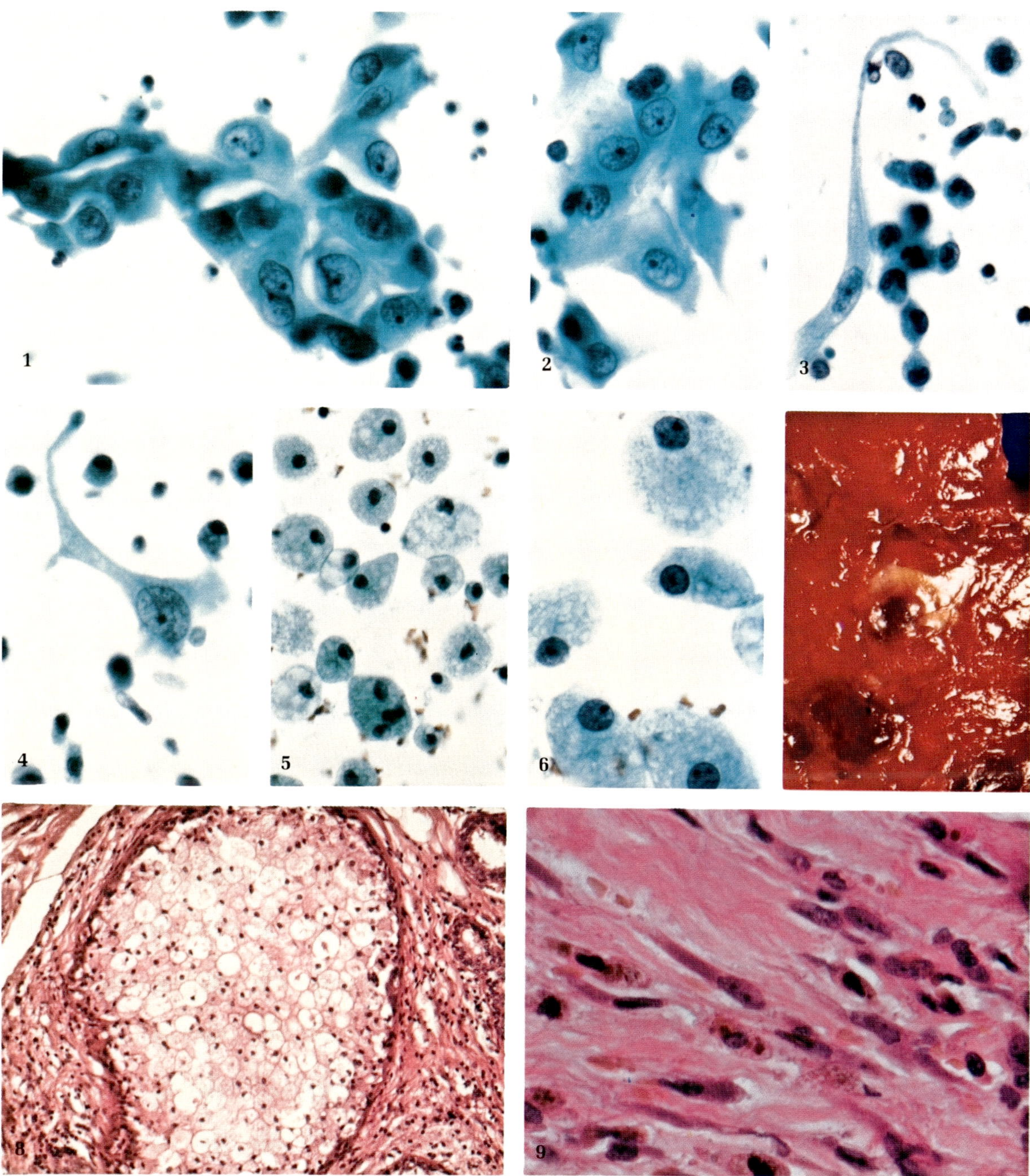

PLATE 3

Fibrocystic Disease with Cellular Atypia

Plate 3–1 to 3–4. Atypical cells in breast FNA smear of fibrocystic disease. Filter preparation of needle washing (Papanicolaou stain, × 400).

Plate 3–5, 3–6. Foam cells in breast FNA smear of fibrocystic disease. Filter preparation of needle washing (Papanicolaou stain; 3–5, × 200; 3–6, × 400).

Plate 3–7. Fibrocystic disease in breast biopsy specimen.

Plate 3–8. Microscopic section of fibrocystic disease containing foam cells (H & E, × 100).

Plate 3–9. Microscopic section of breast tissue showing atypical cells in the cyst wall of fibrocystic disease (H & E, × 400).

PLATE 4

Granular Cell Tumor

Clinical History. A 60-year-old woman noticed a slowly enlarging mass in her left breast and consulted her physician. The physical examination showed a 2-cm, hard, ill-defined mass in her left breast. Her physician felt that the mass was most likely malignant and referred her to the University of Virginia Medical Center for further evaluation and therapy.

Cytologic Findings. An FNA smear stained with the Diff-Quik stain set showed scattered groups of cells with abundant, dense, granular cytoplasm and indistinct cell borders (Plate 4–1, 4–2). The small nuclei were round or oval, uniform in size, and showed even chromatin distribution. Occasional nucleoli were seen in some cells. Because of the characteristic cytoplasmic appearance of these cells, a diagnosis of granular cell tumor was made.

Pathologic Findings. An excisional biopsy confirmed that the lesion was a granular cell tumor. The tumor cells were large with abundant, finely granular, pink cytoplasm and small, dense nuclei (Plate 4–3, 4–4).

Refer to Slide 7 in Optional Slide Set.

PLATE 4

Ductal Hyperplasia

Clinical History. A 43-year-old woman was referred by her family physician to the surgical oncology clinic for the evaluation of a mass in the upper portion of her right breast, first noticed two to three weeks before seeking medical attention. The patient had a family history of breast cancer. Her history also included radiation therapy and excision of a hemangioma on her left breast, which was done during her childhood.

The physical examination revealed an area of thickening and a 2.5-cm mass in the right breast. Her left breast had an area of scar tissue in the upper outer quadrant that was the site of the previous radiation and excision. There were no palpable axillary nodes. Mammograms showed an asymmetric area in the upper outer quadrant of her right breast.

Cytologic Findings. The FNA smears contained cohesive sheets and clusters of uniform cells with scanty basophilic cytoplasm (Plate 4–5 to 4–7). The sheets usually showed good organization and polarity (Plate 4–5); however, nuclear overlapping and crowding were noted in some groups (Plate 4–6). The nuclei of these cells were round or oval, only slightly enlarged, and varied little in size. The chromatin pattern was finely granular and usually evenly distributed. Chromatin clearing with associated thickening of the nuclear membrane was seen in some degenerating forms. Small but distinct nucleoli were seen in almost every cell. These uniform nuclear features and the cohesive sheets were interpreted as consistent with benign ductal hyperplasia.

Pathologic Findings. An open biopsy specimen of the breast showed fibrocystic disease with focal duct hyperplasia without atypia (Plate 4–7 to 4–9). There was no evidence of cancer.

Refer to Slide 8 in Optional Slide Set.

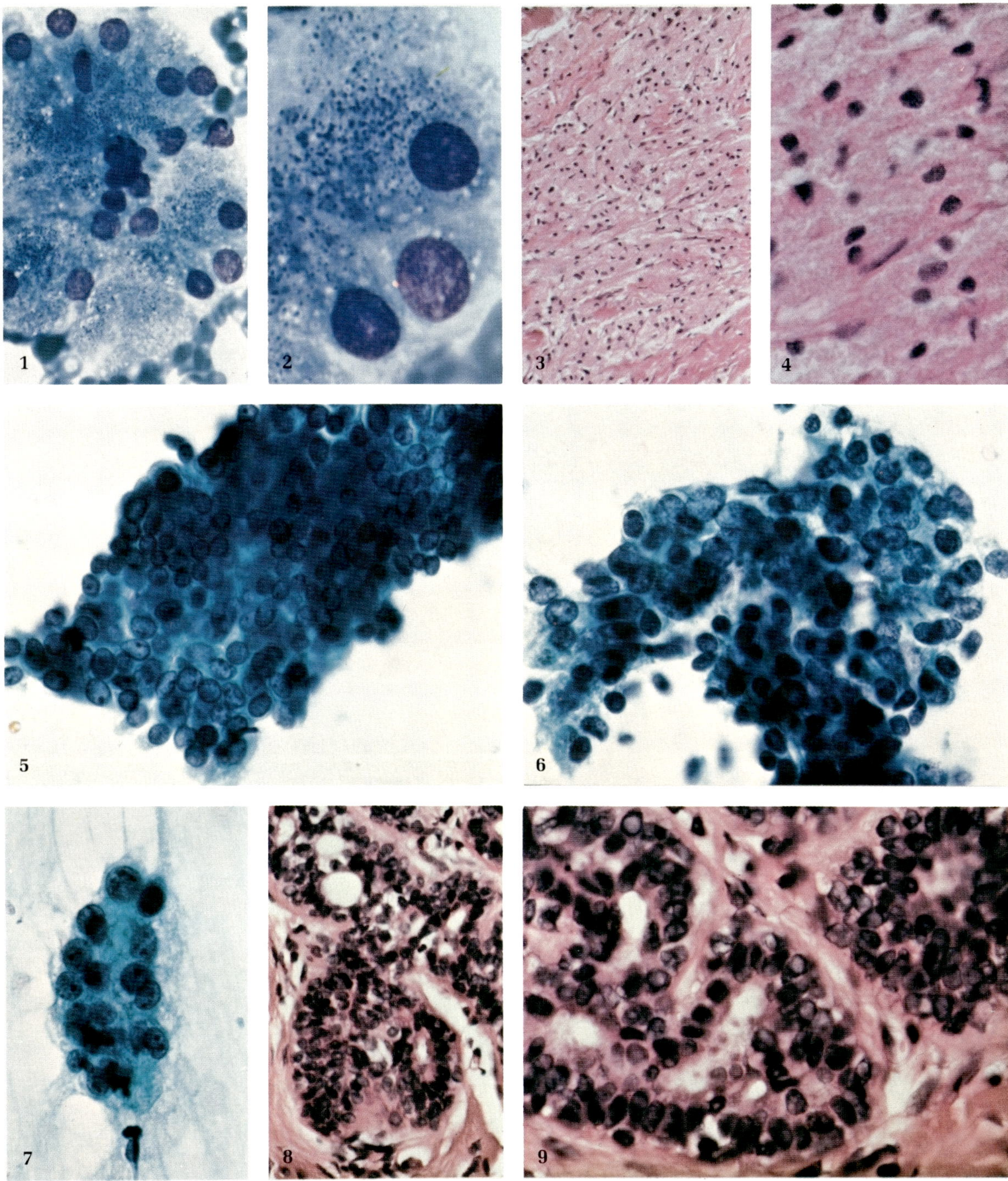

PLATE 4

Granular Cell Tumor

Plate 4–1, 4–2. Granular cell tumor in FNA smear of the breast (Diff-Quik stain set; 4–1, × 400; 4–2, × 1,000).

Plate 4–3, 4–4. Granular cell tumor in excisional biopsy section (H & E; 4–3, × 100; 4–4, × 400).

Ductal Hyperplasia

Plate 4–5 to 4–7. Mildly atypical duct cells from ductal hyperplasia in FNA smear of the breast (Papanicolaou stain, × 400).

Plate 4–8, 4–9. Ductal hyperplasia in microscopic tissue section of breast biopsy specimen (H & E; 4–8, × 200; 4–9, × 400).

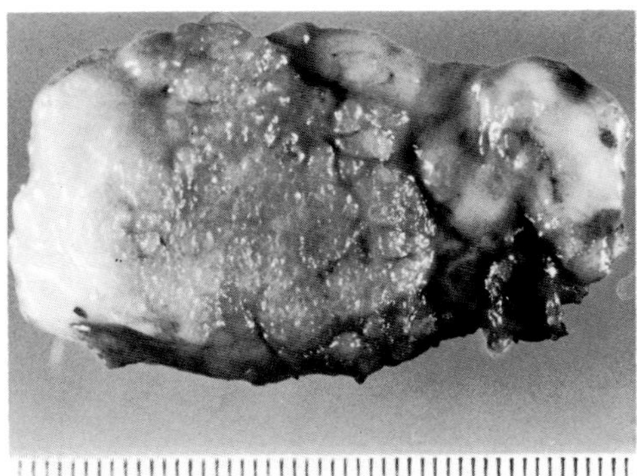

Figure A. Cut surface of breast mass showing finely nodular appearance (scale marked in millimeters).

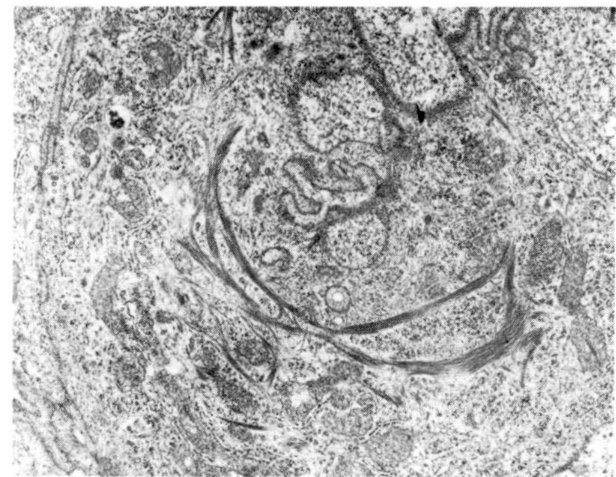

Figure B. Myoepithelial component in duct confirmed by electron microscopy (×7,800).

PLATE 5

Atypical Ductal Hyperplasia

Clinical History. A 17-year-old woman had her first child 17 months before coming to the surgical oncology clinic. Immediately after delivery she went on oral contraceptives for five months, but discontinued them when she noticed a mass developing in her left breast. She monitored the mass for a year and thought that it varied in size with her menstrual cycle. She sought medical attention when, after becoming pregnant for a second time, the mass rapidly tripled in size. She reported no pain, discharge, or bleeding, but had a family history of breast cancer.

The physical examination showed an apparently healthy girl about four months pregnant. Her breast examination showed a 3 × 4–cm, hard, left breast mass that was not fixed to the chest wall, located in the inferior lateral quadrant. Her right breast and axilla were normal.

Cytologic Findings. The breast FNA smears contained many large tissue fragments and sheets of cells (Plate 5–1 to 5–5), which showed good cohesion and distinct cell borders. In general, the cell sheets were well organized and retained normal polarity; however, nuclear overlapping and crowding were seen in some groups (Plate 5–2, 5–3). The slightly enlarged nuclei were round or oval and varied little in size (Plate 5–2, 5–3, 5–5). The chromatin pattern was finely granular and evenly distributed with occasional chromocenters, and the nuclear membranes were smooth and even. Prominent, sometimes multiple, nucleoli were seen in almost every cell. A few groups of stromal cells characterized by their elongated, fiberlike shape and dark, cigar-shaped nuclei were also identified (Plate 5–4). Because of the good cohesion, the uniform organization of the epithelial cell fragments, and the patient's clinical history, the cells were interpreted as benign despite the presence of nuclear atypia. The aspiration was felt to represent a florid hyperplastic process.

Pathologic Findings. Because of the unusual cytologic presentation of this lesion and the patient's family history of breast cancer, a biopsy was recommended for definitive evaluation of the breast mass. The biopsy specimen consisted of a 4 × 3–cm segment of fibrofatty tissue. The cut surface revealed a distinctive, finely nodular appearance and consisted of homogeneous tan tissue intermixed with yellow-white tissue (Figure A). Microscopic sections showed preserved lobular architecture with exuberant adenosis and sclerosis. At higher power there was ductal hyperplasia with proliferation of the epithelial cells that varied from cytologically bland to severely atypical (Plate 5–6, 5–7). A prominent outer myoepithelial component was noted and confirmed by electron microscopy (Figure B).

Refer to Slide 9 in Optional Slide Set.

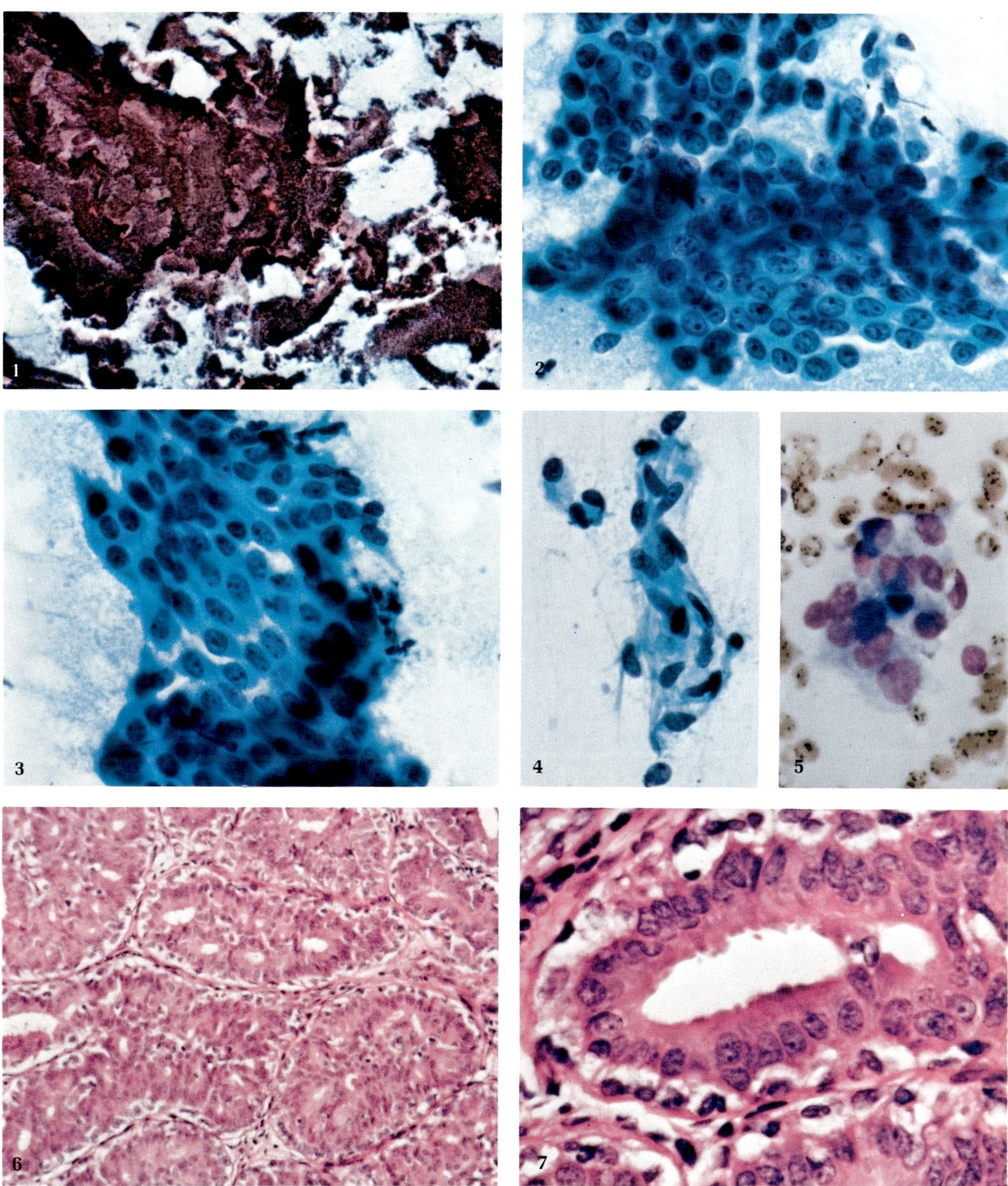

PLATE 5

Atypical Ductal Hyperplasia

Plate 5–1. Florid ductal hyperplasia in FNA smear of the breast (Papanicolaou stain, × 40).

Plate 5–2, 5–3. Sheets of atypical ductal epithelial cells from ductal hyperplasia in FNA smear of the breast (Papanicolaou stain, × 400).

Plate 5–4. Elongated stroma cells from ductal hyperplasia in FNA smear of the breast (Papanicolaou stain, × 400).

Plate 5–5. Atypical duct epithelial cells from ductal hyperplasia in FNA smear of the breast (modified Wright-Giemsa stain, × 400).

Plate 5–6, 5–7. Microscopic section of atypical ductal hyperplasia in excisional biopsy specimen of the breast (H & E; 5–6, × 100; 5–7, × 400).

PLATE 6

Lactating Adenoma

Clinical History. A 23-year-old woman who was 19 weeks pregnant came to the surgery clinic with a two-week history of a mass in the left breast. The physical examination showed a well-circumscribed, mobile, firm, 3 × 4-cm mass in the inferior aspect of the left breast.

Cytologic Findings. The FNA smears contained scattered clusters, sheets, and multilobulated groups of cohesive monomorphic cells (Plate 6–1 to 6–3). The basophilic cytoplasm was moderate in amount and finely vacuolated (Plate 6–2). The enlarged nuclei were vesicular in appearance but contained single, large, round nucleoli (Plate 6–2, 6–3). These clusters were interpreted as consistent with a lactating adenoma; however, the nuclear atypia was unexplained by pregnancy, and biopsy was recommended.

Pathologic Findings. A 4 × 3.5–cm, multilobulated, tan-yellow mass was excised. Microscopic sections demonstrated a lactating adenoma sharply separated from the adjacent breast parenchyma. The adenoma was composed of closely approximated tubular structures lined by a single layer of epithelial cells with prominent cytoplasmic vacuoles. The nuclei were uniform but contained large, single nucleoli (Plate 6–4, 6–5).

Refer to Slide 10 in Optional Slide Set.

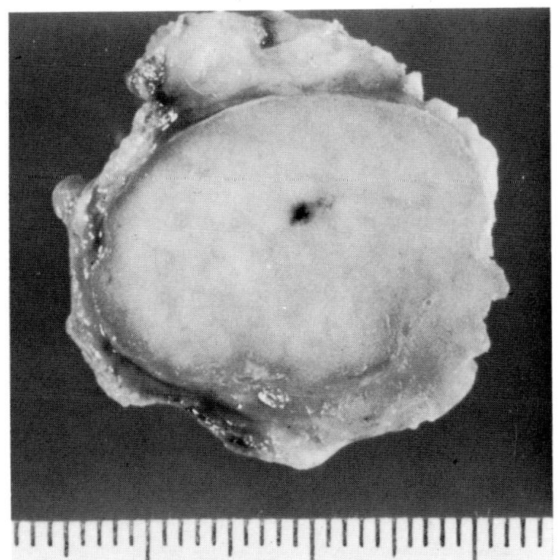

Figure A. Cut section of tubular adenoma (scale marked in millimeters).

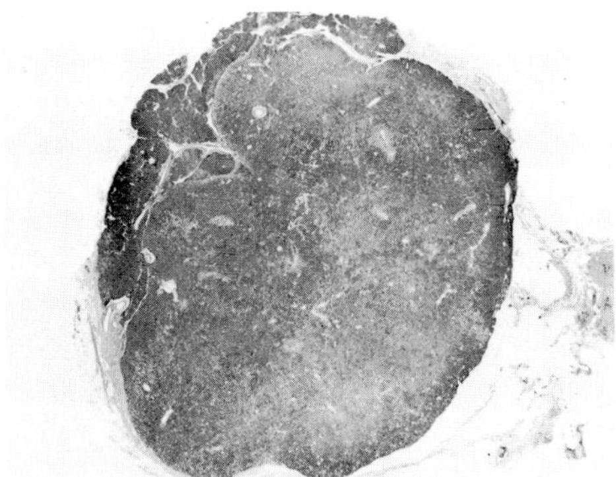

Figure B. Microscopic section of tubular adenoma (× 4).

PLATE 6

Tubular Adenoma

Clinical History. A 26-year-old woman first noticed a small lump in her breast two weeks before admission. The physical examination showed a 1 × 2–cm, firm, nontender, mobile mass just inferior to the nipple in her left breast. There was no nipple discharge and her right breast showed no abnormalities.

Cytologic Findings. The FNA smears contained numerous cohesive ball-like clusters and sheets of benign-appearing epithelial cells with moderate or scant amounts of basophilic cytoplasm (Plate 6–6 to 6–9). Occasional cell clusters showed a layer of flattened myoepithelial cells surrounding them (Plate 6–6, 6–7). The epithelial cell nuclei were somewhat varied in size and shape, but pleomorphism was absent (Plate 6–8, 6–9). The chromatin pattern was finely granular and usually evenly distributed. Occasional chromocenters were seen. Prominent single nucleoli were noted in almost every cell. The characteristic ball-like arrangements of benign cells were indicative of an adenoma.

Pathologic Findings. An excisional biopsy specimen of the mass consisted of an ovoid mass of yellow tissue. The cut section showed a well-demarcated, homogeneous, yellow tumor that measured 2.3 × 2.0 × 0.6 cm (Figure A). Representative microscopic sections showed a tubular adenoma that was composed of uniform, small, tubular structures lined by a single layer of epithelial cells and an attenuated layer of myoepithelial cells. Intervening stroma was sparse (Figure B; Plate 6–10, 6–11).

Refer to Slide 11 in Optional Slide Set.

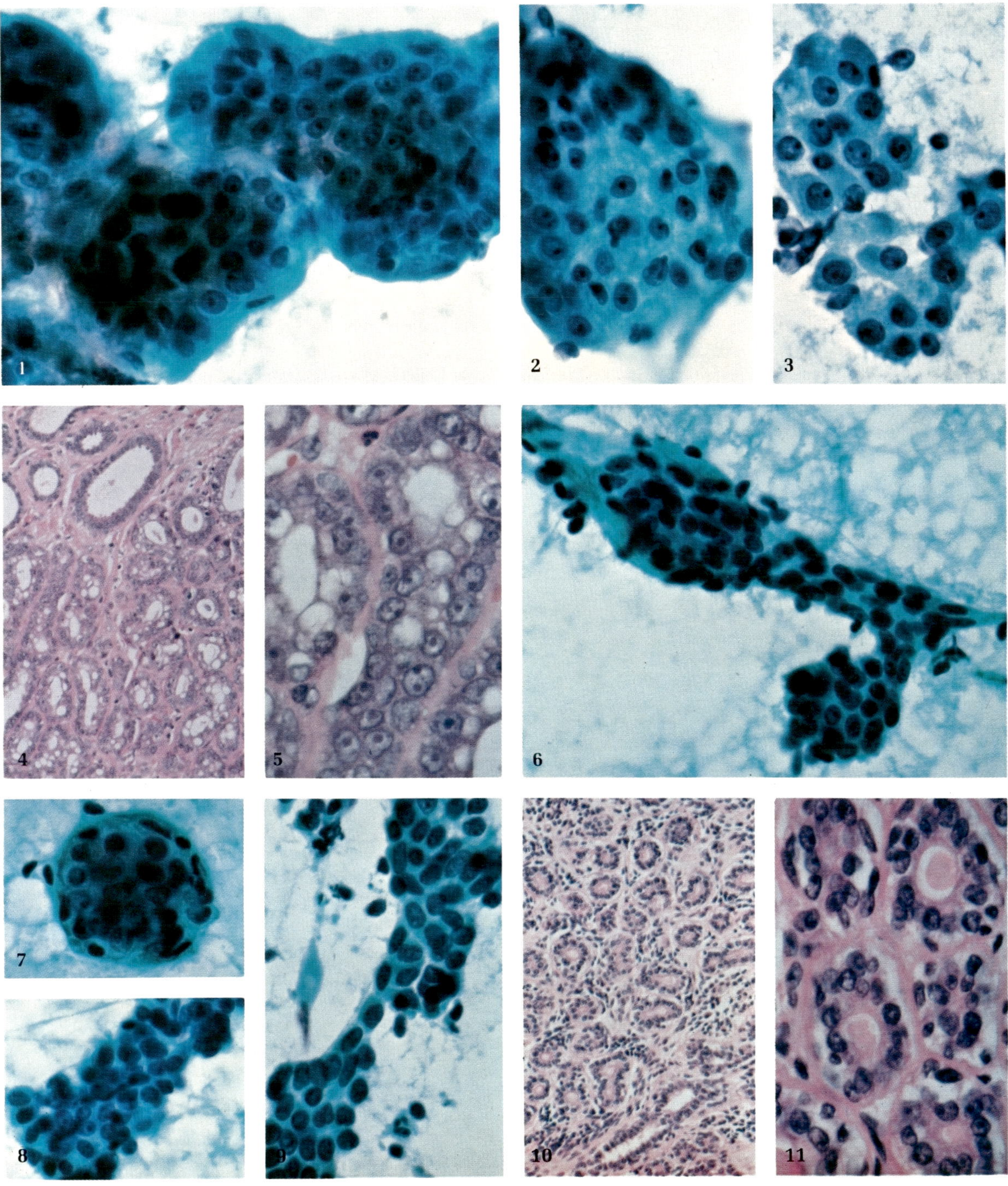

PLATE 6

Lactating Adenoma

Plate 6–1 to 6–3. Lactating adenoma in FNA smear of the breast (Papanicolaou stain, × 400).

Plate 6–4, 6–5. Microscopic tissue section of lactating adenoma in excisional biopsy specimen of the breast (H & E; 6–4, × 100; 6–5, × 400).

Tubular Adenoma

Plate 6–6 to 6–9. Tubular adenoma in FNA smear of the breast (Papanicolaou stain, × 400).

Plate 6–10, 6–11. Microscopic tissue section of tubular adenoma in excisional biopsy specimen of the breast (H & E; 6–10, × 100; 6–11, × 400).

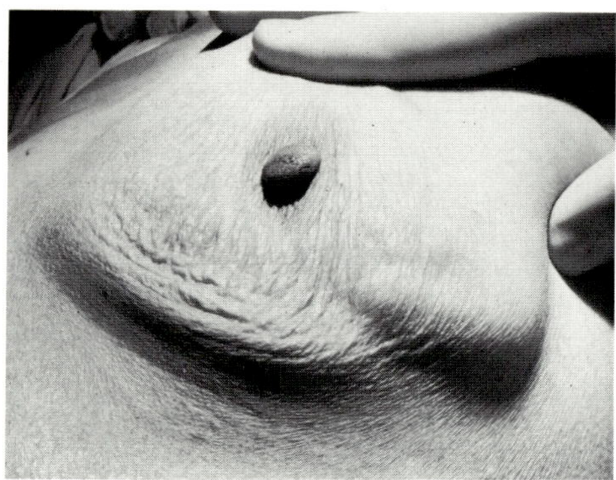

Figure A. Masses (fibroadenomata) visible on breast examination.

PLATE 7
Fibroadenoma

Clinical History. A 65-year-old woman had been aware of several masses in her left breast for several years. She came to the breast clinic when she noticed enlargement of one of the masses. The physical examination showed three nontender, movable masses approximately 1 to 3 cm in her left breast (Figure A).

Cytologic Findings. The FNA smears of the masses showed scattered cohesive sheets and tissue fragments of benign ductal epithelium that often had fingerlike projections (Plate 7–1 to 7–3). The duct cells had uniform, round or oval nuclei with finely granular, evenly distributed chromatin and small nucleoli (Plate 7–4). Their cytoplasm was scant and basophilic, and the cells showed orderly arrangement within the sheets (Plate 7–2, 7–4). The smear background contained numerous oval or elongated, dark-staining bare nuclei (Plate 7–3, 7–5, 7–6). (The exact origin of these cells has not yet been determined. They may represent stromal cells or myoepithelial cells.) Well-defined stroma was also identified. The stroma was characterized by abundant granular cytoplasm containing numerous oval or elongated nuclei. The cytoplasm stained blue-green with the Papanicolaou stain and lavender-pink with the modified Wright-Giemsa stain. Cell borders were not seen (Plate 7–7, 7–8). This cellular pattern was diagnostic of a fibroadenoma.

Pathologic Findings. An excisional biopsy specimen contained three discrete, spherical, 1 to 2–cm masses, which on cut section were gray-white and bulged above the surrounding breast parenchyma. Microscopic tissue sections of the masses showed fibroblastic stroma enclosing glands lined by benign epithelium in a pericanalicular pattern; these features confirmed the FNA diagnosis of fibroadenoma (Plate 7–9). The cells lining the ducts were uniform in size and shape and showed a double-layer arrangement (Plate 7–10).

Refer to Slides 12 and 13 in Optional Slide Set.

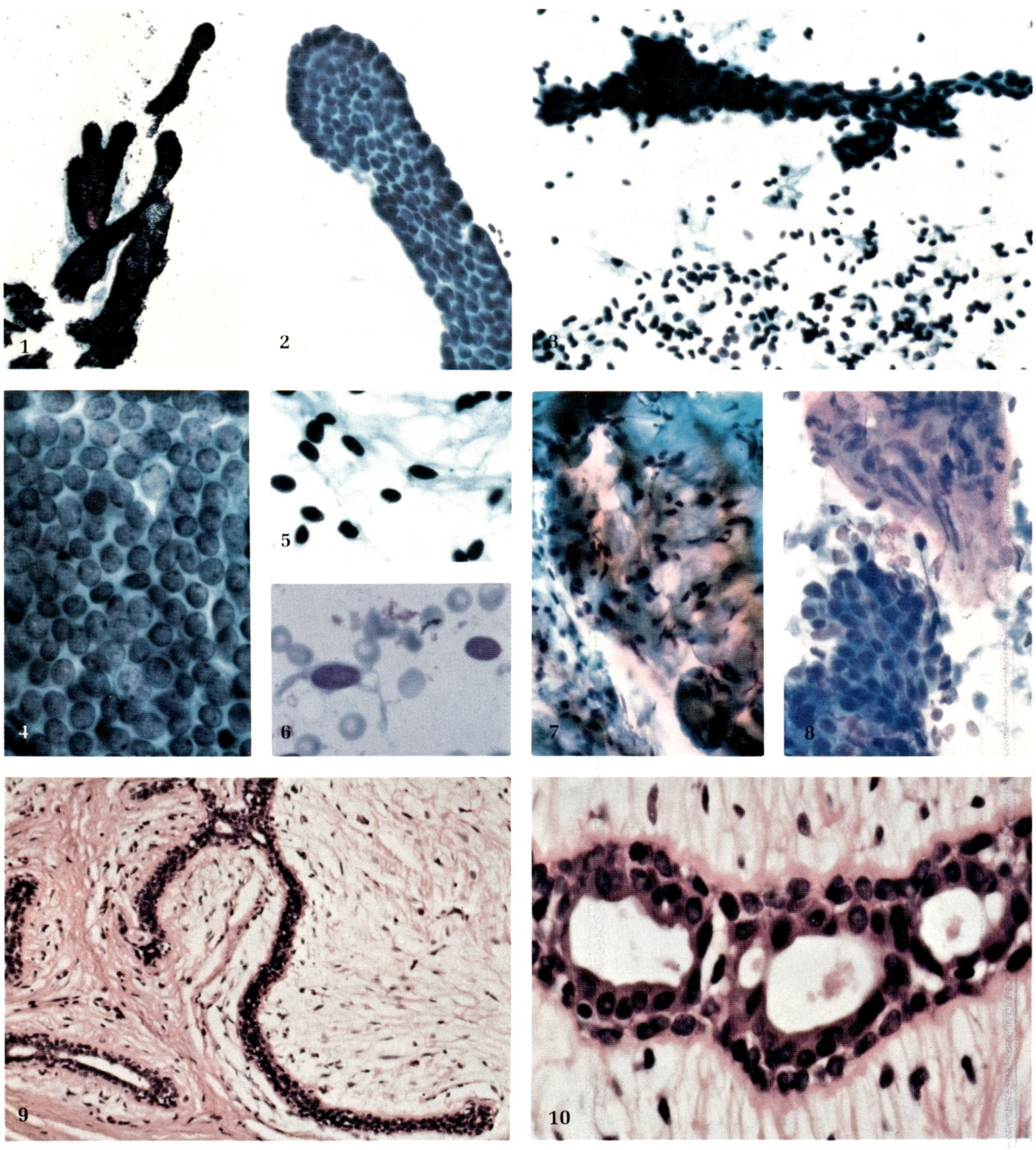

PLATE 7

Fibroadenoma

Plate 7–1, 7–2. Tissue fragments of benign ductal epithelium from fibroadenoma in FNA smears of the breast (Papanicolaou stain; 7–1, × 40; 7–2, × 200).

Plate 7–3. Fragment of benign ductal epithelium and numerous bare nuclei from fibroadenoma in FNA smear of the breast (Papanicolaou stain; × 200).

Plate 7–4. High-power view of benign ductal cells (Papanicolaou stain; × 400).

Plate 7–5. High-power view of bare nuclei (Papanicolaou stain; × 400).

Plate 7–6. High-power view of bare nuclei (modified Wright-Giemsa stain; × 400).

Plate 7–7. Fragment of stroma from fibroadenoma in FNA smear of the breast (Papanicolaou stain; × 200).

Plate 7–8. Benign ductal epithelium and stroma from fibroadenoma in FNA smear of the breast (modified Wright-Giemsa stain; × 200).

Plate 7–9, 7–10. Microscopic sections of fibroadenoma of the breast (H & E; 7–9, × 40; 7–10, × 400).

PLATE 8

Intraductal Papilloma

Clinical History. A 45-year-old woman had a bloody nipple discharge and was seen in the surgery clinic. The physical examination showed an approximately 2-cm, freely movable, soft mass in the subareolar region.

Cytologic Findings. The FNA smears of the breast mass contained numerous sheets and papillary clusters of benign-appearing duct epithelial cells (Plate 8–1). The cells were cuboidal and showed good cohesion and uniform arrangement within the cell groups (Plate 8–2, 8–3). The clusters had smooth, outer contours and a "picket fence" arrangement of the peripheral cells (Plate 8–2). The cell nuclei were generally vesicular and uniform in size and shape. Nucleoli were often visible (Plate 8–3). Occasional groups of elongated cells with dense, pink-staining cytoplasm and small, dark, elongated nuclei were also seen (Plate 8–4). These cells were felt to be of stromal origin. Modified Wright-Giemsa–stained slides clearly showed the papillary nature of this lesion. Papillary groups contained deep blue–staining epithelial cells and well-defined strands of lavender-pink–staining stroma (Plate 8–5, 8–6). Cytoplasmic vacuolization was a common finding in the benign epithelial cells (Plate 8–7).

The presence of uniform, well-oriented duct cells on well-defined stalks of fibrous stroma and the absence of cytologic atypia were compatible with a diagnosis of intraductal papilloma.

Pathologic Findings. Macroscopically, there was a soft, 1.5-cm, friable mass that appeared to originate from a dilated duct. Microscopic sections showed an intraductal papilloma characterized by a complex glandular pattern with a prominent connective tissue component (Plate 8–8). There was a well-developed double layer of benign epithelium separated from adjacent epithelial cells by connective tissue (Plate 8–9, 8–10).

Refer to Slides 14 and 15 in Optional Slide Set.

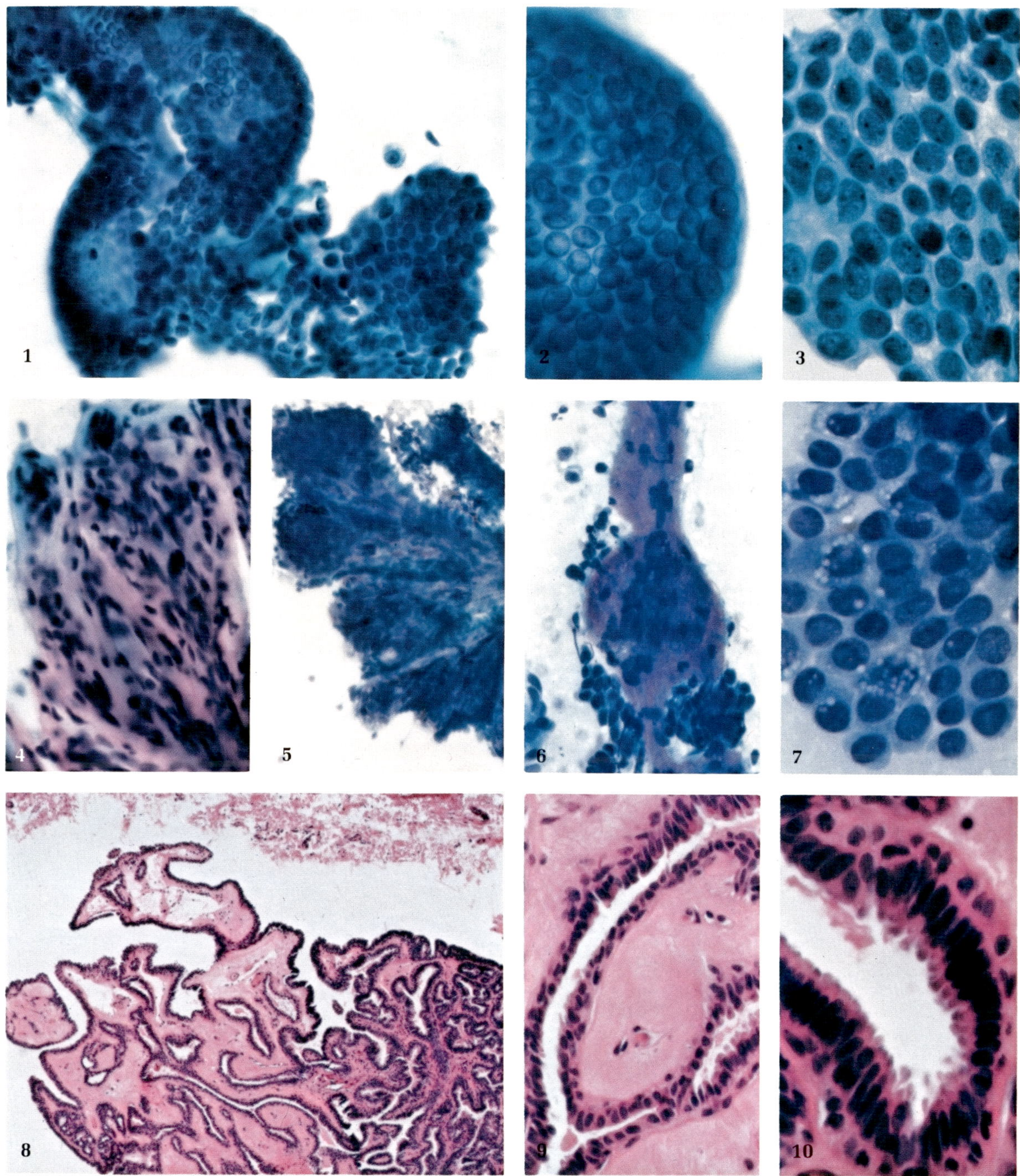

PLATE 8

Intraductal Papilloma

Plate 8–1 to 8–3. Papillary clusters of benign ductal cells from papilloma in FNA smear of the breast (Papanicolaou stain; 8–1, × 200; 8–2, 8–3, × 400).

Plate 8–4. Connective tissue component from papilloma in FNA smear of the breast (Papanicolaou stain; × 200).

Plate 8–5 to 8–7. Benign ductal and stromal cells (modified Wright-Giemsa stain; 8–5, × 100; 8–6, × 200; 8–7, × 400).

Plate 8–8 to 8–10. Microscopic section of intraductal papilloma of the breast (H & E; 8–8, × 40; 8–9, × 200; 8–10, × 400).

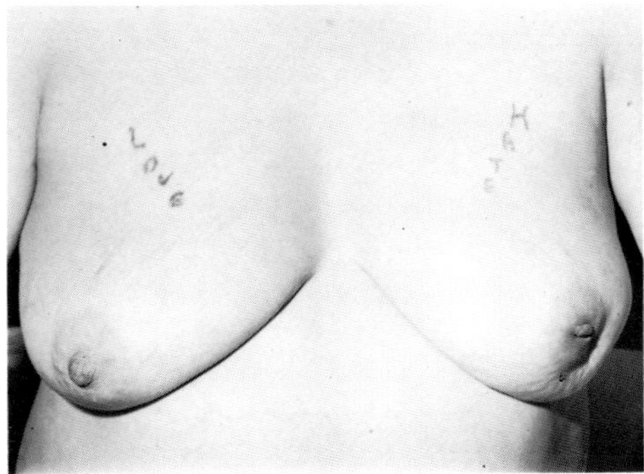

Figure A. Skin dimpling and nipple inversion seen in lower outer quadrant of left breast.

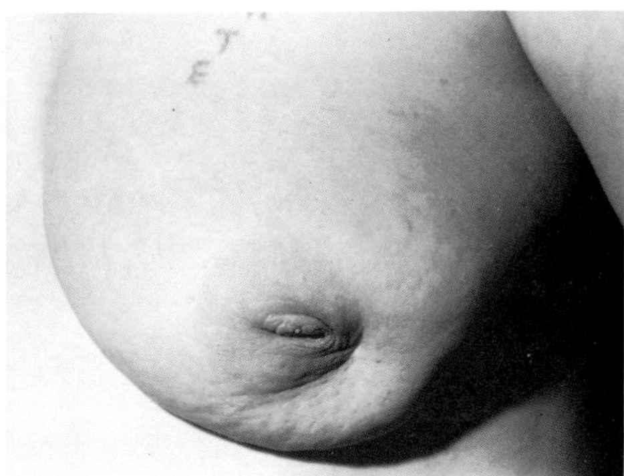

Figure B. Close-up of skin dimpling and nipple inversion seen in Figure A.

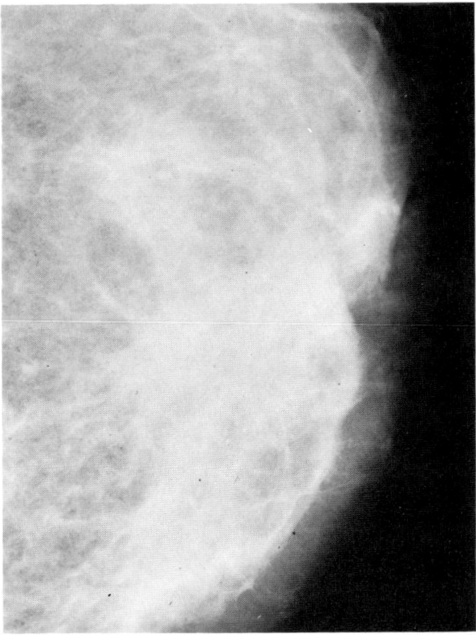

Figure C. Mammogram showing area of increased density and microcalcifications.

PLATE 9

Infiltrating Duct Carcinoma

Clinical History. A 41-year-old woman was admitted to another hospital for an alcohol detoxification program. A breast mass was noted during a physical examination, and she was transferred to the University of Virginia Medical Center for further evaluation.

She first noticed a lump beneath the nipple of her left breast approximately two months before admission. The lump increased in size, and she observed retraction of her nipple. She also gave a history of pain in her left axilla upon abducting her left shoulder. The physical examination showed a 1.5-cm, firm, mobile, slightly tender mass in the lower outer quadrant of the left breast, with overlying skin dimpling and nipple inversion (Figures A, B). Examination of her left axilla disclosed several palpable lymph nodes that were tender but mobile. The remainder of her physical examination showed no abnormalities. A mammogram showed an area of increased density with stranding and microcalcifications suspicious for malignancy (Figure C).

Cytologic Findings. The smears from the FNA of her left breast contained numerous benign ductal cells in sheets and abnormal cells lying singly and in syncytial arrangements (Plate 9–1 to 9–5). The abnormal cells had scant, basophilic cytoplasm and indistinct cell borders. Their nuclei were enlarged, varied in size and shape, and showed mild or moderate hyperchromatism. The chromatin pattern was finely granular and evenly distributed. Nucleoli were prominent, sometimes multiple or irregular, and present in almost every cell (Plate 9–2, 9–3). Infrequent mitotic figures were seen (Plate 9–5). In contrast, the benign ductal cells showed uniform size; cohesive, well-organized sheets; and uniform vesicular nuclei with occasional small nucleoli (Plate 9–4). A diagnosis of infiltrating duct carcinoma was made.

Pathologic Findings. A left modified radical mastectomy was performed, and the specimen contained intraductal and infiltrating duct carcinoma (Plate 9–6, 9–7). The skin from the overlying nipple was involved by the carcinoma in a characteristic pagetoid pattern with 11 of 13 axillary lymph nodes containing metastatic carcinoma.

Refer to Slides 16 and 17 in Optional Slide Set.

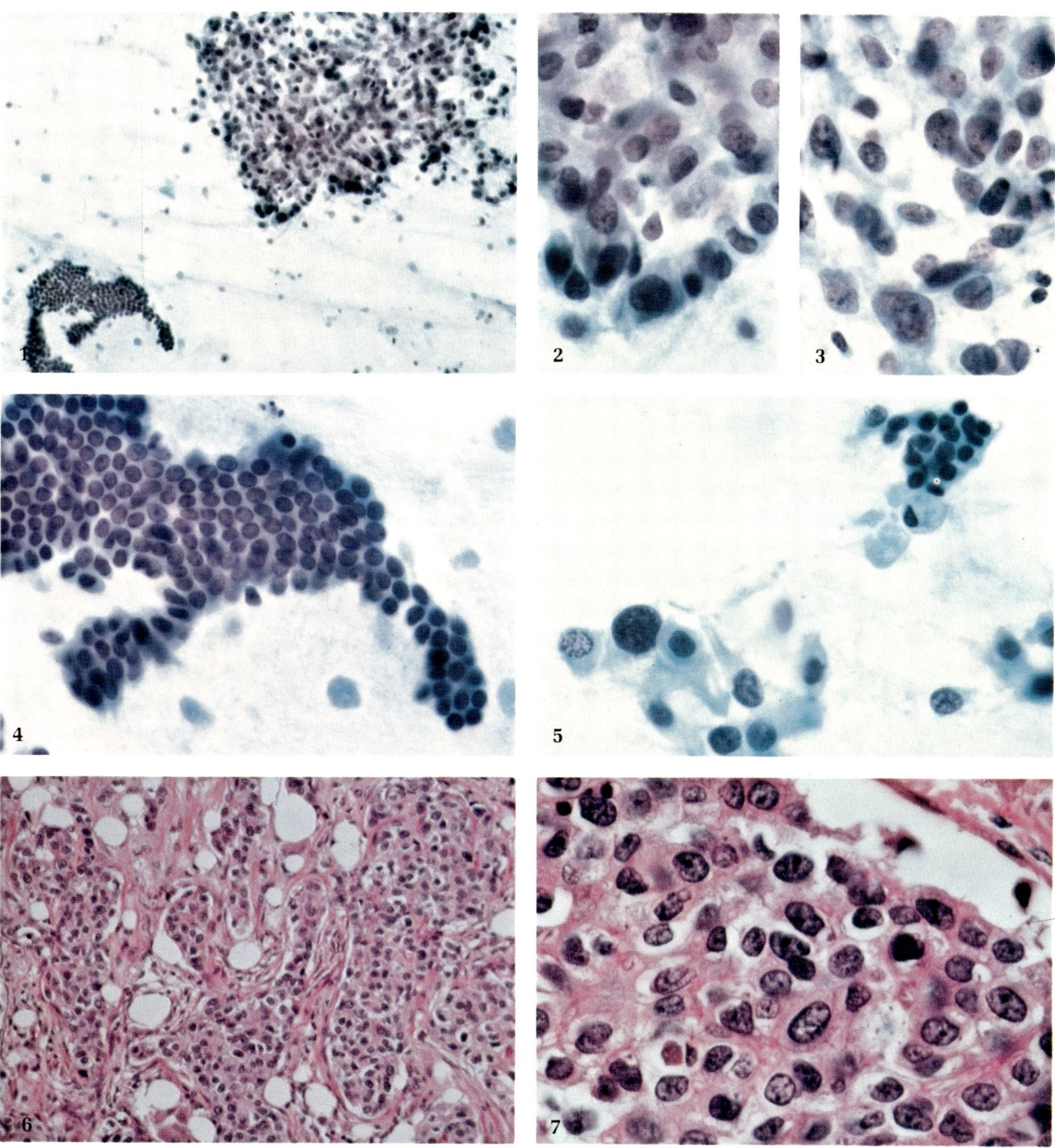

PLATE 9

Infiltrating Duct Carcinoma

Plate 9–1. Benign ductal cells and cells of infiltrating duct carcinoma in FNA smear of the breast (Papanicolaou stain, × 100).

Plate 9–2, 9–3. Infiltrating duct carcinoma in FNA smear of the breast (Papanicolaou stain, × 400).

Plate 9–4. Benign ductal cells in FNA smear of the breast (Papanicolaou stain, × 400).

Plate 9–5. Benign ductal cells and cells of infiltrating duct carcinoma in FNA smear of the breast (Papanicolaou stain, × 400).

Plate 9–6, 9–7. Microscopic tissue section of infiltrating duct carcinoma in mastectomy specimen (H & E; 9–6, × 200; 9–7, × 400).

PLATE 10

Infiltrating Duct Carcinoma

Clinical History. A 53-year-old woman had a three-year history of a painless left breast mass. She thought the mass was cancer but avoided seeing a doctor. There had been some retraction of the skin overlying the mass. The physical examination showed severe skin and nipple retraction overlying an indurated, nontender, 5 × 5–cm mass (Figure A). The right breast was normal. There was no palpable adenopathy in either axilla.

Cytologic Findings. The FNA smears of the breast lesion contained abundant tumor cells lying singly and in syncytial arrangements (Plate 10–1, 10–2). Their cytoplasm was scant, basophilic, and finely granular. Cell borders were indistinct. The cell nuclei varied in size and shape, although a round or oval configuration was common. Occasional nuclear molding was seen within the cell groups (Plate 10–1). The chromatin pattern was finely granular but irregularly distributed, and mild-to-moderate hyperchromatism was noted in many nuclei. Nuclear membrane irregularities were frequently seen. Prominent, sometimes multiple nucleoli were present in almost every cell. These cells were diagnostic of an infiltrating duct carcinoma.

Pathologic Findings. A modified radical mastectomy of the left breast was performed. The skin showed retraction with an underlying stony, hard, 4 × 3 × 2–cm mass. Microscopic sections showed an infiltrating duct carcinoma. Three of 17 axillary lymph nodes contained metastatic carcinoma (Plate 10–3, 10–4).

Refer to Slide 18 in Optional Slide Set.

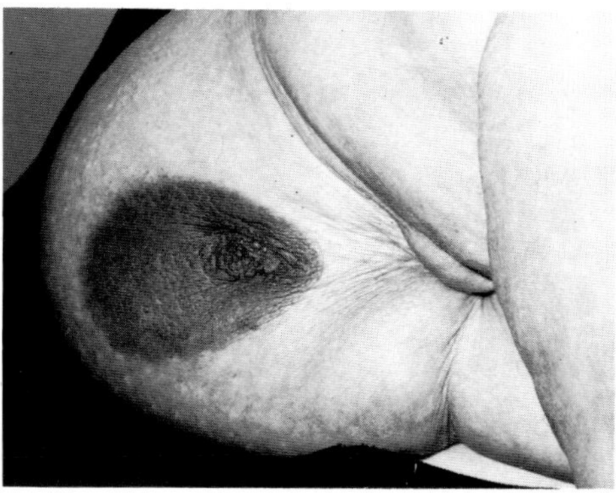

Figure A. Severe skin and nipple retraction of left breast.

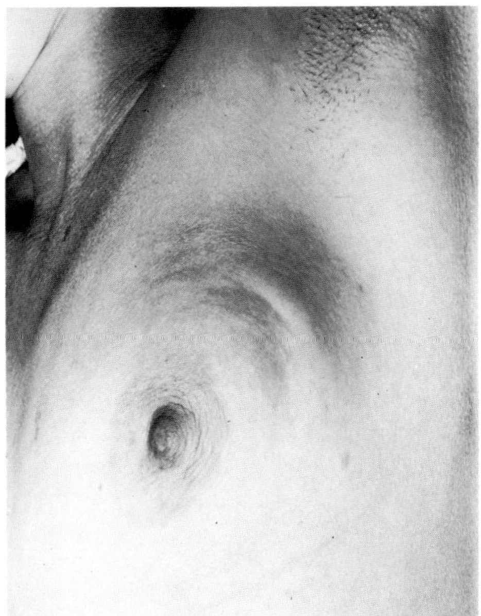

Figure B. Breast mass fixed to overlying skin with dimpling.

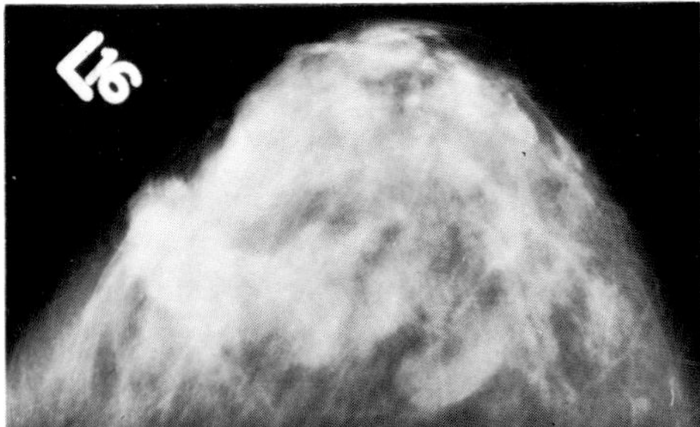

Figure C. Mammogram showing stellate mass with skin retraction interpreted as carcinoma.

PLATE 10

Infiltrating Duct Carcinoma

Clinical History. A 44-year-old woman with schizophrenia had a one-year history of a left breast mass. She had not noticed nipple discharge, tenderness, or skin changes. The physical examination showed a firm, 4 × 4–cm mass in the upper outer quadrant of her left breast. The mass was fixed to the overlying skin with dimpling (Figure B). There was no axillary adenopathy. Mammograms showed a 2-cm stellate mass with skin retraction that was felt to represent a carcinoma (Figure C).

Cytologic Findings. The FNA smears of the breast mass contained numerous abnormal cells of variable size and shape that lay singly, in aggregates, and in "Indian-file" strands. Cellular and nuclear molding were frequently noted within the cell groups. (Plate 10–5 to 10–7). Their cytoplasm was scant, dense, granular, and basophilic. Cell borders were well defined. The nuclei were hyperchromatic and varied in size and shape. Nuclear membrane irregularities were commonly seen, and the chromatin pattern was coarsely granular. No nucleoli were observed; however, they may have been masked by the hyperchromatism. A diagnosis of infiltrating duct carcinoma was made.

Pathologic Findings. A modified radical mastectomy of the left breast was performed, and the tissue removed contained a hard, tan-gray tumor. Microscopic sections showed an infiltrating duct carcinoma with 18 axillary lymph nodes that were free of tumor (Plate 10–8, 10–9).

Refer to Slide 19 in Optional Slide Set.

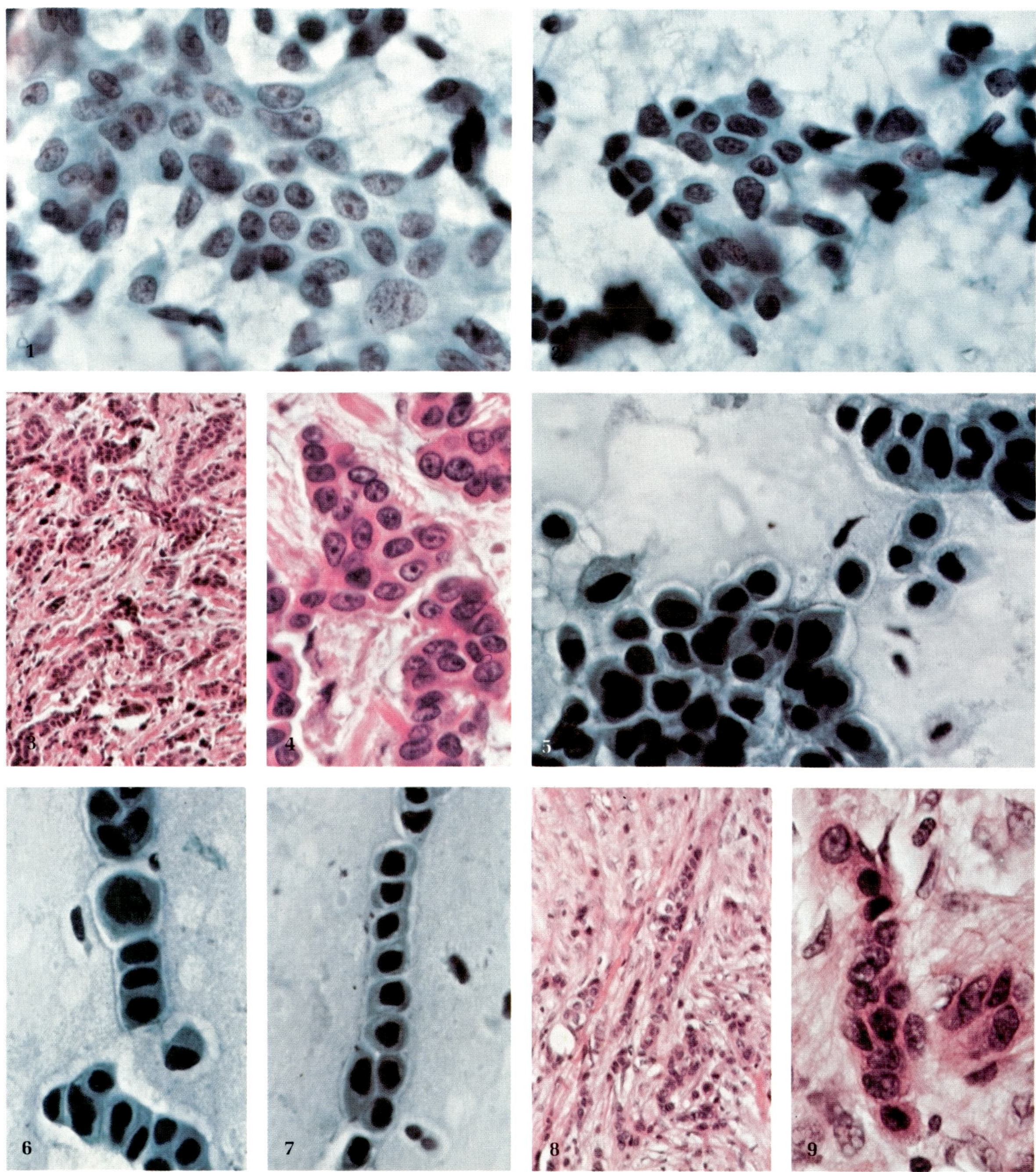

PLATE 10

Infiltrating Duct Carcinoma, Case 1

Plate 10–1, 10–2. Infiltrating duct carcinoma in FNA smear of the breast (Papanicolaou stain; × 400).

Plate 10–3, 10–4. Microscopic section of infiltrating duct carcinoma of the breast (H & E; 10–3, × 100; 10–4, × 400).

Infiltrating Duct Carcinoma, Case 2

Plate 10–5 to 10–7. Infiltrating duct carcinoma in FNA smears of the breast (Papanicolaou stain; × 400).

Plate 10–8, 10–9. Microscopic section of infiltrating duct carcinoma of the breast (H & E; 10–8, × 200; 10–9, × 400).

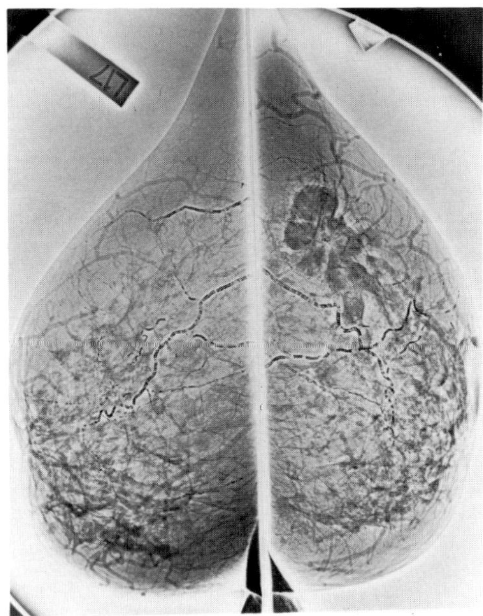

Figure A. Right: Xeromammogram showing lobular mass with irregular borders. *Left:* Normal breast.

PLATE 11

Infiltrating Small-Cell Duct Carcinoma

Clinical History. A 63-year-old woman had a nontender, 4 × 3–cm mass in the upper outer quadrant of her right breast. There was no palpable axillary lymphadenopathy. A xeromammogram of the right breast showed a lobular mass with irregular borders and focal calcifications that was interpreted as cancer. The left breast was normal (Figure A).

Cytologic Findings. The FNA smears of the breast mass contained numerous small cells with a monomorphic appearance at screening magnification. The cells were arranged singly and in syncytial aggregates with some streaming of cells noted (Plate 11–1 to 11–5). Their cytoplasm was scant and basophilic, cell borders were indistinct, and nuclear crowding and overlapping were commonly seen. On high-power examination, subtle nuclear abnormalities were identified (Plate 11–6, 11–7). Although the nuclei were small, there was some variation in size (Plate 11–5). Most nuclei were round or oval; however, occasional irregular shapes were found (Plate 11–5, 11–6). The chromatin pattern was finely granular, and no significant hyperchromatism was noted. Careful study revealed subtle irregularities in chromatin distribution and in the nuclear membranes. Nucleoli were present in almost every cell but no macronucleoli were seen. Despite the lack of obvious malignant criteria in these cells at first glance, close examination provided sufficient cellular features for a definitive diagnosis. They were interpreted as a small cell carcinoma of either duct or lobular type.

Pathologic Findings. A modified radical mastectomy was performed, and the specimen contained a well-circumscribed, firm, pale yellow carcinoma measuring 3.5 × 2.0 × 3.0 cm. Microscopically, the carcinoma was highly cellular and composed of small cells (Plate 11–8). An "Indian-file" arrangement was noted focally and resembled infiltrating lobular carcinoma. However, higher magnification demonstrated an infiltrating duct carcinoma of small-cell type. In contrast to lobular carcinoma, which is characterized by monomorphism, there was variability in the size and shape of cells (Plate 11–9). No metastases were found in 23 axillary lymph nodes.

Refer to Slides 20 and 21 in Optional Slide Set.

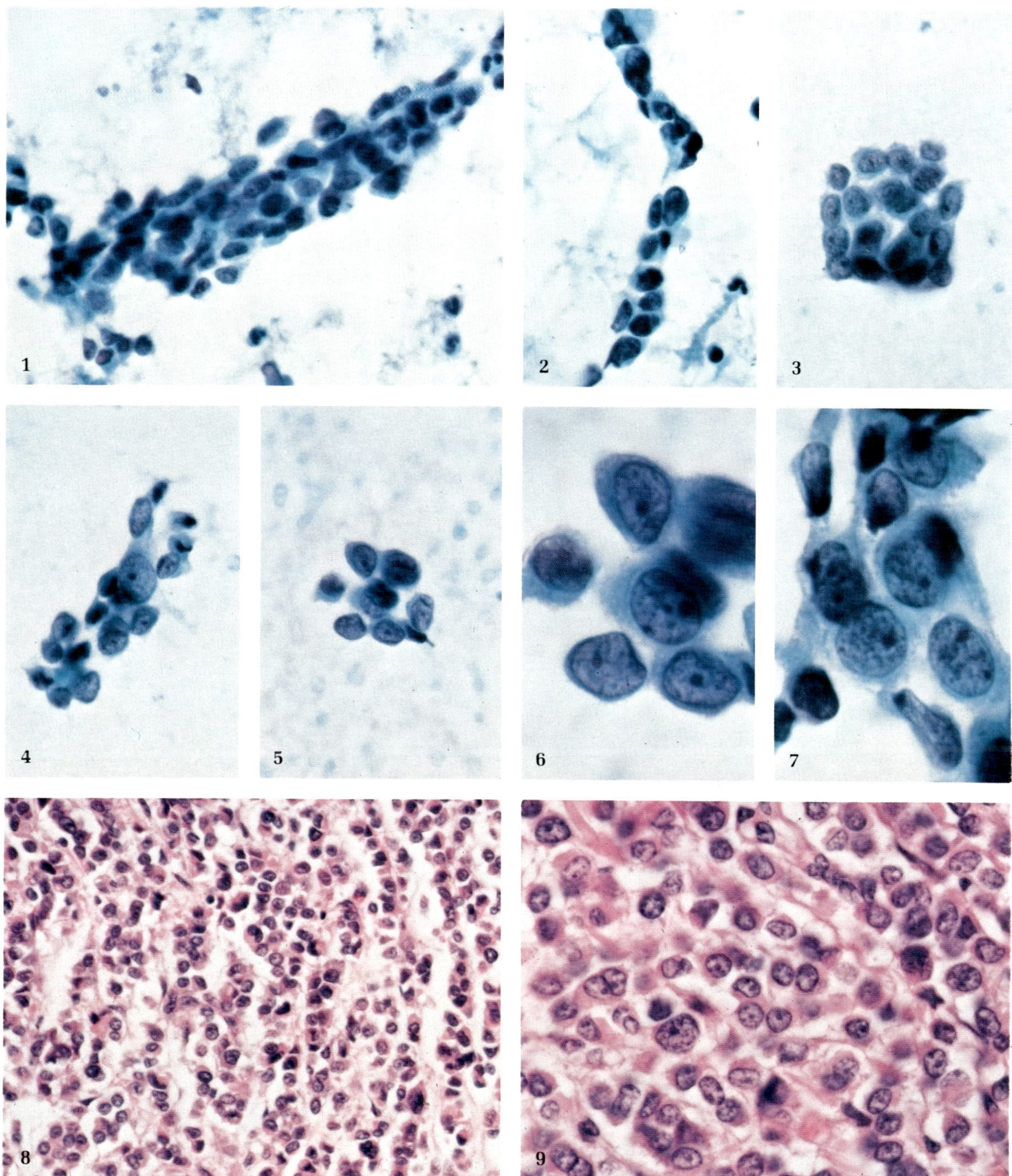

PLATE 11

Infiltrating Small-Cell Duct Carcinoma

Plate 11–1, 11–2. Infiltrating duct carcinoma, small-cell type in FNA smears of the breast (Papanicolaou stain, × 400).

Plate 11–3 to 11–7. Infiltrating duct carcinoma, small-cell type in filter preparation of FNA needle washings (Papanicolaou stain; 11–3 to 11–5, × 400; 11–6, 11–7, × 1,000).

Plate 11–8, 11–9. Infiltrating duct carcinoma, small-cell type in breast tissue section (H & E; 11–8, × 200; 11–9, × 400).

PLATE 12

Infiltrating Comedocarcinoma

Clinical History. A 44-year-old woman noticed a mass in her right breast and was seen in the surgical oncology clinic. During the physical examination, a 2 × 3–cm, firm, movable mass was palpated in the upper outer quadrant of the right breast. No axillary adenopathy was noted on the right side.

Cytologic Findings. The FNA smears of the breast mass contained numerous abnormal cells arranged in papillary clusters and syncytial arrangements or lying singly (Plate 12–1 to 12–5). The cells showed fairly good orientation within the papillary clusters with only occasional cell overlapping and crowding (Plate 12–1 to 12–3). Cells in the syncytial arrangements showed a more haphazard arrangement with frequent overlapping and crowding of the nuclei (Plate 12–4, 12–5). The cytoplasm of these cells was scant, granular, and basophilic. Cell borders were often indistinct. Their mildly hyperchromatic nuclei were enlarged, round, oval or occasionally irregular in shape, and varied in size. The chromatin pattern was finely granular and fairly evenly distributed with frequent chromocenters. Prominent nucleoli were seen in most cells. In addition to the malignant cells, areas of necrotic debris (Plate 12–6) and refractile, pink-staining calcifications (Plate 12–7) were seen. The papillary groupings, necrotic debris, and calcifications were compatible with a diagnosis of comedocarcinoma. However, the more pleomorphic cells present in the syncytial arrangements suggested the possibility of an infiltrating carcinoma.

Pathologic Findings. A modified radical mastectomy of the right breast was performed, and the specimen contained a 3 × 2 × 4–cm, hard mass. When the tumor was compressed, wormlike masses of yellow necrotic tumor extruded from the ducts (Plate 12–8). Microscopic sections showed a comedocarcinoma that was confined to the ducts with central necrosis and calcifications (Plate 12–9 to 12–11). Papillary projections of epithelial cells into the duct lumens (Plate 12–9) corresponded to the papillary configurations seen in the FNA smears (Plate 12–1 to 12–3). In a few foci infiltrating duct carcinoma was present.

Refer to Slides 22 and 23 in Optional Slide Set.

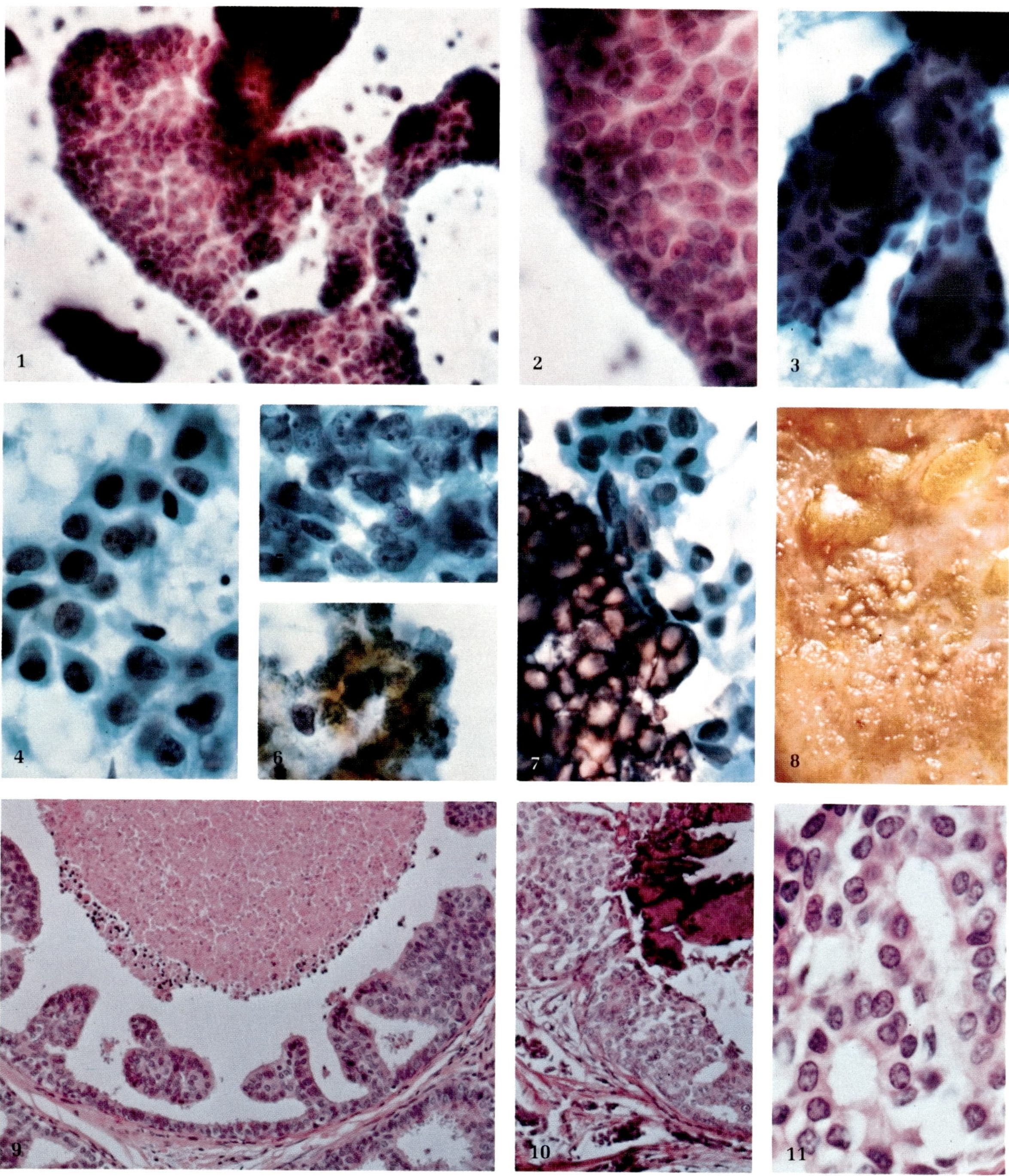

PLATE 12

Infiltrating Comedocarcinoma

Plate 12–1 to 12–3. Papillary clusters of malignant cells from comedocarcinoma in FNA smear of the breast (Papanicolaou stain; 12–1, × 200, 12–2, 12–3, × 400).

Plate 12–4, 12–5. Syncytial arrangements of malignant cells from comedocarcinoma in FNA smear of the breast (Papanicolaou stain; × 400).

Plate 12–6. Area of necrotic debris in smear background of breast FNA (Papanicolaou stain; × 400).

Plate 12–7. Area of calcification and associated malignant cells in FNA smear of the breast (Papanicolaou stain, × 400).

Plate 12–8. Gross appearance of tumor in mastectomy specimen.

Plate 12–9 to 12–11. Microscopic section of infiltrating comedocarcinoma of the breast (H & E; 12–9, × 100; 12–10, × 200; 12–11, × 400).

PLATE 13

Well-Differentiated Tubular Carcinoma

Clinical History. A 72-year-old woman observed a discrete, firm mass in her right breast and saw her family physician. The physical examination showed a 1.5 × 2–cm nodule in the upper outer quadrant of her right breast.

Cytologic Findings. The FNA smears of the breast nodule contained abundant cells arranged in ball-like and tubular structures (Plate 13–1 to 13–5). Various cell levels could be observed by changing the level of focus. The individual cells within these formations were small and fairly uniform in size and arrangement (Plate 13–4). The cytoplasm was scant and basophilic. The nuclei of these cells were small and showed only mild variation in size and shape (Plate 13–2). The chromatin pattern was finely granular and evenly distributed with occasional chromocenters. Nucleoli were present in many cells. The uniformity of the cells and their particular arrangement suggested the diagnosis of well-differentiated tubular carcinoma.

Pathologic Findings. Because of the unusual nature of these cells, a frozen section was requested to substantiate the diagnosis. Though frozen section was performed, the diagnosis was deferred until permanent sections were made; the permanent sections revealed a tubular carcinoma. The patient had a modified radical mastectomy, and the specimen contained a poorly circumscribed, hard, 2-cm, gray-white mass. Microscopic sections showed a haphazard arrangement of well-differentiated glands with an absence of necrosis and significant cytologic atypia (Plate 13–6 to 13–8). This pattern was diagnostic of a well-differentiated tubular carcinoma. Axillary lymph nodes were free of tumor.

Refer to Slides 24 and 25 in Optional Slide Set.

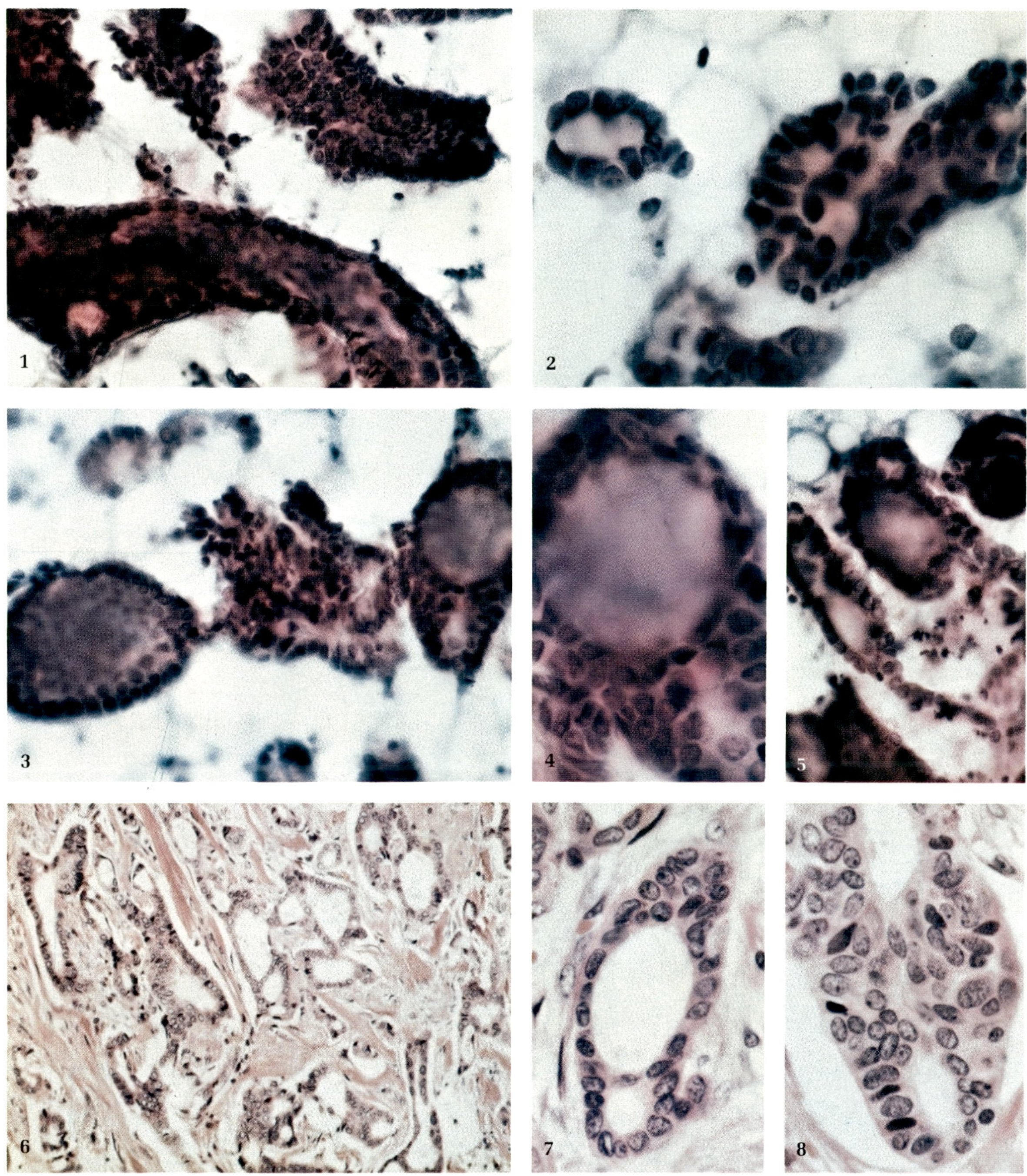

PLATE 13

Well-Differentiated Tubular Carcinoma

Plate 13–1 to 13–5. Ball-like and tubular structures from tubular carcinoma in FNA smear of the breast (Papanicolaou stain; 13–1, 13–3, 13–5, × 200; 13–2, 13–4, × 400).

Plate 13–6 to 13–8. Well-differentiated tubular carcinoma in mastectomy tissue sections (H & E; 13–6, × 200; 13–7, 13–8, × 400).

PLATE 14

Inflammatory Carcinoma

Clinical History. A 54-year-old woman first noticed a lump in her right breast seven months before consulting her physician. The mass continued to increase in size, and the skin of her right breast became reddened. She finally visited her physician, topical antibiotics were administered without improvement; she was referred to the University of Virginia Medical Center for further evaluation.

The physical examination showed that her right breast was swollen, warm, and red (Plate 14–1). A hard mass was palpable just inferior to the nipple. The mass extended 2 to 4 cm circumferentially.

Cytologic Findings. The smears from the FNA of the right breast contained numerous abnormal cells arranged singly and in syncytial arrangements in a background of cellular debris (Plate 14–2, 14–3). The cells had scant or moderate basophilic, dense cytoplasm and indistinct cell borders. Their enlarged nuclei were round or oval with finely granular, irregularly distributed chromatin. There was some thickening of the nuclear membranes. Nucleoli were present in almost every cell. A diagnosis of infiltrating duct carcinoma was made.

Pathologic Findings. A biopsy specimen of the right breast confirmed the clinical diagnosis of an inflammatory carcinoma by the presence of tumor emboli in the dermal lymphatics (Plate 14–4, 14–5). An infiltrating duct carcinoma was present in the underlying breast tissue (Plate 14–6). The patient received radiation therapy to her breast.

Ten months later, a malignant pleural effusion developed; and she was treated with chemotherapy. Four months following completion of therapy, she died with clinical evidence of extensive metastatic disease. An autopsy was denied.

Refer to Slide 26 in Optional Slide Set.

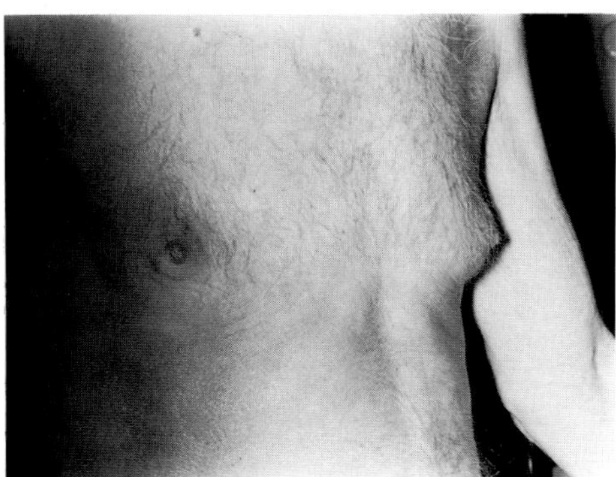

Figure A. Enlargement of left breast in male patient.

PLATE 14

Male Breast Carcinoma

Clinical History. A 70-year-old man noticed swelling of his left breast for one year before seeking medical advice (Figure A). A nonbloody nipple discharge was periodically observed, but he was unaware of a breast mass. He was receiving no medication and had no problems related to his prostate. The physical examination showed an approximately 2.5-cm mass in the left breast just lateral to the areola at the 3-o'clock position. The right breast was normal.

Cytologic Findings. The FNA smears of the breast mass contained aggregates of abnormal cells with indistinct cell borders and overlapping cell nuclei (Plate 14–7, 14–8). The cytoplasm was scant, basophilic, and finely granular. The enlarged nuclei varied in size but were usually round or oval. Occasional nuclear membrane irregularities were noted. The chromatin pattern was finely granular and fairly evenly distributed with some chromocenters present. Nucleoli were seen in almost every cell. A diagnosis of adenocarcinoma was made.

Pathologic Findings. A modified radical mastectomy of the right breast was performed. The specimen contained a 2-cm, firm, yellow-white tumor that on microscopic examination showed an infiltrating duct carcinoma (Plate 14–9).

Refer to Slide 27 in Optional Slide Set.

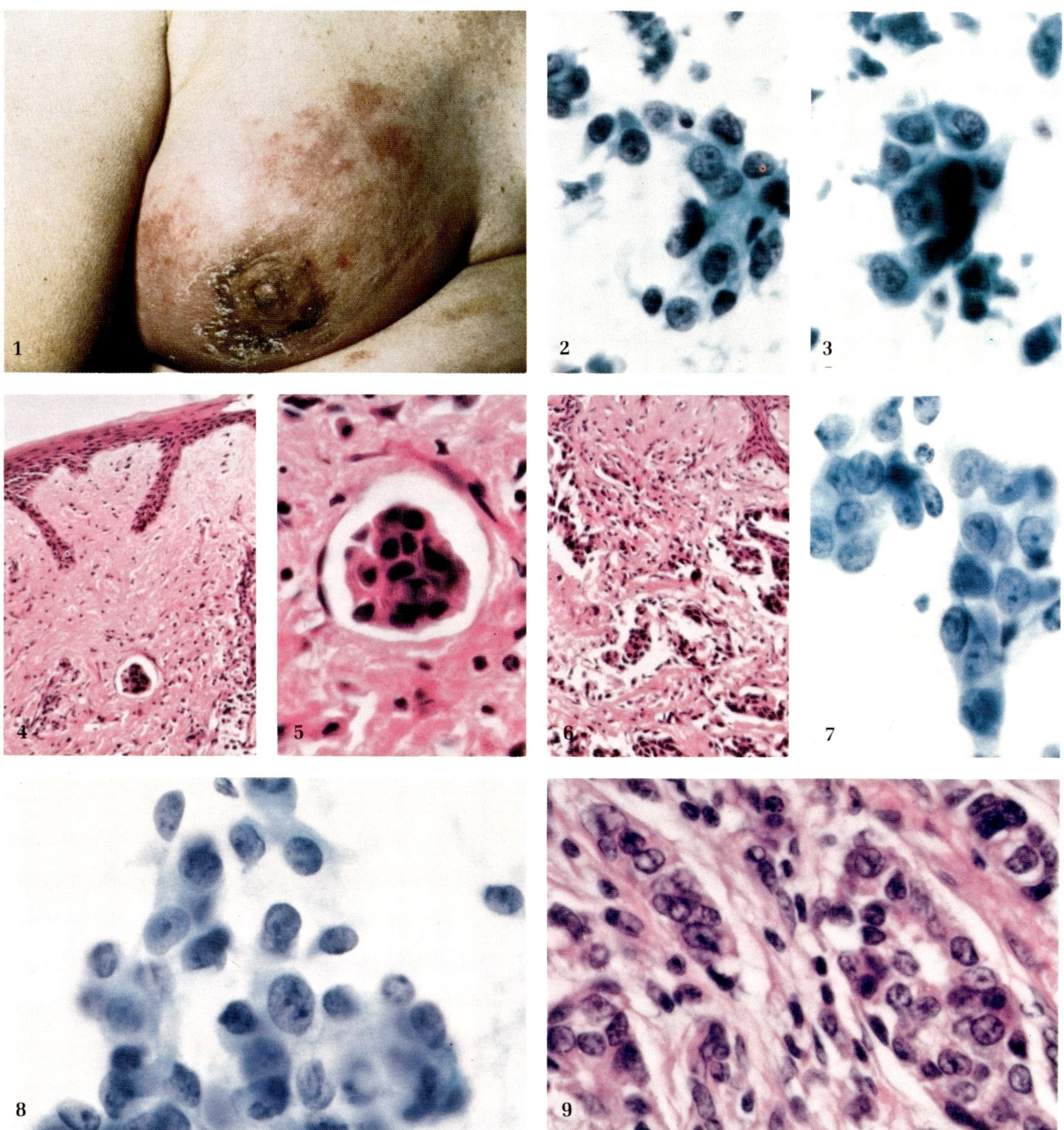

PLATE 14

Inflammatory Carcinoma

Plate 14–1. Patient with inflammatory carcinoma of the breast.

Plate 14–2, 14–3. Malignant cells from inflammatory carcinoma in filter preparation of FNA needle washings (Papanicolaou stain; × 400).

Plate 14–4, 14–5. Tumor embolus present in dermal lymphatic from inflammatory carcinoma of the breast (H & E; 14–4, × 100; 14–5, × 400).

Plate 14–6. Infiltrating duct carcinoma in microscopic section of the breast (H & E, × 100).

Male Breast Carcinoma

Plate 14–7, 14–8. Infiltrating duct carcinoma in FNA smears of the male breast (Papanicolaou stain; × 400).

Plate 14–9. Microscopic section of an infiltrating duct carcinoma of the breast in male patient (H & E, × 400).

PLATE 15

Paget's Disease

Clinical History. A 78-year-old woman consulted her surgeon because of bleeding and discharge from the left nipple. The physical examination showed the nipple was hyperemic and crusted (Plate 15–1). A sanguineous discharge was collected and Papanicolaou-stained smears were prepared. These smears contained abundant cells with obvious malignant criteria, and a diagnosis of carcinoma was made (Plate 15–2). The patient's breast was reexamined in an effort to identify a palpable mass. Examination of her left breast in various positions showed a firm mass underlying the diseased nipple. An FNA of this mass was performed.

Cytologic Findings. The FNA smears of the breast mass contained innumerable abnormal cells lying singly and in syncytial arrangements (Plate 15–3 to 15–6). Their mildly or moderately hyperchromatic nuclei were enlarged and varied in size and shape. Irregularities in the nuclear membrane were seen in many cells. The chromatin pattern was finely granular but often irregularly distributed with parachromatin clearing. Prominent, sometimes multiple nucleoli were seen in almost every cell. The cytoplasm was scant or moderate, basophilic, and finely granular. Occasional cytoplasmic vacuoles were present. The smear background contained blood, inflammatory cells, and cellular debris. These cytologic features were interpreted as malignant and, together with the clinical presentation, were diagnostic of Paget's disease.

Pathologic Findings. A modified radical mastectomy of the left breast was performed. The breast contained a well-circumscribed, homogeneous, gray-white neoplasm measuring 2.5 cm (Plate 15–7). Histologic sections from the nipple showed Paget's cells involving the epidermis (Plate 15–8, 15–9). Microscopically, the underlying breast mass consisted of an intraductal and infiltrating duct carcinoma (Plate 15–10, 15–11). A connection between the carcinoma within the ducts and the carcinoma in the overlying nipple was shown (Plate 15–10). The malignant cells present within the epidermis were identical to those seen within the ducts (Plate 15–9, 15–11).

Refer to Slides 28 and 29 in Optional Slide Set.

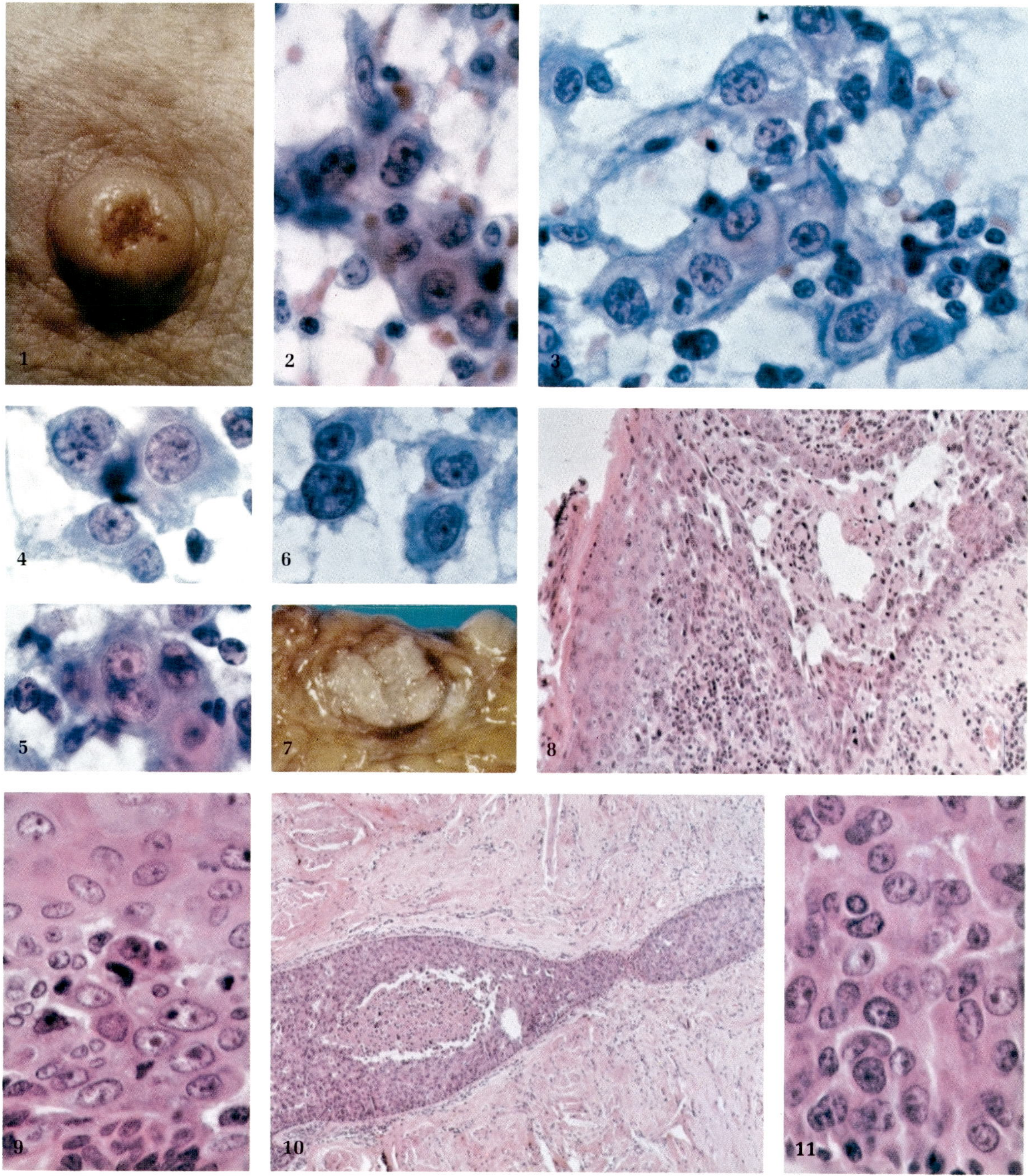

PLATE 15

Paget's Disease

Plate 15–1. Ulcerated lesion of the nipple.

Plate 15–2. Malignant cells from Paget's disease present in nipple discharge smear (Papanicolaou stain, × 400).

Plate 15–3 to 15–6. Malignant cells from Paget's disease and duct carcinoma in FNA smears of the breast (Papanicolaou stain, × 400).

Plate 15–7. Tumor mass underlying the nipple in the mastectomy specimen.

Plate 15–8. Malignant cells extending into the epidermis in histologic sections of the nipple (H & E, × 100).

Plate 15–9. High-power view of 15–8 showing malignant Paget's cells with overlying benign squamous epithelium (H & E, × 400).

Plate 15–10. Intraductal carcinoma filling the ducts in microscopic sections of the breast (H & E, × 40).

Plate 15–11. Infiltrating duct carcinoma in microscopic section from tumor mass (H & E, × 400).

PLATE 16

Apocrine Cell Carcinoma

Clinical History. A 50-year-old woman was seen in the medical clinic because of symptoms related to her myasthenia gravis. During the physical examination, a firm 2-cm mass was detected in her left breast.

Cytologic Findings. The FNA smears from this mass contained numerous, large abnormal cells lying singly and in syncytial arrangements (Plate 16–1 to 16–4). The cells were often polygonal, but varied greatly in size. Their cytoplasm was abundant, basophilic, and finely granular. Cell borders were often indistinct. The nuclei were large, round or oval, and varied greatly in size. The chromatin pattern was finely granular and evenly distributed with occasional chromocenters. Prominent nucleoli or macronucleoli were present in every cell. Diff-Quik-stained slides emphasized the granularity of the cytoplasm and the prominent nucleoli (Plate 16–5, 16–6). A diagnosis of apocrine cell carcinoma was made.

Pathologic Findings. A modified radical mastectomy of the left breast was performed, and the specimen contained a 1.5 × 2-cm mass. Microscopic sections showed an infiltrating carcinoma with apocrine features. The carcinoma cells were characterized by abundant, finely granular, pink cytoplasm and nuclear features identical to those seen in the FNA smears (Plate 16–7, 16–8).

Refer to Slides 30 and 31 in Optional Slide Set.

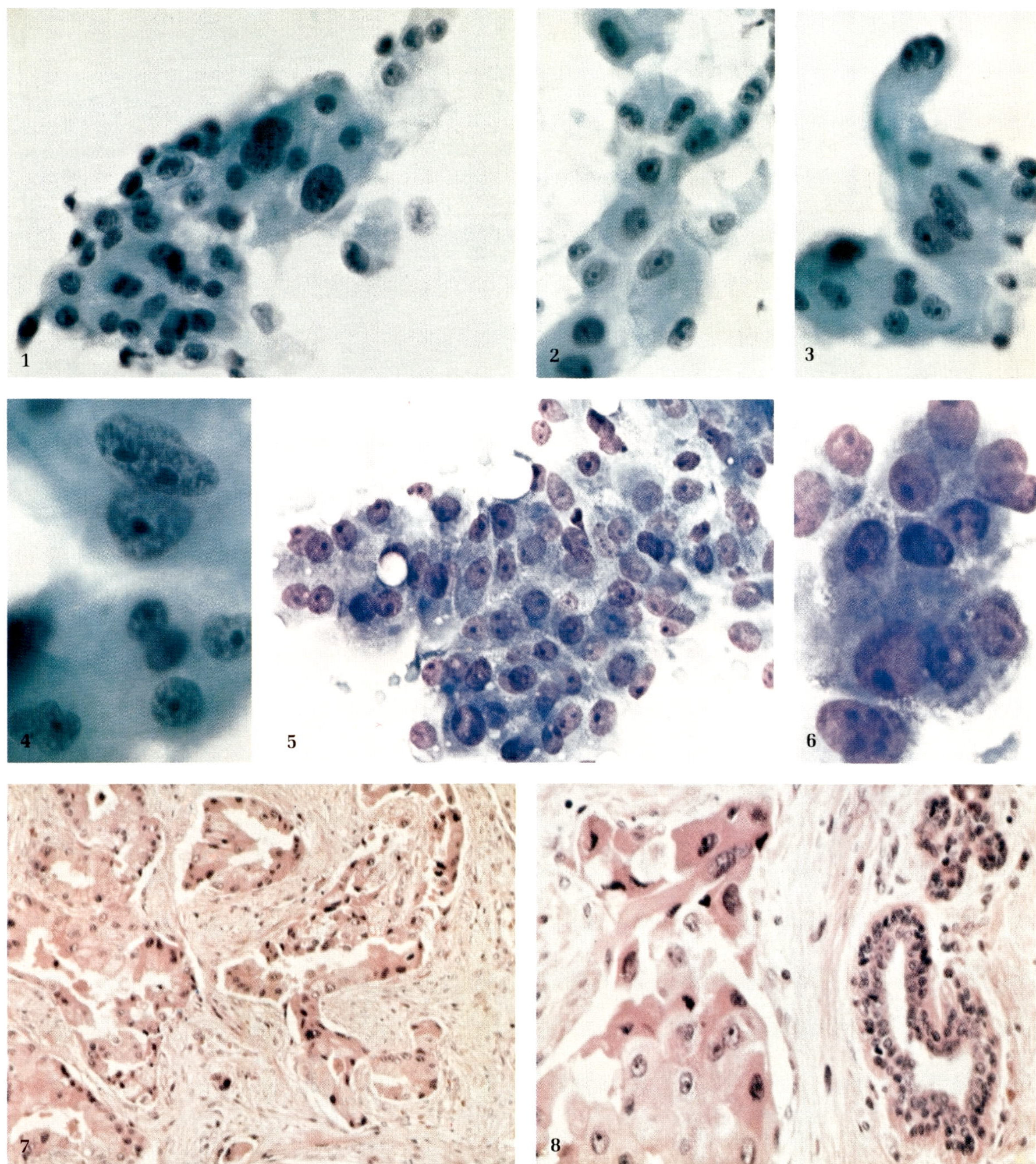

PLATE 16

Apocrine Cell Carcinoma

Plate 16–1 to 16–3. Apocrine cell carcinoma in FNA smears of the breast (Papanicolaou stain, × 200).

Plate 16–4. High-power view of 16–3 (Papanicolaou stain, × 400).

Plate 16–5, 16–6. Apocrine cell carcinoma in FNA smears of the breast (Diff-Quick stain set; 16–5, × 200; 16–6, × 400).

Plate 16–7, 16–8. Microscopic sections of infiltrating carcinoma with apocrine features in the mastectomy specimen. Note normal ductal structures adjacent to tumor cells (H & E; 16–7, × 100; 16–8, × 200).

PLATE 17

Colloid (Mucinous) Carcinoma

Clinical History. An 80-year-old woman noticed a painless mass in her left breast. She was seen by her physician and then referred to the University of Virginia Medical Center for evaluation and treatment. The physical examination showed a firm, 3 × 3–cm, mobile mass immediately adjacent and superior to the left nipple. There was no skin retraction, and the left axilla was normal.

Cytologic Findings. The FNA smears of the breast mass contained numerous pleomorphic tumor cells and pools of translucent, basophilic mucus (Plate 17–1). The tumor cells varied in size and had scant-to-abundant, basophilic, frequently vacuolated cytoplasm (Plate 17–2, 17–3). Their round or oval nuclei varied in size and were hyperchromatic and often eccentrically placed, especially in those cells with cytoplasmic vacuolization. The chromatin pattern was finely granular and evenly distributed with occasional chromocenters seen. The nucleoli were prominent, round to irregular, and sometimes multiple. Scattered mitotic figures were noted (Plate 17–3). A modified Wright-Giemsa–stained slide showed abundant purple-blue mucin and associated malignant cells (Plate 17–4). A diagnosis of colloid (mucinous) carcinoma was made.

Pathologic Findings. A simple mastectomy of the left breast was performed. The specimen contained a soft, gray, glistening, gelatinous tumor that measured 3.3 × 2.0 × 2.0 cm (Plate 17–5). Microscopic sections showed a colloid carcinoma characterized by islands of tumor cells within lakes of mucin (Plate 17–6, 17–7, 17–8). An alcian-blue stain demonstrated copious amounts of extracellular mucin with scanty intracellular mucin (Plate 17–9).

Refer to Slides 32 and 33 in Optional Slide Set.

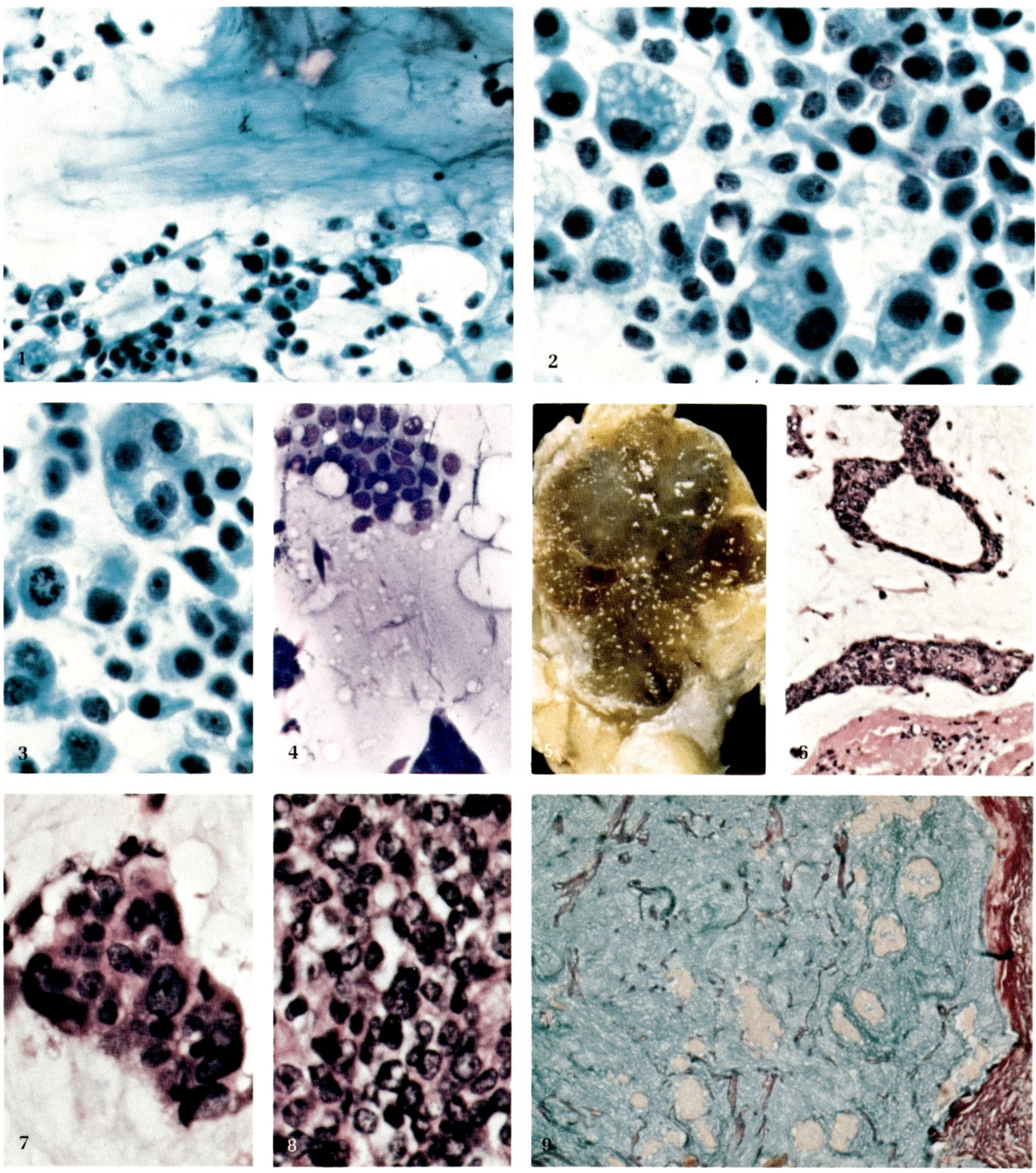

PLATE 17

Colloid (Mucinous) Carcinoma

Plate 17–1. Pool of mucin with adjacent malignant cells in FNA smear of the breast (Papanicolaou stain, × 200).

Plate 17–2, 17–3. Malignant cells of colloid carcinoma in FNA smears of the breast (Papanicolaou stain, × 400).

Plate 17–4. Abundant mucin admixed with malignant cells (modified Wright-Giemsa stain, × 400).

Plate 17–5. Gross appearance of colloid carcinoma in the mastectomy specimen.

Plate 17–6 to 17–8. Colloid carcinoma in microscopic section of the breast (H & E; 17–6, × 100; 17–7, 17–8, × 400).

Plate 17–9. Microscopic tissue section from colloid carcinoma of the breast (alcian-blue stain, × 40).

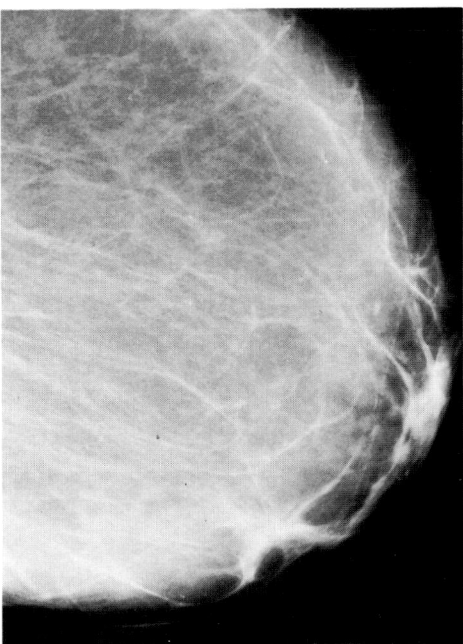

Figure A. Mammogram showing area of increased density in lower outer aspect of right breast.

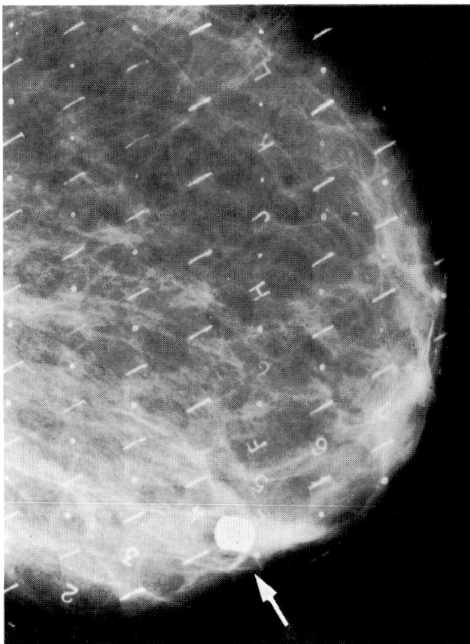

Figure B. Compression cone localization of breast mass.

PLATE 18

Signet-Ring Carcinoma

Clinical History. A 59-year-old woman had left breast pain for approximately three months before coming to the surgery clinic. The physical examination demonstrated that her breasts were large and pendulous with no palpable masses. The remainder of her examination showed no abnormalities. Mammograms showed an area of increased density in the lower outer aspect of her right breast (Figure A). An FNA of this region was performed under roentgenographic guidance (Figure B).

Cytologic Findings. The FNA smears of the breast mass contained numerous pleomorphic cells lying singly and occasionally in aggregates (Plate 18–1 to 18–5). The cells varied widely in size and shape. The enlarged nuclei were round or oval but varied in size. Nuclear membrane irregularities were seen in some cells, and the chromatin pattern was finely granular and evenly distributed. Single, rounded macronucleoli were present in almost every cell. The basophilic cytoplasm was moderate or abundant and frequently contained small-to-large, hyperdistended cytoplasmic vacuoles (Plate 18–1, 18–3, 18–4). The vacuolated cells showed eccentric nuclear placement and nuclear molding, giving the cells a signet-ring appearance (Plate 18–1, 18–4). Polymorphonuclear leukocytes were occasionally seen within the vacuoles (Plate 18–5). A mucicarmine-stained slide was positive for mucin (Plate 18–6). A diagnosis of signet-ring adenocarcinoma was made.

Pathologic Findings. A modified radical mastectomy of the right breast was performed, and the specimen contained a 1.5 × 2.0–cm, gray, gelatinous tumor. Microscopic sections showed a signet-ring carcinoma composed of sheets of signet-ring cells (Plate 18–7, 18–8). Intracellular mucin was abundant and mucicarminophilic (Plate 18–9). Multiple sections disclosed a histologic pattern characterized exclusively of signet-ring cells; therefore, the cancer was a pure signet-ring carcinoma.

Refer to Slides 34 and 35 in Optional Slide Set.

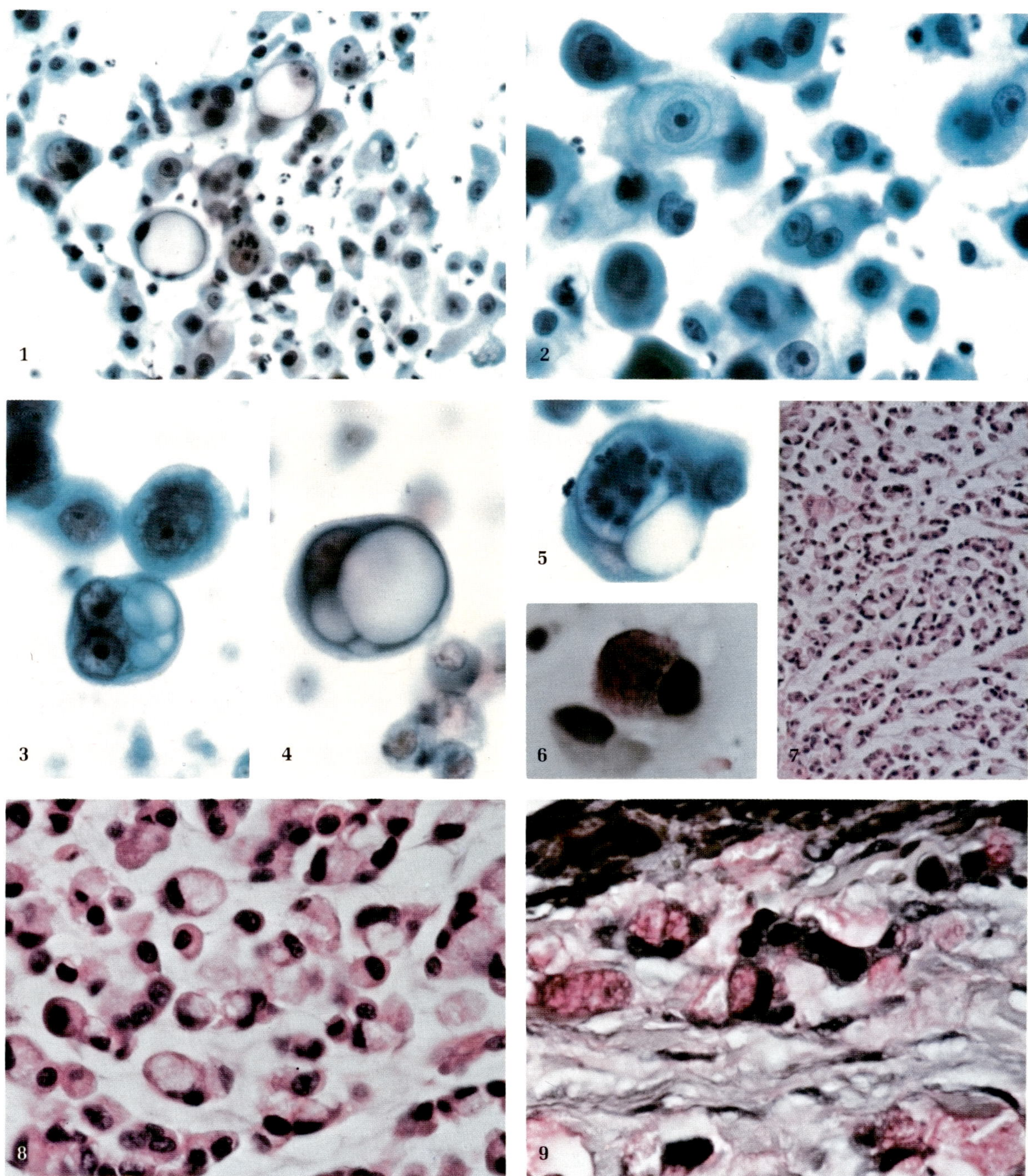

PLATE 18

Signet-Ring Carcinoma

Plate 18–1 to 18–5. Signet-ring carcinoma in FNA smear of the breast (Papanicolaou stain; 18–1, × 200; 18–2 to 18–5, × 400).

Plate 18–6. Mucin-positive malignant cell in FNA smear of the breast (mucicarmine stain, × 400).

Plate 18–7, 18–8. Signet-ring carcinoma in microscopic sections of the mastectomy specimen (H & E; 18–7, × 100; 18–8, × 400).

Plate 18–9. Mucin-positive tissue section of signet-ring carcinoma (mucicarmine stain, × 400).

PLATE 19
Papillary Carcinoma

Clinical History. A 58-year-old woman was admitted with the chief complaint of hoarseness. Laryngoscopy showed a vocal cord mass, and a biopsy specimen demonstrated a granular cell tumor. A firm, 1 × 2–cm, mobile mass was found in the upper outer quadrant of the right breast during the physical examination. Mammograms showed a 1.5-cm lobular mass with smooth but indistinct borders in the upper outer quadrant of the right breast, and FNA was performed.

Cytologic Findings. The FNA smears of the breast mass contained numerous papillary clusters of variably sized cells with scanty basophilic cytoplasm (Plate 19–1, 19–2). The nuclei were enlarged, round, oval or occasionally irregular in shape and varied in size. Nuclear crowding and overlapping were frequently seen within the papillary clusters. The chromatin pattern was finely granular and evenly distributed. Subtle irregularities were found in the nuclear membranes of some cells. Small, sometimes multiple nucleoli were seen in almost every cell. A diagnosis of papillary carcinoma was made.

Pathologic Findings. A modified radical mastectomy of the right breast was performed. The excised tissue contained a 2.0 × 0.6–cm, firm, tan lesion located in the upper outer quadrant. Microscopically, there was an intraductal papillary carcinoma composed of multilayered papillary formations protruding into the ducts. The epithelial cells were focally pleomorphic (Plate 19–3, 19–4). All 16 axillary lymph nodes were free of tumor.

Refer to Slides 36 and 37 in Optional Slide Set.

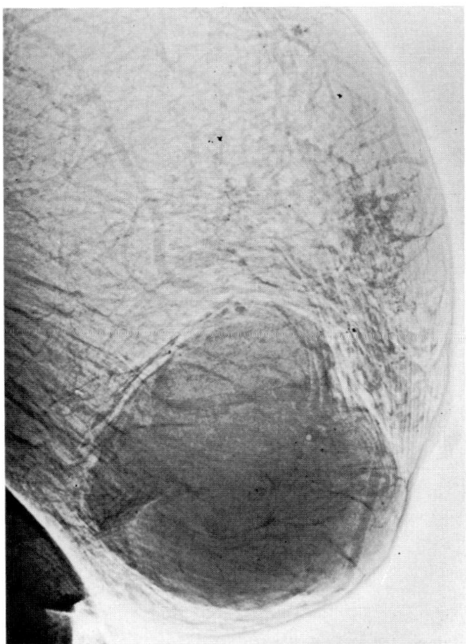

Figure A. Xeromammogram showing large, right breast mass.

PLATE 19

Intracystic Carcinoma

Clinical History. An 82-year-old woman went to her physician with a one-year history of a nonpainful lump in her right breast and a five-day history of a small bleeding lesion on her right breast. She was referred to the surgical oncology clinic. During the physical examination, a hard, mobile, 5 to 6-cm mass was found in the lower outer quadrant of her right breast. The skin overlying the mass was darkened with an 8-mm ulcer. The left breast was without masses. A xeromammogram showed a 7.5 × 8-cm mass in the right breast (Figure A).

Cytologic Findings. An FNA of the breast mass yielded a cloudy, brown fluid that rapidly filled the syringe. This fluid was centrifuged, and filters were prepared. A second needle pass was performed on the residual mass, and smears were made. The filters and smears contained abundant hemosiderin, red blood cells, and scattered papillary clusters of small cells with scanty or moderate cytoplasm (Plate 19–5 to 19–8). The nuclei of these cells were round, oval, or irregular in shape and variable in size. Nuclear overlapping within the groups was a common finding. The chromatin pattern was finely granular and evenly distributed. Occasional chromocenters were seen. Subtle nuclear membrane irregularities were observed in some cells. Micronucleoli were present in almost every cell. A diagnosis of adenocarcinoma was made.

Pathologic Findings. A modified radical mastectomy of the right breast was performed, and the specimen contained a firm, indurated area just lateral to the nipple. A small fistulous tract in this region communicated with a 5 × 5 × 3-cm necrotic cystic cavity that was filled with brown coagulated fluid (Plate 19–9). There were numerous, firm nodules located around the periphery of this cavity, principally in the lower outer quadrant. Microscopically, the cyst cavity was partially lined by a low-grade papillary carcinoma that was cytologically identical to the clusters of cells seen in the FNA (Plate 19–10, 19–11). In situ and infiltrating duct carcinoma was present in the adjacent breast parenchyma. All 35 axillary lymph nodes were free of tumor. The patient was alive and without evidence of tumor 43 months after mastectomy.

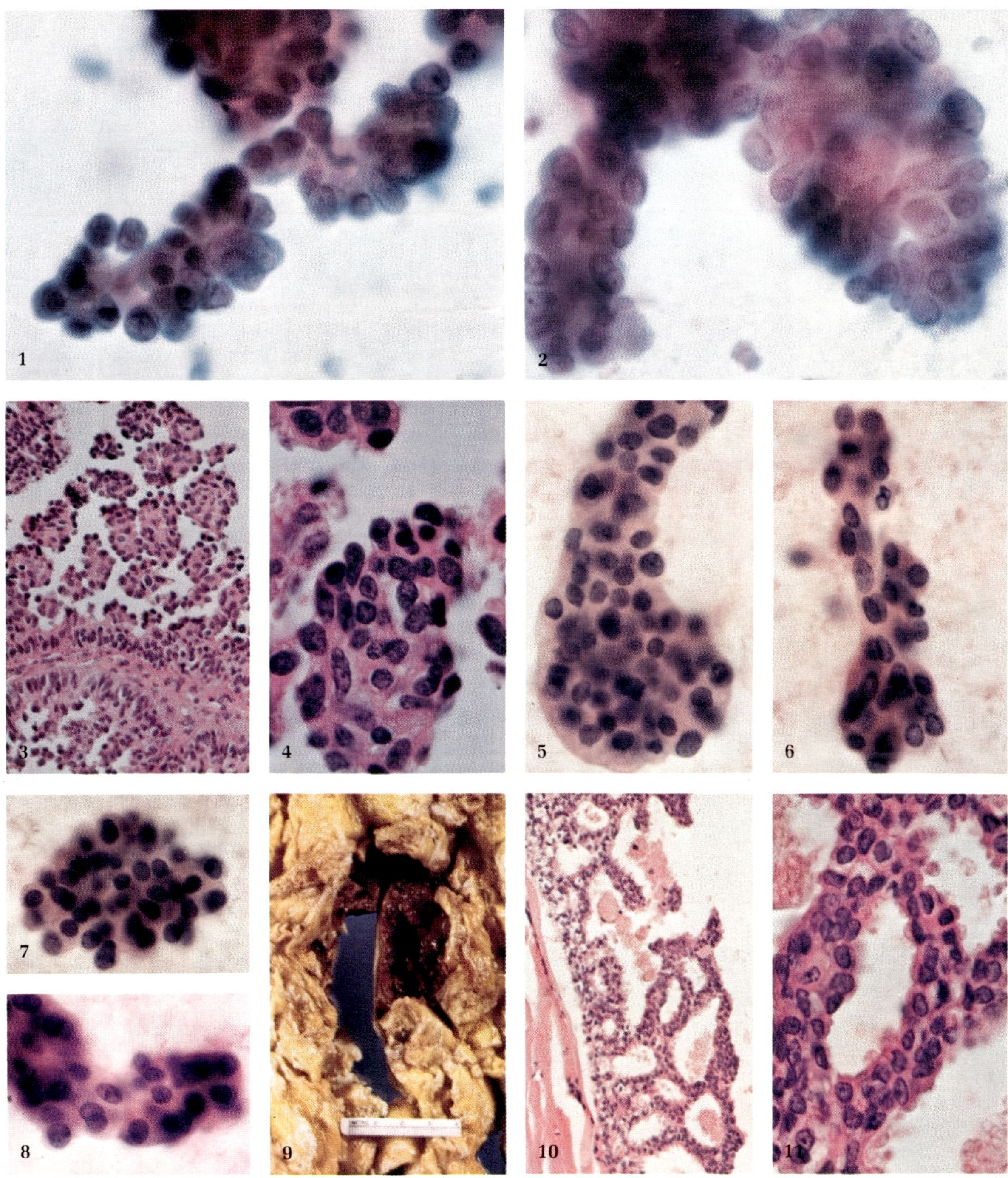

PLATE 19

Papillary Carcinoma

Plate 19–1, 19–2. Papillary carcinoma in FNA smears of the breast (Papanicolaou stain, × 400).

Plate 19–3, 19–4. Intraductal papillary carcinoma in microscopic sections of the breast (H & E; 19–3, × 100; 19–4, × 400).

Intracystic Carcinoma

Plate 19–5 to 19–8. Papillary clusters from intracystic carcinoma in FNA smears of the breast (Papanicolaou stain, × 400).

Plate 19–9. Intracystic carcinoma in the mastectomy specimen.

Plate 19–10, 19–11. Low-grade papillary carcinoma lining the cystic space in microscopic sections of the breast (H & E; 19–10, × 100; 19–11, × 400).

PLATE 20

Medullary Carcinoma

Clinical History. A 64-year-old woman noticed a lump in her left breast while performing a breast self-examination and was subsequently seen in the surgery clinic. The physical examination of her left breast revealed a 2 × 2–cm, firm, irregular, freely movable mass medial to the nipple.

Cytologic Findings. The FNA of the breast mass contained abundant, large malignant cells lying singly and in syncytial arrangements with numerous inflammatory cells, primarily lymphocytes, in the background (Plate 20–1 to 20–6). The cytoplasm of the abnormal cells was basophilic, dense, and moderate or scant. The mildly hyperchromatic nuclei varied greatly in size but were generally round or oval. Occasional binucleated cells were seen (Plate 20–6). The chromatin pattern was granular and irregularly distributed. Prominent, sometimes multiple nucleoli were seen in almost every cell. Because of the presence of obviously malignant, pleomorphic cells and numerous lymphocytes, a diagnosis of medullary carcinoma was made.

Pathologic Findings. A modified left radical mastectomy was performed; and in the inferior medial quadrant of the breast there was a 1.9-cm, soft, well-circumscribed, tan-pink tumor (Plate 20–7). Microscopic examination showed a medullary carcinoma characterized by a syncytial growth pattern with large pleomorphic nuclei, numerous mitoses, and indistinct cytoplasmic margins. Nucleoli were large and frequently multiple. A prominent lymphoid infiltrate was present between nests of carcinoma cells (Plate 20–8, 20–9).

Refer to Slides 38 and 39 in Optional Slide Set.

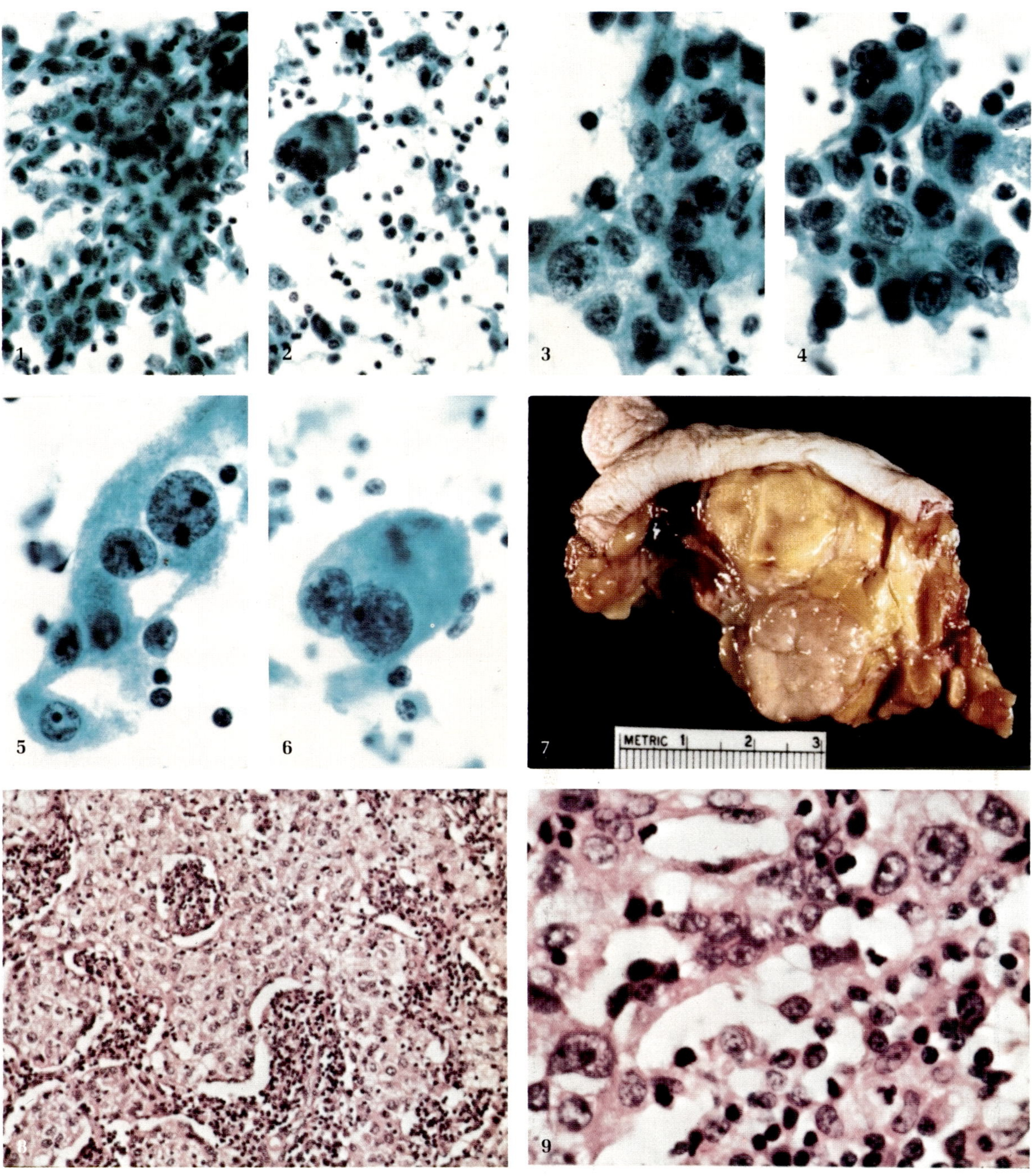

PLATE 20

Medullary Carcinoma

Plate 20–1, 20–2. Numerous malignant cells in background rich with lymphocytes from medullary carcinoma in FNA smears of the breast (Papanicolaou stain, × 200).

Plate 20–3 to 20–6. Large tumor cells of medullary carcinoma in FNA smears of the breast (Papanicolaou stain, × 400).

Plate 20–7. Gross appearance of medullary carcinoma in mastectomy specimen.

Plate 20–8, 20–9. Microscopic sections of medullary carcinoma of the breast (H & E; 20–8, × 200; 20–9, × 400).

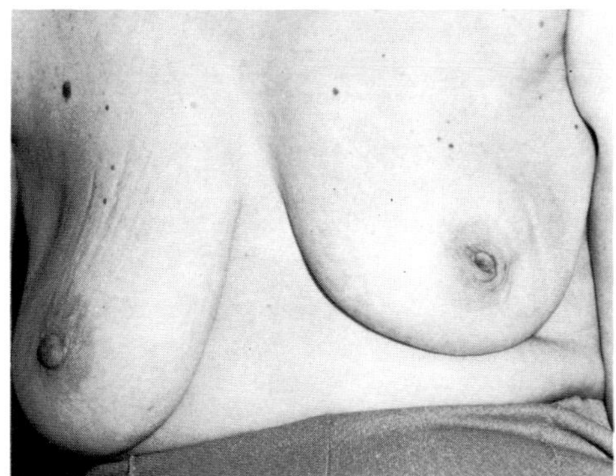

Figure A. Nipple retraction and skin dimpling seen in left breast.

PLATE 21

Tubular-Lobular Carcinoma

Clinical History. A 54-year-old woman first noticed a mass in her left breast during routine breast self-examination. Because of its "small" size and lack of pain, she deferred seeking medical attention for several months. She then consulted her family physician who noticed the breast mass and referred her to the surgery clinic at the University of Virginia Medical Center. The physical examination showed a 4 × 4–cm, nontender mass near the midline in the upper outer quadrant of the left breast. Some nipple retraction and skin dimpling were present (Figure A). The axillae were free from adenopathy, and the right breast was normal.

Cytologic Findings. The FNA smears of the breast mass contained innumerable, uniform, round-to-cuboidal, small cells lying singly and in aggregates (Plate 21–1 to 21–4). Their cytoplasm was scant, dense, granular, and basophilic with well-defined cytoplasmic borders. Small cytoplasmic vacuoles were noted on the modified Wright-Giemsa–stained slides (Plate 21–3, 21–4). The nuclei were enlarged, round or oval, and showed moderate hyperchromatism. The chromatin pattern was finely granular and evenly distributed. Prominent nucleoli were identified in some cells. This cytologic pattern of a monomorphic cell population of abundant abnormal cells was diagnostic of a lobular carcinoma.

Pathologic Findings. A modified radical mastectomy of the left breast was performed. The specimen contained a hard mass that measured approximately 3.8 cm at its greatest dimension and was located beneath the nipple (Plate 21–5). Microscopic sections showed a mixed pattern with tubular carcinoma (Plate 21–6, 21–7) and in situ and infiltrating lobular carcinoma (Plate 21–8, 21–9). All 26 axillary lymph nodes were negative for malignancy.

The tubular component of this lesion was not identified in the breast FNA.

Refer to Slides 40 and 41 in Optional Slide Set.

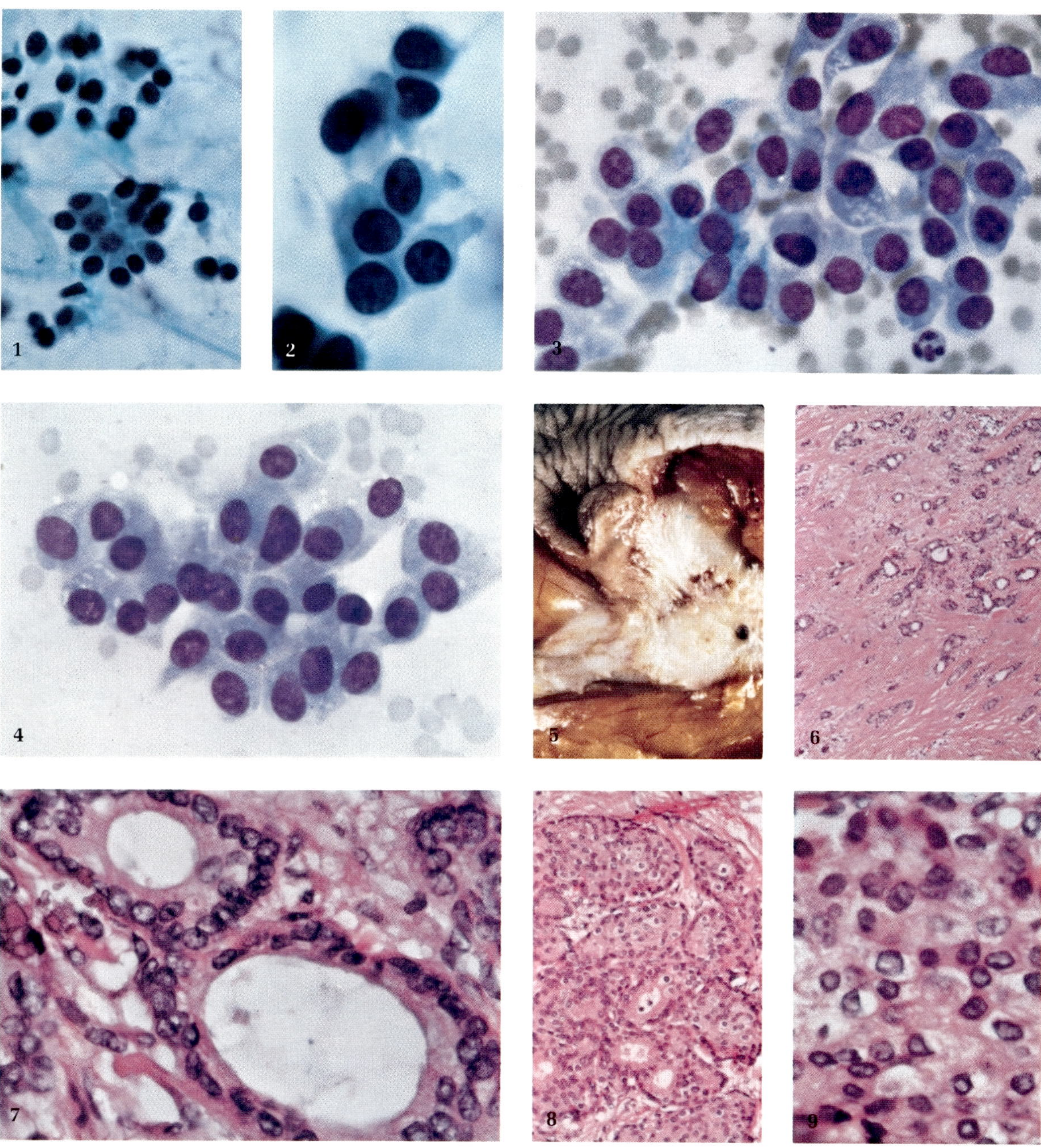

PLATE 21

Tubular-Lobular Carcinoma

Plate 21–1, 21–2. Lobular carcinoma in FNA smears of the breast (Papanicolaou stain; 21–1, × 400; 21–2, × 1,000).

Plate 21–3, 21–4. Lobular carcinoma in FNA smears of the breast (modified Wright-Giemsa stain, × 400).

Plate 21–5. Gross tumor in the mastectomy specimen.

Plate 21–6, 21–7. Tubular carcinoma in microscopic sections of the breast (H & E; 21–6, × 100; 21–7, × 400).

Plate 21–8, 21–9. Lobular carcinoma in microscopic sections of the breast (H & E; 21–8, × 200; 21–9, × 400).

PLATE 22

Invasive Lobular Carcinoma

Clinical History. An 86-year-old woman was admitted for evaluation and treatment of an enlarging, nontender breast mass. The patient stated that the lesion had been there for eight to nine years. The physical examination showed skin retraction overlying a 2 × 5-cm mass in the lower outer quadrant of the left breast (Figure A). There was no axillary adenopathy.

A bilateral mammogram revealed a dominant mass adjacent to the chest wall in the lower quadrant of the left breast (Figure B). Diagnostic studies, including brain and bone scans, showed no evidence of metastatic disease.

Cytologic Findings. The FNA smears of the breast mass contained numerous uniform small cells arranged singly, in clusters, and in "Indian-file" strands (Plate 22–1 to 22–3). Their nuclei were small, uniform, and round or oval. Nuclear molding was seen in some cells, especially those arranged in strands. The chromatin material was finely granular and evenly distributed. Micronucleoli were found in many cells. The cytoplasm was scant and basophilic. Cell borders were indistinct, and nuclear overlapping was common within the cell groups. The cytologic picture showed monomorphic small cells in an infiltrating pattern. A diagnosis of lobular carcinoma was made.

Pathologic Findings. A modified radical mastectomy of the right breast was performed, and the specimen contained a 1.3-cm hard tumor. Microscopic sections showed infiltrating lobular carcinoma with an "Indian-file" pattern (Plate 22–4, 22–5).

Refer to Slide 42 in Optional Slide Set.

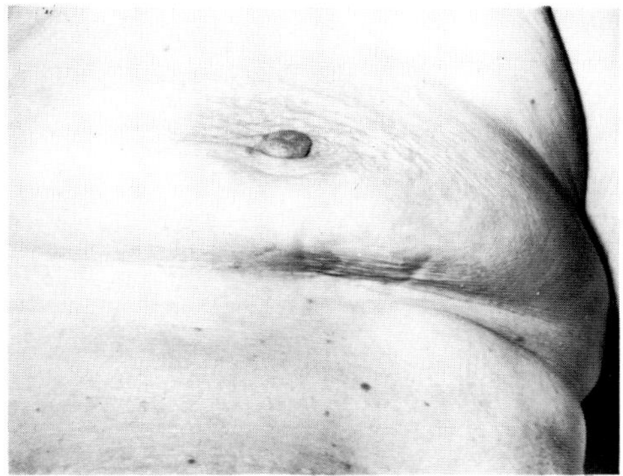

Figure A. Skin retraction seen in lower outer quadrant of left breast.

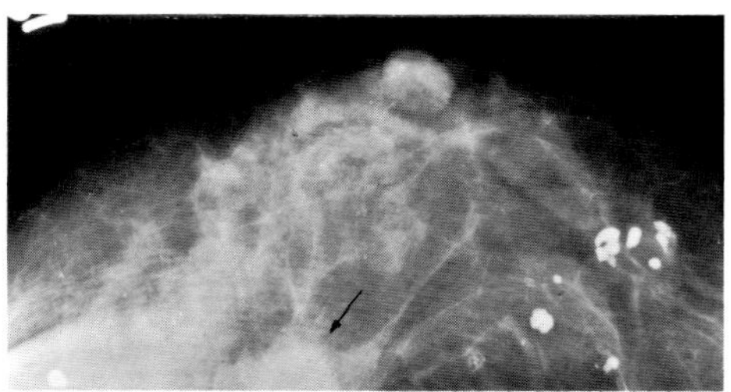

Figure B. Mammogram showing mass adjacent to chest wall.

PLATE 22

Invasive Lobular Carcinoma with Signet-Ring Pattern

Clinical History. A 60-year-old woman noticed aching pain in her left breast three months before her clinic visit. The pain temporarily resolved with administration of moist heat, but had recently increased. The physical examination showed an approximately 2.5-cm, fixed mass in the lower inner quadrant of the left breast.

Cytologic Findings. The smears from the FNA of the breast mass contained numerous, small, abnormal cells arranged singly, in loose aggregates and in strands (Plate 22–6 to 22–10). The small but variably sized nuclei had finely granular, evenly distributed chromatin with occasional chromocenters. The nuclei were round, oval, or irregular. Prominent nucleoli were present in almost every cell. The cytoplasm was scant and basophilic. Some cells showed large single cytoplasmic vacuoles. They had eccentrically placed nuclei that were molded around the vacuole, giving a signet-ring appearance (Plate 22–9, 22–10). A diagnosis of adenocarcinoma was made.

Pathologic Findings. A modified radical mastectomy of the left breast was performed, and the specimen contained a 2-cm, firm mass. Microscopic sections showed an infiltrating lobular carcinoma (Plate 22–11) with a signet-ring pattern in a few foci (Plate 22–12).

Refer to Slide 43 in Optional Slide Set.

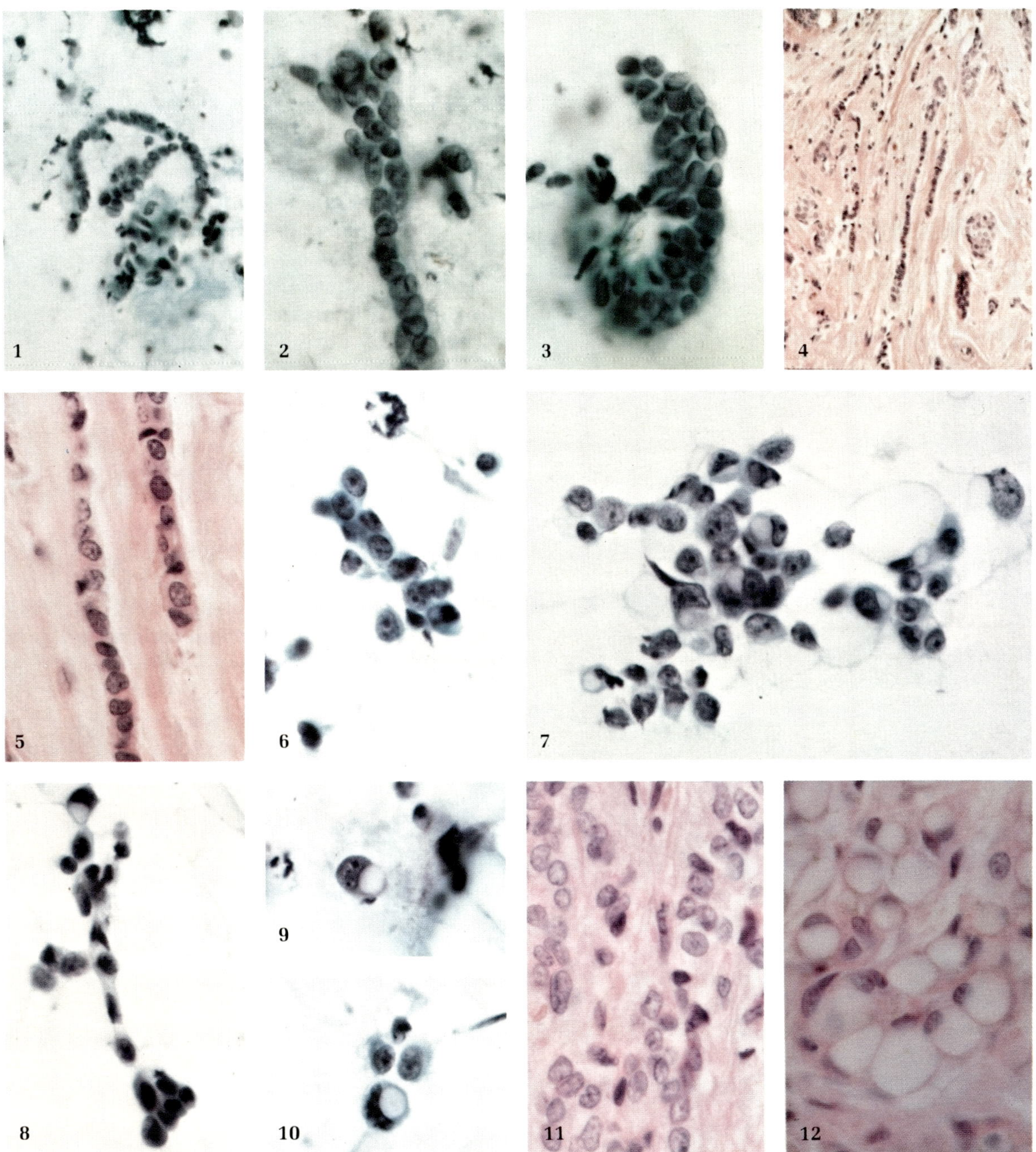

PLATE 22

Invasive Lobular Carcinoma

Plate 22–1 to 22–3. "Indian-file" pattern of lobular carcinoma in FNA smears of the breast (Papanicolaou stain; 22–1, × 200; 22–2, 22–3, × 400).

Plate 22–4, 22–5. Infiltrating lobular carcinoma in microscopic sections of the breast (H & E; 22–4, × 100; 22–5, × 400).

Invasive Lobular Carcinoma with Signet-Ring Pattern

Plate 22–6 to 22–10. Lobular carcinoma with signet-ring cells in FNA smears of the breast (Papanicolaou stain, × 400).

Plate 22–11. Infiltrating lobular carcinoma in microscopic sections of the breast (H & E, × 400).

Plate 22–12. Focus of signet-ring pattern in microscopic sections of infiltrating lobular carcinoma of the breast (H & E, × 400).

PLATE 23

Malignant Cystosarcoma Phyllodes

Clinical History. A 50-year-old woman with a long history of fibrocystic disease first noticed a small lump in her right breast five to six years before she saw a physician. It remained relatively quiescent until approximately one year before she sought medical attention. During that year, the lump began to gradually increase in size and then it increased quite rapidly during the last few months before she came to the surgery clinic. Physical examination showed that the right breast was greatly enlarged, and a firm nodular mass was palpated (Plate 23–1).

Cytologic Findings. The FNA smears of the breast were highly cellular and showed a wide range of cellular features (Plate 23–2, 23–3). There were numerous groups of elongated or spindle-shaped cells with varying degrees of nuclear atypia (Plate 23–4 to 23–7). These spindle-shaped cells had basophilic cytoplasm and cigar-shaped, mildly or moderately hyperchromatic nuclei with finely granular, irregularly distributed chromatin. They were felt to represent a sarcoma. Other cells had a more rounded appearance with a moderate amount of basophilic cytoplasm (Plate 23–3). Their nuclei were round or oval in shape, uniform in size, and had prominent, single nucleoli. The chromatin pattern was finely granular and evenly distributed. These cells were interpreted as benign duct cells. This cytologic pattern in conjunction with the clinical findings was suggestive of cystosarcoma phyllodes.

Pathologic Findings. A simple mastectomy of the right breast was performed, and just beneath the skin of the entire breast there was a firm, multinodular, gray-white mass that measured 20.5 cm at its greatest dimension. Sectioning showed cleftlike spaces (Plate 23–8) and numerous cysts up to 5.0 cm that contained dark brown fluid. Microscopic sections of the breast demonstrated malignant cystosarcoma phyllodes with a benign ductal component and a sarcomatous stroma having up to 12 mitoses per 10 high-power fields (HPF) (Plate 23–9 to 23–11).

Refer to Slides 44 and 45 in Optional Slide Set.

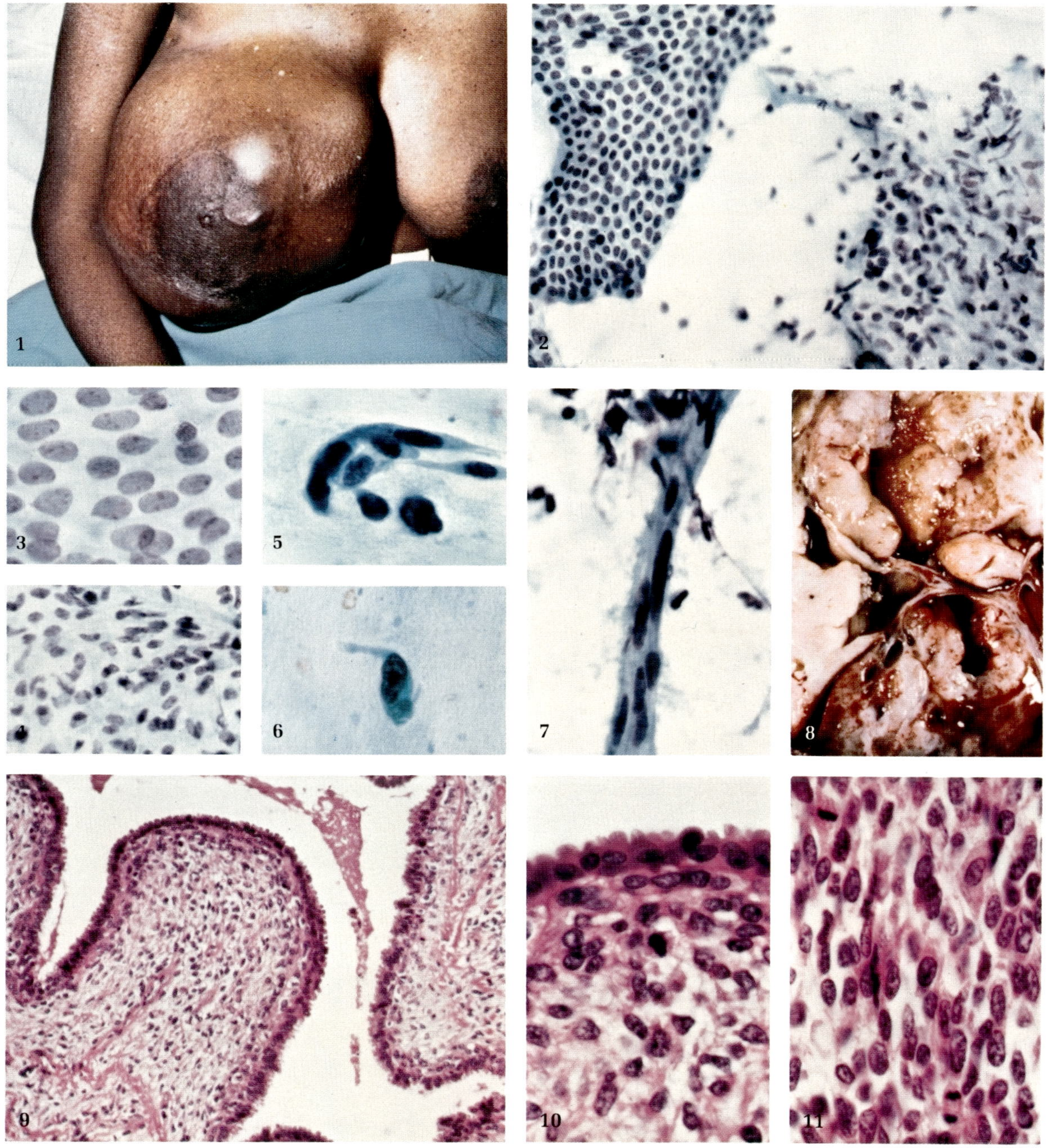

PLATE 23

Malignant Cystosarcoma Phyllodes

Plate 23–1. Patient with cystosarcoma phyllodes of the breast.

Plate 23–2. Benign duct cells and sarcomatous cells of malignant cystosarcoma phyllodes in FNA smear of the breast (Papanicolaou stain, × 200).

Plate 23–3. Benign duct cells from cystosarcoma phyllodes in FNA smear of the breast (Papanicolaou stain, × 400).

Plate 23–4 to 23–7. Sarcomatous component of cystosarcoma phyllodes in FNA smears of the breast (Papanicolaou stain, × 400).

Plate 23–8. Gross appearance of cystosarcoma phyllodes in the mastectomy specimen.

Plate 23–9 to 23–11. Microscopic sections of malignant cystosarcoma phyllodes of the breast (H & E; 23–9, × 100; 23–10, 23–11, × 400).

PLATE 24

Angiosarcoma

Clinical History. A 37-year-old woman (gravida VII, para VII) was in her usual state of good health and six months pregnant when she noticed a small mass in the lower aspect of her right breast. Her physician thought that the lesion was benign and decided to monitor its growth. The mass slowly enlarged and became tender; she then consulted another physician. The physical examination showed a 4-cm, freely movable, soft mass in the lower outer quadrant of her right breast.

Cytologic Findings. The FNA smears of the breast mass contained numerous syncytial masses of round-to-spindle-shaped cells in a bloody background (Plate 24–1 to 24–5). The cytoplasm was basophilic and scant. The nuclei had round, oval, elongated, or irregular shapes. The chromatin material was finely granular, but irregularly distributed; and many chromocenters were visible. Significant hyperchromatism was absent. Prominent single nucleoli were seen in many cells. These cells were interpreted as malignant and consistent with a sarcoma.

Pathologic Findings. The aspiration was thought to be malignant, but because of the unusual nature of the cells, tissue verification was recommended before therapy was started. An excisional biopsy was done; and the specimen disclosed a soft, spongy, hemorrhagic tumor. Microscopically, the tumor was composed of anastamosing vascular channels lined by atypical endothelial cells characteristic of an angiosarcoma (Plate 24–6 to 24–8).

A total mastectomy was recommended but the patient and her husband opposed further surgery. As part of her evaluation, numerous studies (chest x-ray films, bone scan, bone marrow biopsy, etc) were done; and the results showed no evidence of metastatic disease. In the absence of known metastases and inconclusive evidence that chemotherapy has a role in the treatment of angiosarcomas, it was felt that chemotherapy was not indicated. However, because of the high propensity of angiosarcomas to recur locally, radiation therapy was indicated and 5000 rads were given to her breast and chest wall.

Refer to Slides 46 and 47 in Optional Slide Set.

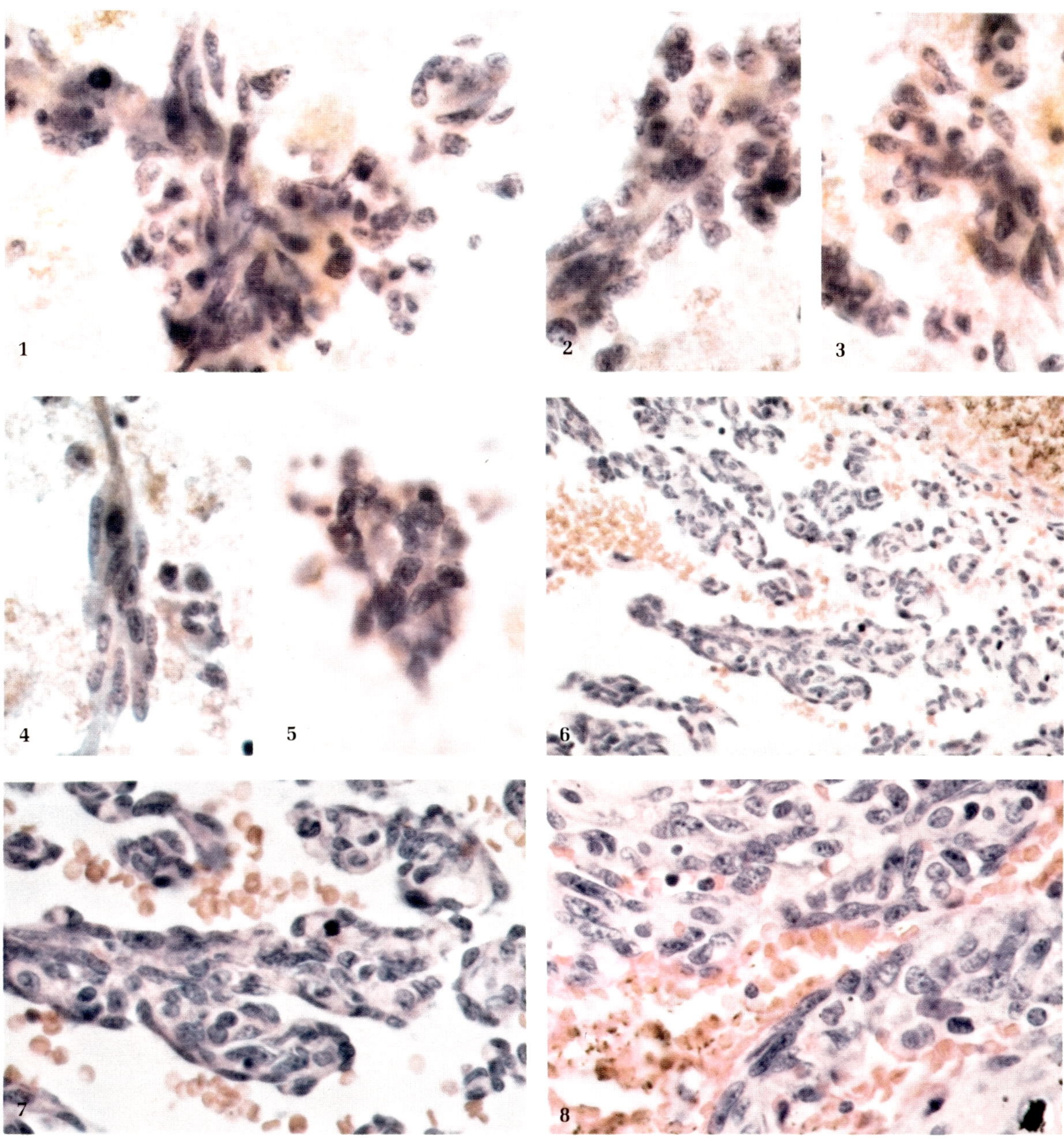

PLATE 24

Angiosarcoma

Plate 24–1 to 24–5. Malignant cells consistent with angiosarcoma in FNA smears of the breast (Papanicolaou stain, × 400).

Plate 24–6 to 24–8. Microscopic sections of angiosarcoma of the breast (H & E; 24–6, × 200; 24–7, 24–8, × 400).

PLATE 25

Osteosarcoma with Intraductal and Infiltrating Duct Carcinoma

Clinical History. A 69-year-old woman noticed a lump in her right breast six months before admission to the University of Virginia Hospital. She reported a one-month history of a watery nipple discharge. The physical examination showed a normal left breast, but a 2 × 3-cm, firm, irregular, mobile mass was found adjacent to the areola in the upper outer quadrant of her right breast. The results of the examination of the axilla on both sides were normal. Mammograms revealed dense tissue that contained several calcifications and a 1-cm area of round, amorphous calcifications (Figure A). These findings were suspicious for carcinoma, but a calcified intraductal papilloma could also have this appearance. During FNA of the mass, a gritty sensation was encountered as the needle entered the tumor.

Cytologic Findings. The FNA smears contained a pleomorphic cell population of three different cell types. There were numerous multinucleated giant cells with many round or oval, uniform, vesicular nuclei and prominent nucleoli (Plate 25–1 to 25–4). Their cytoplasm was dense, granular, and well defined. These cells appeared cytologically benign and resembled osteoclasts.

The second cell population consisted of pleomorphic cells with a moderate amount of dense, granular, basophilic cytoplasm and sharply defined cell borders, lying singly in the smear background (Plate 25–3 to 25–5). Their nuclei were round, oval, or irregular and frequently eccentrically placed. A clear space was adjacent to the nucleus in the cytoplasm of many cells. The chromatin pattern was granular and sometimes irregularly distributed, with mild or moderate hyperchromatism. Prominent nucleoli or macronucleoli were found in almost every cell of this type. These cells were interpreted as malignant and resembled osteoblasts.

The third cell population was composed of abnormal cells lying singly and in syncytial arrangements (Plate 25–3, 25–6), with moderate or scant, finely granular, and basophilic cytoplasm. Cell borders were indistinct. The nuclei were generally round or oval in shape but varied widely in size. Finely granular, but irregularly distributed chromatin and mild hyperchromatism were common nuclear features. Prominent, sometimes multiple nucleoli were noted in most cells. This final cell type was consistent with the classic cytologic presenta-

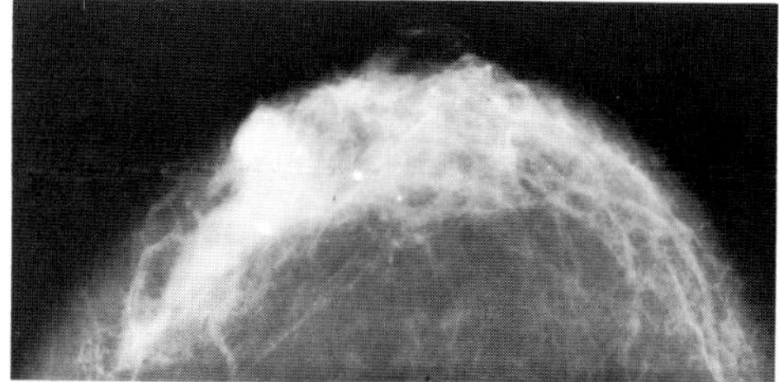

Figure A. Mammogram demonstrating dense tissue and calcifications.

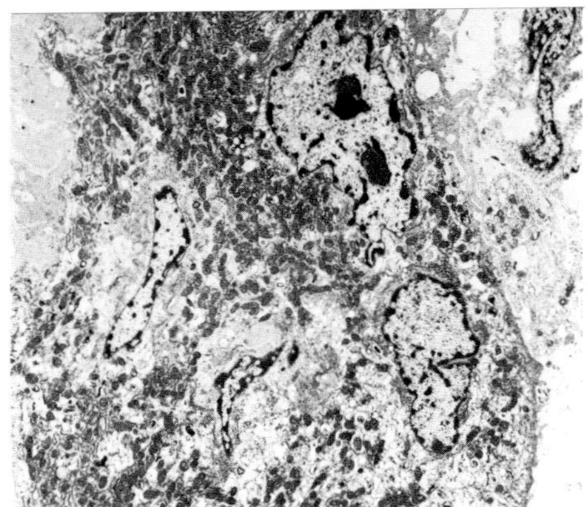

Figure B. Electron micrograph of large, multinucleated giant cell with ruffled border (×2,730).

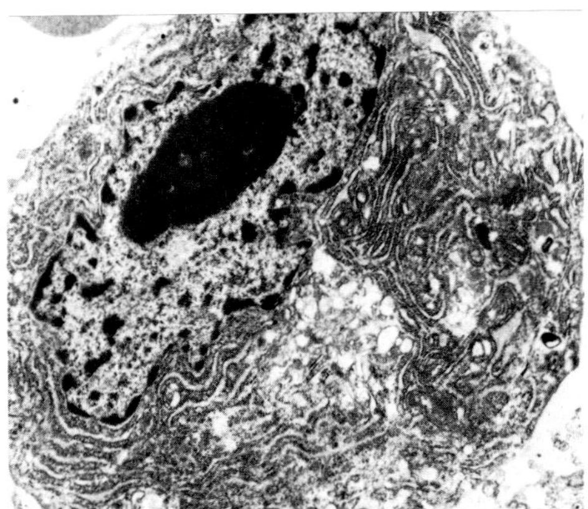

Figure C. Electron micrograph of osteoblastlike cell with eccentric nucleus and prominent nucleolus (×13,000).

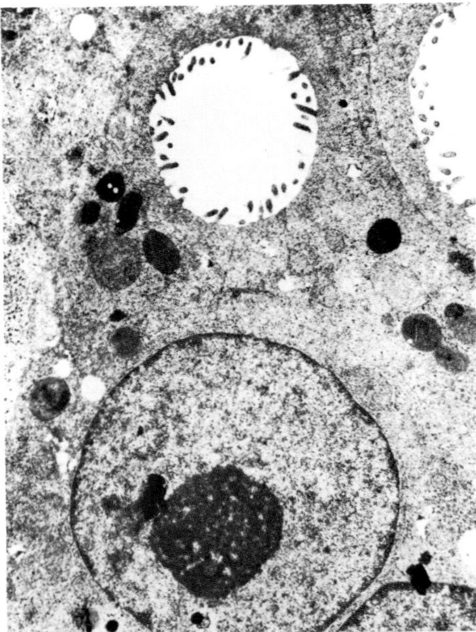

Figure D. Electron micrograph of carcinoma cell with intracytoplasmic lumen (×6,500).

PLATE 25

Osteosarcoma with Intraductal and Infiltrating Duct Carcinoma *(continued)*

tion of a duct carcinoma. The cytologic pattern was interpreted to represent an infiltrating duct carcinoma with a coexisting malignant neoplasm of uncertain type. The differential diagnosis included metaplastic carcinoma and osteosarcoma.

Pathologic Findings. A frozen section specimen was obtained before the mastectomy due to the unusual nature of the FNA. The specimen was a 3 × 2-cm segment of tan tissue. Sectioning showed that it was hard and gritty. Microscopic sections demonstrated what appeared to be an osteosarcoma. Because this type of tumor is rare in the breast, the diagnosis was deferred until permanent sections confirmed osteosarcoma.

There were osteoid deposits among the malignant osteoblasts and well-formed calcified trabeculae (Plate 25–7). Osteoclastlike giant cells with benign nuclei were interspersed among the osteoblasts (Plate 25–8). Higher magnification showed a few wisps of osteoid surrounded by osteoblasts with a variety of nuclear shapes (Plate 25–9). Additional sections showed intraductal and infiltrating duct carcinoma (Plate 25–10, 25–11).

A modified radical mastectomy of the right breast was performed, and the specimen contained a 3.0 × 1.0-cm mass adjacent to the biopsy site. Microscopic sections contained an infiltrating duct carcinoma with no evidence of the sarcomatous component of the tumor. Thirteen axillary lymph nodes were free of tumor.

Electron microscopic studies of tissue from the breast biopsy demonstrated three cell types. The first type was scattered, large multinucleated giant cells with a ruffled border (Figure B). Nuclei varied in size. The cytoplasm contained numerous mitochondria with sparse endoplasmic reticulum. The second type was numerous osteoblastlike cells with eccentric nuclei and prominent nucleoli (Figure C). Adjacent to the nucleus was a well-developed Golgi apparatus consisting of smooth membranous lamellae, small vesicles, and vacuoles. Rough endoplasmic reticulum and free ribosomes were abundant. The third type was carcinoma cells that contained intracytoplasmic lumina (Figure D). Nuclei varied in size and shape and had prominent nucleoli. *Note:* Robert E. Fechner, MD, at the University of Virginia Medical Center, concurred with the diagnosis of osteosarcoma combined with areas of duct carcinoma.

Refer to Slides 48 and 49 in Optional Slide Set.

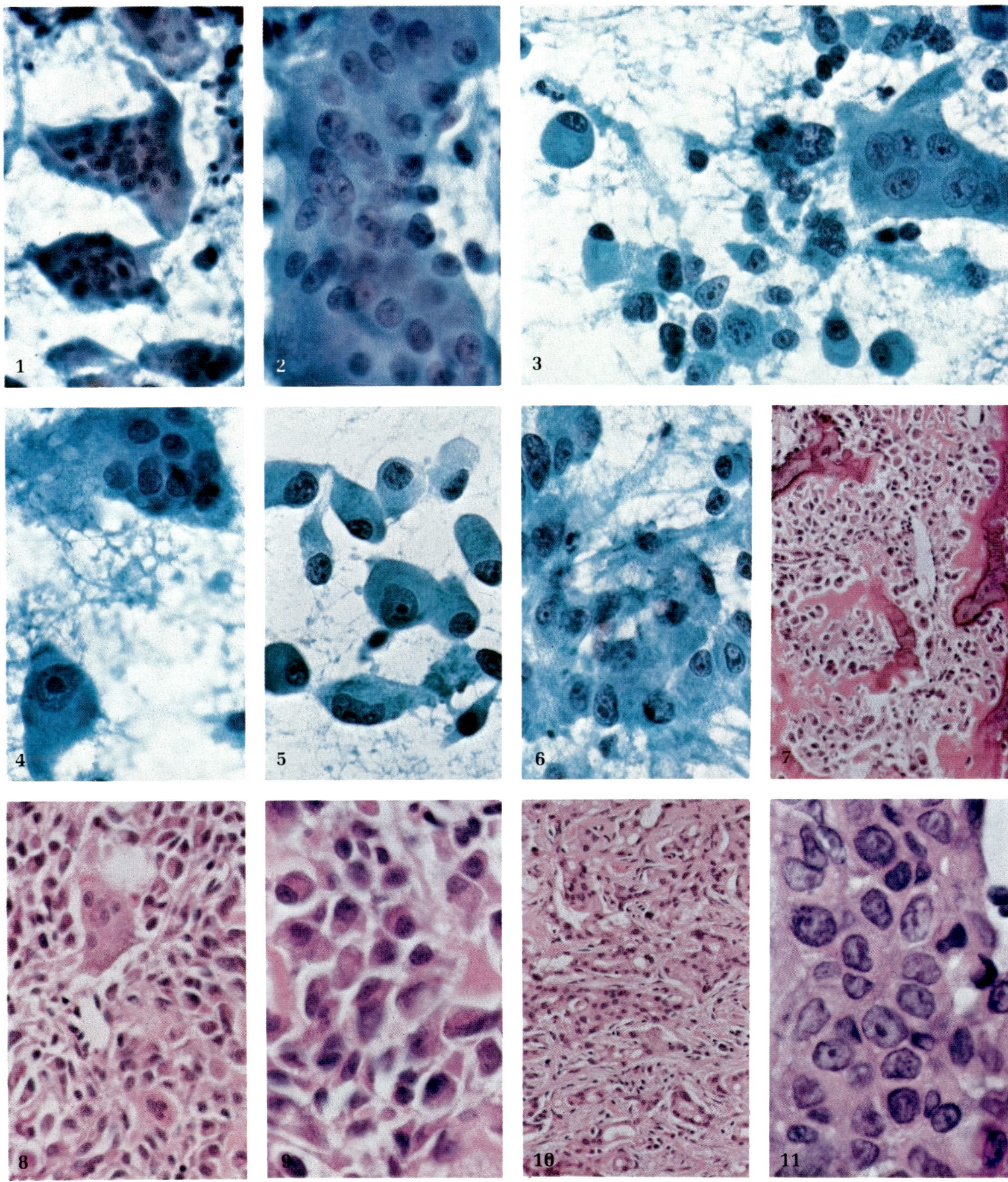

PLATE 25

Osteosarcoma with Intraductal and Infiltrating Duct Carcinoma

Plate 25–1, 25–2. Benign osteoclasts in FNA smear of the breast (Papanicolaou stain; 25–1, × 200; 25–2, × 400).

Plate 25–3. Benign osteoclast, malignant osteoblasts, and duct carcinoma cells in FNA smear of the breast (Papanicolaou stain, × 400).

Plate 25–4. Benign osteoclast and malignant osteoblast from osteosarcoma in FNA smear of the breast (Papanicolaou stain, × 400).

Plate 25–5. Malignant osteoblasts from osteosarcoma in FNA smear of the breast (Papanicolaou stain, × 400).

Plate 25–6. Duct carcinoma component of the osteosarcoma in FNA smear of the breast (Papanicolaou stain, × 400).

Plate 25–7 to 25–9. Osteosarcoma in microscopic sections of the breast (H & E; 25–7, × 100; 25–8, × 200; 25–9, × 400).

Plate 25–10, 25–11. Infiltrating duct carcinoma component in microscopic sections of the breast (H & E; 25–10, × 100; 25–11, × 400).

PLATE 26

Metastatic Small-Cell Undifferentiated (Oat Cell) Carcinoma

Clinical History. A 42-year-old woman with a 20-pack year smoking history was admitted to another hospital for evaluation of fever, chest pain, and productive cough. Chest x-ray films at that time revealed consolidation of the lower lobe of the right lung. Her physical examination on admission showed a large, hard, supraclavicular lymph node. A biopsy specimen of the lymph node showed metastatic small-cell undifferentiated carcinoma. A friable, obstructing lesion was seen along the medial border of the right bronchus intermedius during bronchoscopy. Bronchial biopsy specimens of the lesion were interpreted as necrotic material but no identifiable tumor was present. Two months after admission, the patient was referred to the medical center for palliative radiation therapy and chemotherapy. One month after completion of therapy, she developed multiple masses in both breasts.

Cytologic Findings. The FNA smears of the breast lesions contained numerous abnormal small cells with scant, basophilic cytoplasm lying singly and in syncytial masses. (Plate 26–1 to 26–4). The cell nuclei were small, variably sized, and frequently irregular in shape. Nuclear molding was a common finding within the cell groups. The chromatin pattern was finely granular but irregularly distributed (Plate 26–2) with chromatin clumping and parachromatin clearing (Plate 26–4). Irregularities in the nuclear membranes were also visible. Occasional nucleoli were seen. These cells showed the classic cytologic features of a small-cell undifferentiated carcinoma of the lung and were identical to those seen in the previous lymph node biopsy specimen (Plate 26–5). A diagnosis of metastatic small-cell undifferentiated carcinoma was made.

Follow-up. Because of the rapid progression of the disease and because the disease failed to respond to the previous therapy, the patient elected to forego further therapy. She died three months later at another hospital, and no autopsy was performed.

Refer to Slide 50 in Optional Slide Set.

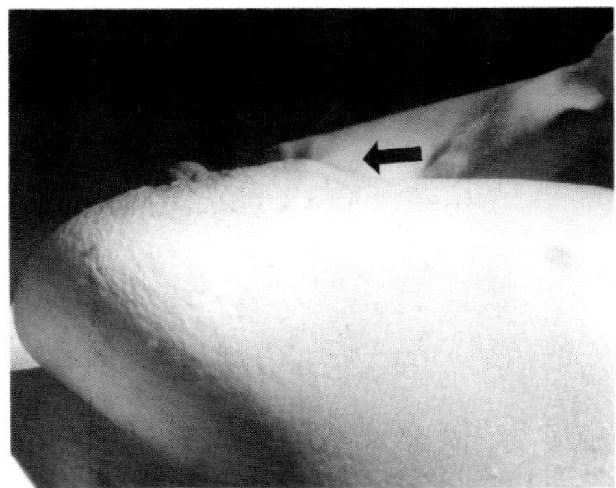

Figure A. Palpable mass *(see arrow)* in superior periareolar area of right breast.

PLATE 26

Metastatic Ovarian Carcinoma

Clinical History. A 61-year-old woman first noticed a lump in her right breast two weeks before admission to the University of Virginia Hospital. A 2 × 1.5-cm mass in the superior periareolar area of her right breast was palpated during the physical examination (Figure A). The mass was firm, freely movable, and not associated with any tenderness or nipple discharge. Palpation of her left breast revealed a 1 × 1.5–cm mass. No axillary adenopathy was noted.

Her past medical history included ovarian carcinoma diagnosed and treated eight years earlier and perineal resection with vaginectomy for squamous cell carcinoma.

Mammograms showed a 2-cm mass in her right breast that had benign characteristics.

Cytologic Findings. The FNA smears of the breast mass contained many pleomorphic cells lying singly, in syncytial arrangements, or in ball-like clusters (Plate 26–6 to 26–9). Cell borders within the groups were indistinct. The cytoplasm of these cells was basophilic, moderate in amount, and often finely vacuolated (Plate 26–7, 26–9). Their nuclei were of various sizes and shapes, and nuclear membrane irregularities were frequently seen. The chromatin pattern was finely granular but irregularly distributed with parachromatin clearing. Prominent, single nucleoli were seen in most cells. A diagnosis of adenocarcinoma was made. Comparison of the FNA material with tissue sections from the patient's previous ovarian carcinoma showed marked similarity of malignant cytologic features (Plate 26–10). The FNA results were interpreted as consistent with metastatic ovarian carcinoma.

Follow-up. The chest x-ray film, taken at the time of admission, revealed multiple nodular densities in the lungs compatible with metastatic tumor. She was discharged on chemotherapy but died four weeks later. An autopsy was denied.

Refer to Slide 50 in Optional Slide Set.

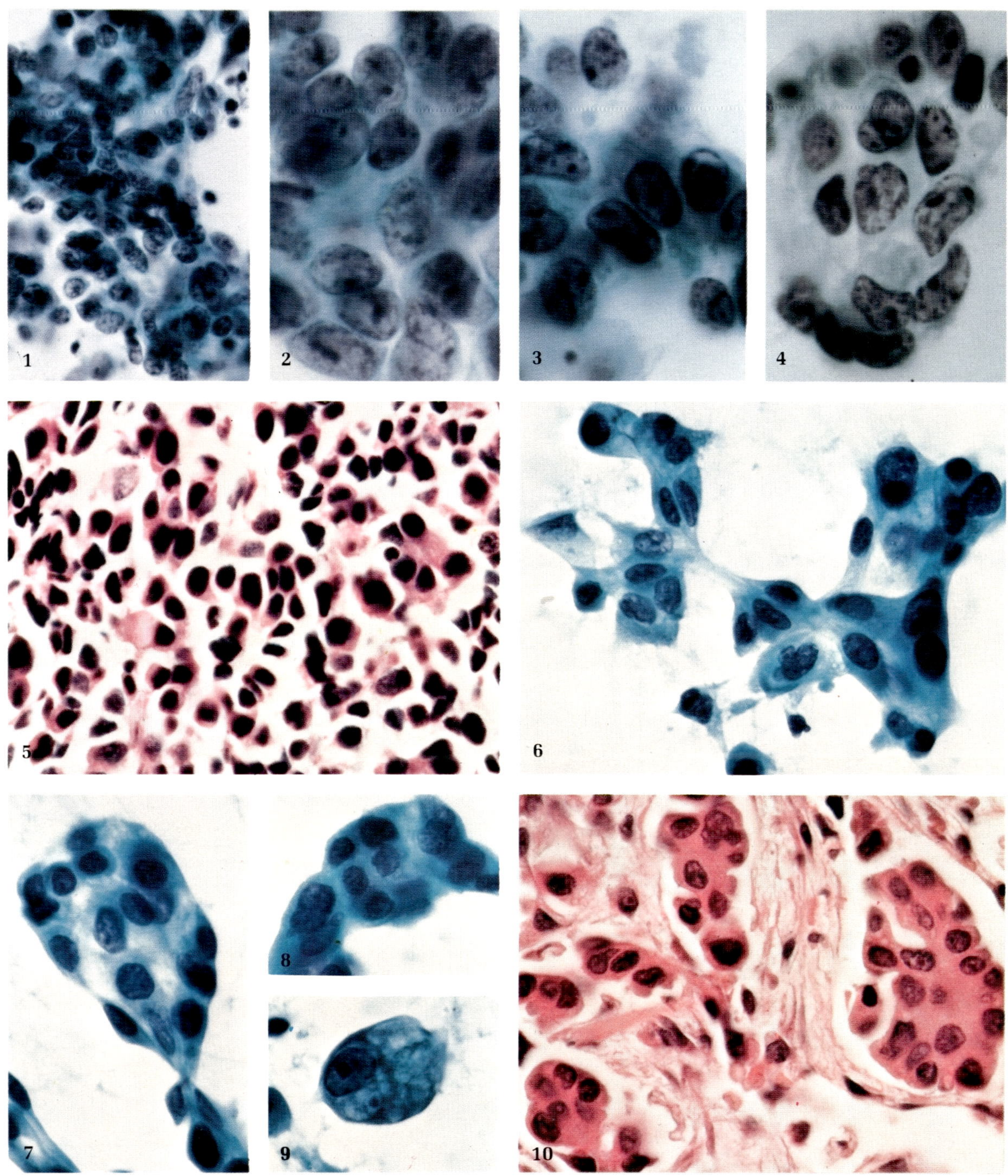

PLATE 26

Metastatic Small-Cell Undifferentiated (Oat Cell) Carcinoma

Plate 26–1 to 26–4. Metastatic small-cell undifferentiated carcinoma in FNA smears of the breast (Papanicolaou stain; 26–1, × 400; 26–2 to 26–4, × 1,000).

Plate 26–5. Metastatic small-cell undifferentiated carcinoma in lymph node biopsy (H & E, × 400).

Metastatic Ovarian Carcinoma

Plate 26–6 to 26–9. Metastatic ovarian carcinoma in FNA smears of the breast (Papanicolaou stain, × 400).

Plate 26–10. Microscopic sections of the primary lesion, papillary serous cystadenocarcinoma of the ovary (H & E, × 400).

Suggested Readings

Angiosarcoma

Azzopardi JG: *Problems in Breast Pathology.* Philadelphia, WB Saunders Co, 1979.

Masin M, Masin F: Cytology of angiosarcoma of the breast—A case report. *Acta Cytol* 1978;22(3):162–164.

Apocrine Cell Carcinoma

Azzopardi JG: *Problems in Breast Pathology.* Philadelphia, WB Saunders Co, 1979.

Frable WJ: *Thin Needle Aspiration Biopsy.* Philadelphia, WB Saunders Co, 1983.

Zajicek J: *Aspiration Biopsy Cytology. Part I: Cytology of Supradiaphragmatic Organs,* in Wied GL (ed): Monographs in Clinical Cytology. New York, Karger, 1974, vol 4.

Breast Abscess/Fat Necrosis/Gynecomastia

Bannayan GA, Hajdu SI: Gynecomastia: Clinicopathologic study of 351 cases. *Am J Clin Pathol* 1972;57:431–437.

Carlson HE: Gynecomastia. *N Eng J Med* 1980;303:795–799.

Kline TS: *Handbook of Fine Needle Aspiration Biopsy Cytology.* St. Louis, CV Mosby Co, 1981.

Colloid (Mucinous) Carcinoma

Azzopardi JG: *Problems in Breast Pathology.* Philadelphia, WB Saunders Co, 1979.

Frable WJ: *Thin Needle Aspiration Biopsy.* Philadelphia, WB Saunders Co, 1983.

Kaminsky DB: *Aspiration Biopsy for the Community Hospital.* New York, Masson Publishing Co, 1981.

Zajicek J: *Aspiration Biopsy Cytology. Part I: Cytology of Supradiaphragmatic Organs,* in Wied GL (ed): Monographs in Clinical Cytology. New York, Karger, 1974, vol 4.

Ductal Hyperplasia

Azzopardi JG: *Problems in Breast Pathology.* Philadelphia, WB Saunders Co, 1979.

Kern WH, Dermer GB: The cytopathology of hyperplastic and neoplastic mammary duct epithelium. *Acta Cytol* 1972;16:120–129.

Kline TS: *Handbook of Fine Needle Apiration Biopsy Cytology.* St. Louis, CV Mosby Co, 1981.

McDivitt RW: Breast carcinoma. *Human Pathol* 1978;9:3–21.

Fibroadenoma

Azzopardi JG: *Problems in Breast Pathology.* Philadelphia, WB Saunders Co, 1979.

Franzen S, Zajicek J: Aspiration biopsy in diagnosis of palpable lesions of the breast. *Acta Radiol Ther Physics Biol* 1968;7:241–262.

Linsk J, Kreuzer G, Zajicek J: Cytologic diagnosis of mammary tumors from aspiration biopsy smears. II. Studies on 210 fibroadenomas and 210 cases of benign dysplasia. *Acta Cytol* 1972;16:130–138.

Zajicek J: *Aspiration Biopsy Cytology. Part I: Cytology of Supradiaphragmatic Organs,* in Wied GL (ed): Monographs in Clinical Cytology. New York, Karger, 1974, vol 4.

Fibrocystic Disease

Franzen S, Zajicek J: Aspiration biopsy in diagnosis of palpable lesions of the breast. *Acta Radiol* 1968;7:241–262.

Johnston JH Jr: Aspiration as diagnostic and therapeutic procedure in cystic disease of the breast. *Ann Surg* 1954;139(5):635–643.

Kreuzer G: Aspiration biopsy cytology in proliferative benign mammary dysplasia. *Acta Cytol* 1978;22(3):128–132.

Linsk J, Kreuzer G, Zajicek J: Cytologic diagnosis of mammary tumors from aspiration biopsy smears. II. Studies on 210 fibroadenomas and 210 cases of benign dysplasia. *Acta Cytol* 1972;16:130–138.

Zajicek J: *Aspiration Biopsy Cytology. Part I: Cytology of Supradiaphragmatic Organs,* in Wied GL (ed): Monographs in Clinical Cytology. New York, Karger, 1974, vol 4.

Fibrocystic Disease with Cellular Atypia

Frable WJ: *Thin Needle Aspiration Biopsy.* Philadelphia, WB Saunders Co, 1983.

Granular Cell Tumor

Lowhagen T, Rubio CA: The cytology of the granular cell myoblastoma of the breast. *Acta Cytol* 1977;21(2):314–315.

Sussman EB, Hajdu SI, Gray GF: Granular cell myoblastoma of the breast. *Am J Surg* 1973;126:669–670.

Infiltrating Comedocarcinoma

Frable WJ: *Thin Needle Aspiration Biopsy.* Philadelphia, WB Saunders Co, 1983.

Infiltrating Duct Carcinoma

Frable WJ: *Thin Needle Aspiration Biopsy.* Philadelphia, WB Saunders Co, 1983.

Franzen S, Zajicek J: Aspiration biopsy in diagnosis of palpable lesions of the breast. *Acta Radiol* 1968;7:241–262.

Zajicek J: *Aspiration Biopsy Cytology. Part I: Cytology of Supradiaphragmatic Organs,* in Wied GL (ed): Monographs in Clinical Cytology. New York, Karger, 1974, vol 4.

Infiltrating Small-Cell Duct Carcinoma

Frable WJ: *Thin Needle Aspiration Biopsy.* Philadelphia, WB Saunders Co, 1983.

Franzen S, Zajicek J: Aspiration biopsy in diagnosis of palpable lesions of the breast. *Acta Radiol* 1968;7:241–262.

Zajicek J: *Aspiration Biopsy Cytology. Part I: Cytology of Supradiaphragmatic Organs,* in Wied GL (ed): Monographs in Clinical Cytology. New York, Karger, 1974, vol 4.

Inflammatory Carcinoma

Azzopardi JG: *Problems in Breast Pathology.* Philadelphia, WB Saunders Co, 1979.

Frable WJ: *Thin Needle Aspiration Biopsy.* Philadelphia, WB Saunders Co, 1983.

Intracystic Carcinoma

Gatchell FG, Dockerty MB, Clagett OT: Intracystic carcinoma of the breast. *Surg Gynecol Obstet* 1958; 106:347–352.

Squires JE, Betsill WL: Intracystic carcinoma of the breast. *Acta Cytol* 1981;25:267–271.

Intraductal Papilloma

Frable WJ: *Thin Needle Aspiration Biopsy.* Philadelphia, WB Saunders Co, 1983.

Franzen S, Zajicek J: Aspiration biopsy in diagnosis of palpable lesions of the breast. *Acta Radiol* 1968;7:241–262.

Zajicek J: *Aspiration Biopsy Cytology. Part I: Cytology of Supradiaphragmatic Organs,* in Wied GL (ed): Monographs in Clinical Cytology. New York, Karger, 1974, vol 4.

Invasive Lobular Carcinoma

Frable WJ: *Thin Needle Aspiration Biopsy.* Philadelphia, WB Saunders Co, 1983.

Kaminsky DB: *Aspiration Biopsy for the Community Hospital.* New York, Masson Publishing Co, 1981.

Kline TS: *Handbook of Fine Needle Aspiration Biopsy Cytology.* St. Louis, CV Mosby Co, 1981.

Zajicek J: *Aspiration Biopsy Cytology. Part I: Cytology of Supradiaphragmatic Organs,* in Wied GL (ed): Monographs in Clinical Cytology. New York, Karger, 1974, vol 4.

Invasive Lobular Carcinoma with Signet-Ring Pattern

Azzopardi JG: *Problems in Breast Pathology.* Philadelphia, WB Saunders Co, 1979.

Frable WJ: *Thin Needle Aspiration Biopsy.* Philadelphia, WB Saunders Co, 1983.

Steinbrecher JS, Silverberg SG: Signet-ring cell carcinoma of the breast. *Cancer* 1976;37:828–840.

Lactating Adenoma

Azzopardi JG: *Problems in Breast Pathology.* Philadelphia, WB Saunders Co, 1979.

Hertel BF, Zaloudek C, Kompson RI: Breast adenomas. *Cancer* 1976;37:2891–2905.

Male Breast Carcinoma

Azzopardi JG: *Problems in Breast Pathology.* Philadelphia, WB Saunders Co, 1979.

Crichlow RW: Carcinoma of the male breast. *Surg Gynecol Obstet* 1972;134:1011–1019.

Kaminsky DB: *Aspiration Biopsy for the Community Hospital.* New York, Masson Publishing Co, 1981.

Malignant Cystosarcoma Phyllodes

Azzopardi JG: *Problems in Breast Pathology.* Philadelphia, WB Saunders Co, 1979.

Degrell I: Fine-needle biopsy of sarcomas of the breast. *Acta Med Acad Sci Hung* 1980;37(1):73–81.

Lester, J, Stout AP: Cystosarcoma Phyllodes. *Cancer* 1954;7:335–353.

Stawickl ME, Hsiu JG: Malignant cystosarcoma phyllodes report with cytologic presentation. *Acta Cytol* 1979;23:61–64.

Medullary Carcinoma

Azzopardi JG: *Problems in Breast Pathology.* Philadelphia, WB Saunders Co, 1979.

Frable WJ: *Thin Needle Aspiration Biopsy.* Philadelphia, WB Saunders Co, 1983.

Kaminsky DB: *Aspiration Biopsy for the Community Hospital.* New York, Masson Publishing Co, 1981.

Ridolfi RL, Rosen PP, Porta KD, et al: Medullary carcinoma of the breast. A clinicopathologic study with 10 year follow-up. *Cancer* 1977;40:1365–1385.

Metastatic Ovarian Carcinoma

Royen PM, Ziter FMH: Case reports. Ovarian carcinoma metastatic to the breast. *Br J Radiol* 1974;47:356–357.

Metastatic Small-Cell Undifferentiated (Oat Cell) Carcinoma

Azzopardi JG: *Problems in Breast Pathology.* Philadelphia, WB Saunders Co, 1979.

McIntosh IH, Hooper AA, Mills RR, et al: Metastatic carcinoma within the breast. *Clin Oncol* 1976;2:393–401.

Zajdela A, Ghossein NA, Pilleron JP, et al: The value of aspiration cytology in the diagnosis of breast cancer: Experience at the Fondation Curie. *Cancer* 1975; 35(2):499–506.

Osteosarcoma with Intraductal and Infiltrating Duct Carcinoma

Azzopardi JG: *Problems in Breast Pathology.* Philadelphia, WB Saunders Co, 1979.

Benediktsdottir K, Lagerberg F, Lundell L, et al: Osteogenic sarcoma of the breast. Report of a case. *Acta Pathol Microbiol Scand* 1980;88A(3):161–165.

Frable WJ: *Thin Needle Aspiration Biopsy.* Philadelphia, WB Saunders Co, 1983.

Harris M, Persaud V: Carcinosarcoma of the breast. *J Pathol* 1974;112:99–105.

Kaminsky DB: *Aspiration Biopsy for the Community Hospital.* New York, Masson Publishing Co, 1981.

Kennedy T, Bitgart JD: Sarcoma of the breast. *Br J Cancer* 1967;21:635–644.

Mertens HH, Langnickel D, Staedtler F: Primary osteogenic sarcoma of the breast. *Acta Cytol* 1982;26:512–516.

Rottino A, Howley CP: Osteoid sarcoma of the breast: A complication of fibroadenoma. *Arch Pathol* 1945; 40:44–50.

Paget's Disease

Azzopardi JG: *Problems in Breast Pathology.* Philadelphia, WB Saunders Co, 1979.

Eisen MJ, Taft RH: Cytologic diagnosis of mammary cancer associated with incipient Paget's disease of the nipple. *Cancer* 1951;4:150–153.

Zajicek J: *Aspiration Biopsy Cytology. Part I: Cytology of Supradiaphragmatic Organs,* in Wied GL (ed): Monographs in Clinical Cytology. New York, Karger, 1974, vol 4.

Papillary Carcinoma

Azzopardi JG: *Problems in Breast Pathology.* Philadelphia, WB Saunders Co, 1979.

Fisher ER, Gregorio RM, Fisher B: The pathology of invasive breast cancer. *Cancer* 1975;36:1–263.

Kline TS: *Handbook of Fine Needle Aspiration Biopsy Cytology.* St. Louis, CV Mosby Co, 1981.

Signet-Ring Carcinoma

Azzopardi JG: *Problems in Breast Pathology.* Philadelphia, WB Saunders Co, 1979.

Frable WJ: *Thin Needle Aspiration Biopsy.* Philadelphia, WB Saunders Co, 1983.

Hull M, Seo IS, Battersby JS, et al: Signet-ring cell carcinoma of the breast. *Am J Clin Pathol* 1980;73:31–35.

Steinbrecher JS, Silverberg SG: Signet-ring cell carcinoma of the breast. *Cancer* 1976;37:828–840.

Tubular Adenoma

Azzopardi JG: *Problems in Breast Pathology.* Philadelphia, WB Saunders Co, 1979.

Hertel BF, Zaloudek C, Kempson RI: Breast adenomas. *Cancer* 1976; 37:2891–2905.

Tubular-Lobular Carcinoma

Frable WJ: *Thin Needle Aspiration Biopsy.* Philadelphia, WB Saunders Co, 1983.

Kaminsky DB: *Aspiration Biopsy for the Community Hospital.* New York, Masson Publishing Co, 1981.

Kline TS: *Handbook of Fine Needle Aspiration Biopsy* Cytology. St. Louis, Missouri, CV Mosby Co, 1981.

Zajicek J: *Aspiration Biopsy Cytology. Part I: Cytology of Supradiaphragmatic Organs,* in Wied GL (ed): Monographs in Clinical Cytology. New York, Karger, 1974, vol 4.

Well-Differentiated Tubular Carcinoma

Carstens PHB, Huvos AB, Foote FW, et al: Tubular carcinoma of the breast: a clinicopathologic study of 35 cases. *Am J Clin Pathol* 1972;58:231–238.

Frable WJ: *Thin Needle Aspiration Biopsy.* Philadelphia, WB Saunders Co, 1983.

PART THREE

Fine Needle Aspiration of the Lung

5

Technique and Interpretation

Introduction

Needle aspiration of the lung is not a new procedure as it dates back to the nineteenth century. In 1853, Pravaz developed a metallic syringe used originally in the treatment of vascular diseases and subsequently for lung punctures.[1] In 1882, Günther used a Pravaz syringe for a lung puncture to obtain organisms from a patient with pneumonia.[1] Six months later, Leyden used this method to obtain bacteria from a pneumonic lung.[1] In 1884, Krönig was the first to establish the histologic diagnosis of lung cancer by means of a needle aspirate.[2] Two years later Ménétrier diagnosed a lung carcinoma using the lung puncture technique.[3] Towards the end of the nineteenth and first two decades of the twentieth centuries, additional reports documented the diagnostic advantages of lung aspiration.[4–8]

Early reports emphasized the use of pulmonary needle aspiration to obtain organisms from patients with pneumonia.[4–9] Large caliber needles were used with serious complications.[10,11] Subsequently, the use of lung needle aspiration was accepted reluctantly and with skepticism.

In 1930, Martin and Ellis, at the Memorial Hospital for Cancer and Allied Diseases (Memorial Sloan-Kettering Cancer Center) in New York City, reported their findings with needle aspirations from 65 malignant tumors, two from the lung.[12] They used 18-gauge needles and aspirated cellular material rather than a tissue core biopsy specimen, which required diagnosis by cytologic rather than histologic criteria. They are credited with establishing and popularizing the needle aspiration technique. Within the next four years, Martin and Ellis obtained positive diagnoses of cancer by aspiration biopsy[13] in more than 1,400 cases. Forty-one cancers from this series were diagnosed by results obtained by lung aspirations.

By 1937, the experience at Memorial Hospital had expanded to 92 needle aspirations of pulmonary lesions.[14–16] With improved technique and roentgenographic guidance, the percentage of lung tumors correctly diagnosed on the basis of needle aspirations increased from 40% in 1931 to 90% in 1937.[16] Encouraged by the success at Memorial, other physicians began publishing reports of their experiences with lung needle aspirations. Between 1937 and 1948, Gledhill et al[17] and Rosemond et al[18] published their successful series on lung aspirations. It appeared that needle aspiration of the lung was off to a great start, and the future of this technique was most promising.

Ochsner and DeBakey, in 1939, stated that a lung aspiration was a useful procedure and could be "performed with relative safety and with a fair degree of accuracy."[19] Unfortunately, in 1947, they condemned this procedure because three of their patients developed tumor implants at the site of the needle biopsy.[20] Similarly, others strongly denounced needle biopsies of the lung because of the risk of disseminating tumor cells along the needle tract.[21,22] In the United States, this fear of implanting tumor cells resulted in a sharp decline in the use of pulmonary needle biopsies. However, this criticism was proved invalid, as all but one of the cases of tumor implants resulted from the use of large cutting needles (14-gauge) and not the 18-gauge or smaller aspirating needles.[20–27] See chapter 1 for a detailed discussion of the history and development of needle aspiration.

In 1966, Dahlgren and Nordenström's monograph on transthoracic needle biopsy resulted in a resurgence of interest in lung fine needle aspiration (FNA).[28] They summarized their experience with 519 lung aspirations performed during 1963 and 1964 on 365 patients; their diagnostic accuracy was 89%. Factors responsible for their more accurate results were as follows: (1) improved image-intensified fluoroscopic guidance of their fine needle aspirations; and (2) the use of narrow-gauge needles (outside diameter of 0.9 to 1.1 mm).

The merit of lung FNA has since been reported in numerous series.[29–45] The experience reported from many of the early series and more recent, larger series is summarized in Tables 7 and 8. Although a direct comparison of these results would be very useful, the variation in the aspiration techniques used in each study (needle size, patient populations, indications, etc) make such comparisons infeasible.

Indications

On the basis of clinical information and roentgenographic findings, a clinician can form an educated opinion as to the nature of a lung lesion. However, a definitive diagnosis must be established by either tissue section or cytologic evaluation before appropriate therapy can begin. Any patient with a localized pulmonary lesion undiagnosed by conventional methods (eg, sputum cytology, bronchoscopy with washings or brushings, or biopsy) is a candidate for FNA of the lung, provided there are no contraindications.

Suspected Malignant Lesions

In our experience, the most frequent indication for a lung FNA has been in patients who have a solitary lung nodule of undetermined cause in which malignancy is included in the differential diagnosis, and for whom results from routine cytologic evaluation have been nondiagnostic. This is especially true of peripheral lesions in asymptomatic patients in whom a lung mass was detected on routine chest x-ray films. Some patients may be inoperable or refuse surgery, and it is essential to obtain either a cytologic or tissue diagnosis before initiating therapy. We believe that a percutaneous FNA takes precedence over a cutting-needle biopsy or thoracotomy-directed biopsy in this situation, since the morbidity and mortality rates are much lower with FNA.[37,46,47]

The second most frequent indication for a lung aspiration is in patients who have a known extrathoracic primary malignancy and a solitary lung mass detected on chest x-ray film. If results from routine noninvasive procedures are negative, FNA of the mass is indicated. One should *not* assume that the solitary lung mass is a metastasis without further investigation. The possibility of a new primary cancer in the lung or even a benign lung process must be included in the differential diagnosis. Cahan et al discussed the significance of a solitary lung nodule in 54 patients with colon carcinoma.[48] Of these patients, 46% had metastatic disease, but 54% had a new primary lung cancer.

Recently at our institution, a patient with poorly differentiated lymphocytic lymphoma had a solitary lung mass. The differential diagnosis included the following possibilities: an inflammatory process, a lymphoma, or a primary lung carcinoma. The FNA of the mass revealed the last of these—adenocarcinoma of the lung. Moertel and Hagedorn suggested that "any patient with leukemia or lymphoma who presents signs or symptoms of a focal malignant lesion should be regarded as having another primary lesion until proven otherwise on pathologic examination."[49] In particular, primary lung cancer should be included in the differential diagnosis when a pulmonary lesion is observed in patients with lymphoma.[41]

The possibility of a benign inflammatory process must also be considered. Our series included a 34-year-old woman in whom a mass in the right lung developed three months after diagnosis of sarcoma of the arm with axillary node involvement. The FNA of the mass indicated benign granulomatous inflammation with *Histoplasma capsulatum* and not sarcoma. Cahan et al reported results from a series of 465 patients with an extrathoracic malignancy in whom either a synchronous or metachronous solitary lung mass developed. Of these patients, 28% had a solitary metastasis; 70%, a primary bronchogenic carcinoma; and 2%, a benign pulmonary disease.[50]

Occasionally, a patient who has metastases in the lung where the site of the primary malignancy is unknown is a candidate for FNA. Percutaneous aspiration of one of the metastases may help determine the site of the primary malignancy, for example, skin (ie, melanoma) or kidney.

Inflammatory Disease

Lung aspirations have been used primarily to diagnose malignant tumors. However, when conventional methods are inconclusive in the diagnosis of

TABLE 7. Accuracy of Diagnosis Based on Results of Fine Needle Aspiration: Malignant Lung Lesions

Author	Year	Needle Size*	Total Patients	Total FNA Procedures	Histologic Dx: Malignant	FNA Diagnoses: Positive	FNA Diagnoses: False-Negative†	FNA Diagnoses: False-Positive‡
Craver & Binkley[15]	1939	17.0–18.0	92	ND	66	60 (91)	6 (9)	7
Gledhill et al[17]	1949	18.0	56	75	56	44 (79)	12 (21)	0
Rosemond et al[18]	1949	18.0	231	272	163	135 (83)	28 (17)	1
Lauby et al[29]	1965	18.0	520	626	326	235 (72)	91 (28)	0
Dahlgren & Nordenström[28]	1966	0.9–1.1 mm	365	519	156	139 (89)	17 (11)	3
Cardozo et al[42]	1967	1.5 mm	139	ND	139	121 (87)	18 (13)	ND
Dahlgren[97]	1967	0.9–1.1 mm	667	912	217	188 (87)	29 (13)	4
Stevens et al[30]	1968	18.0	100	126	62	52 (84)	10 (16)	2
Fontana et al[31]	1970	18.0	100	ND	83	65 (78)	18 (22)	ND
Sanders et al[43]	1971	19.0–20.0	164	182	77	64 (83)	13 (17)	ND
Dick et al[44]	1974	18.0	223	227	180	138 (77)	42 (23)	ND
Sargent et al[32]	1974	16.0–18.0	350	410	230	190 (83)	40 (17)	ND
Sagel et al[34]	1978	18 0	1,153	ND	896	860 (96)	36 (4)	2
Lalli et al[33]	1978	18.0	1,223	1,296	945	801 (85)	144 (15)	1
Sinner[36]	1979	0.9–1.1 mm	2,726	5,300	2,726	2,472 (91)	254 (9)	127 (2.4)§
Flower & Verney[35]	1979	19.0–20.0 or Rotex	287	300	201	162 (81)	39 (19)	3
Stitik[37]	1979	16.0–18.0	200	226	109	93 (85)	16 (15)	0
Westcott[40]	1980	20.0	422	432	293	284 (97)	9 (3)	4
Poe & Tobin[45]	1980	18.0 or Rotex	95	103	77	69 (90)	8 (10)	1
Berquist et al[38]	1980	18.0	430	ND	420	343 (82)	77 (18)	ND
Jackson et al[39]	1980	20.0 or Nordenström screw	199	299	180	146 (81)	34 (19)	1
Feldman & Covell	1983	22.0 or Rotex	296	307	221	193 (87)	28 (13)	0

NOTE: Numbers in parentheses are percentages of cases in "Histologic Dx: Malignant" column that were also diagnosed using the results of fine needle aspiration.

ABBREVIATIONS: Dx = diagnoses; ND = no data.

*Size of needles used for the fine needle aspiration procedures is given in gauge, unless the unit "mm" appears. The measurements in millimeters indicate the outside diameter of the needle. Rotex screw needle is manufactured by Surgimed, Inc., Summerville, SC.

†"False-Negative" category includes all patients who had lesions that were diagnosed as not malignant, based on results of fine needle aspiration.

‡Cases in "False-Positive" column are not among the cases with malignant histologic diagnoses.

§Percentage of the total number of fine needle needle aspirations.

TABLE 8. Complications of Lung Fine Needle Aspiration

Author	Year	Needle Size*	Total FNA Procedures	Pneumothorax: Total PTX Patients	Pneumothorax: Spontaneously Resolved	Pneumothorax: Required Therapy	Hemoptysis	Hemorrhage	No., Cause of Death
Lauby et al[29]	1965	18.0	626	39 (6)	30 (77)	9 (23)	17 (3)	ND	1, tension PTX
Stevens et al[30]	1968	18.0	126	39 (31)	30 (77)	9 (23)	6 (5)	ND	0
Fontana et al[31]	1970	18.0	100†	57 (57)	40 (70)	17 (30)	6 (6)	ND	0
Sanders et al[43]	1971	19.0–20.0	182	55 (30)	52 (95)	3 (5)	9 (5)	0	0
Sargent et al[32]	1974	16.0–18.0	410	109 (27)	79 (72)	30 (28)	4 (1)	2 (<1)	2, PTX/hemorrhage
Dick et al[44]	1974	18.0	227	43 (19)	32 (74)	11 (26)	7 (3)	1 (<1)	0
Sinner[46]	1976	0.9–1.1 mm	5,300	1,431 (27)	1,317 (92)	114 (8)	371 (7)	583 (11)	0
Lalli et al[33]	1978	18.0	1,223†	296 (24)	247 (83)	54 (18)	22 (2)	0	1, unknown
Sagel et al[34]	1978	18.0	1,153†	292 (25)	125 (43)	167 (57)	73 (6)	48 (4)	0
Flower & Verney[35]	1979	19.0–20.0 or Rotex	300	82 (27)	61 (74)	21 (26)	uncommon	ND	0
Stitik[37]	1979	16.0–18.0	200†	54 (27)	44 (81)	10 (19)	27 (19)	ND	0
Jackson et al[39]	1980	20.0 or Nordenström screw	229	101 (44)	74 (73)	27 (27)	14 (6)	rare	0
Westcott[40]	1980	20.0	432	118 (27)	73 (62)	45 (38)	36 (8)	ND	0
Poe & Tobin[45]	1980	18.0 or Rotex	103	36 (35)	30 (83)	6 (17)	2 (2)	uncommon	0
Berquist et al[38]	1983	18.0	430†	211 (49)	121 (57)	90 (43)	47 (11)	112 (26)	2, pulmonary hemorrhage
Feldman & Covell	1983	22.0 or Rotex	240	90 (38)	47 (52)	43 (48)	14 (6)	8 (3)	0

NOTE: Numbers in parentheses in "Total PTX Patients" and "Hemoptysis" columns are percentages of "Total FNA Procedures." Numbers in parentheses in "Spontaneously Resolved" and "Required Therapy" columns are percentages of "Total PTX Patients."

ABBREVIATIONS: ND = no data; PTX = pneumothorax.

*Size of needles used for the fine needle aspiration procedures is given in gauge,unless the unit "mm" appears. The measurements in millimeters indicate the outside diameter of the needle. Rotex screw needle is manufactured by Surgimed, Inc., Summerville, SC.

†Number of patients, not the number of procedures.

inflammatory disease, FNA can be used by combining bacteriologic and cytologic diagnoses of aspirated material. Jackson et al reported a 75% success rate in identifying microorganisms from lung aspirations in their series of 229 FNAs.[39] Sargent et al were also able to diagnose 39 of 51 inflammatory lesions (76%) by FNA.[32]

In immunocompromised patients, pneumonia caused by opportunistic infection is a major complication; and in these cases, lung FNA has proved to be a rapid, safe, and effective method to identify the specific etiologic agent (for example, *Pneumocystis carinii*). Castellino and Blank reported their 73% success rate (79/108) with pulmonary FNA of immunocompromised patients.[51] Sagel et al obtained a 77% success rate (24/31) in a similar series.[34] In patients with *P carinii,* Castellino observed an 80% diagnostic accuracy on the first FNA and close to 100% if the FNA was repeated after inconclusive results on the first attempt.[52] Chaudhary et al reported their results from FNAs of 202 patients suspected of having pneumocystic pneumonia.[53] This diagnosis was established in 121 patients (60%) by demonstrating *Pneumocystis* organisms in the stained smears of lung aspirations.[53] All of these patients were studied before fluoroscopy was used as a guidance technique for FNA. Since the introduction of fluoroscopically guided FNA, no cases of pneumocystic pneumonia have gone undetected.

Sporadic reports have indicated that preoperative radiation treatment of Pancoast's tumors followed by surgical resection improves survival rates.[37,54] Since there are many malignant and benign neoplasms as well as inflammatory processes that can produce Pancoast's syndrome, it is essential that histologic or cytologic diagnosis is obtained before initiation of radiation therapy.[54] Walls et al achieved excellent results with FNA of Pancoast's tumors, whereas their results from other diagnostic procedures (sputum cytology, bronchoscopy, and lymph node biopsy) were extremely poor.[54] They concluded that the most appropriate method to diagnose these neoplasms was transthoracic FNA. Stitik's experience agreed with that of Walls et al, and he recommended FNA as the first procedure of choice to diagnose Pancoast's tumors.[37]

If conventional diagnostic methods have failed, FNA may be useful even under nonoptimal conditions because it involves less risk than thoracotomy. The benefits versus the potential risks for each patient must be carefully weighed.

Contraindications

Severely debilitated patients are at high risk for complications resulting from FNA. Patients selected for FNA must be alert enough to clear their secretions and blood clots. Meyer et al reported a fatality due to a lung aspiration when the patient had been oversedated and could not clear the airway of blood.[55]

Suspected vascular lesions are not aspirated in our hospital because of the potential for serious bleeding. However, this complication from FNA of the lung may be more theoretical than real. For example, Lalli et al reported "needling (18-gauge) the pulmonary artery and vein many times, the aorta, and an aortic aneurysm with no resulting complications. Experience with translumbar aortograms also indicates that large vessels such as the aorta can be punctured safely with only a rare incidence of hemorrhage."[56] Despite these results, the potential for hemorrhage still exists.

Suspicion of an *Echinococcus* cyst in the lung is an absolute contraindication to FNA because the aspiration may release highly antigenic cystic fluid and result in anaphylaxis. Fortunately, hydatid disease is usually apparent from the clinical picture, radiologic findings, and results of serologic and skin tests. However, in places where the disease is not endemic, physicians may be unfamiliar with its clinical presentation. Stewart aspirated a lung nodule in a patient whose serologic test results for the presence of *Echinococcus granulosus* had been negative.[14] Daughter cysts of *Echinococcus* organisms were aspirated, and the patient had a considerable immediate reaction following the procedure. The diagnosis of echinococcosis can be established from evaluation of sputum, bronchial washings, and pleural fluid cytology.[57,58]

The patient must be cooperative during the FNA. If the patient is uncooperative (eg, will not suspend respiration when indicated), the procedure must be discontinued. Some centers recommend administration of general anesthesia during FNA, but we have not resorted to this procedure.[37] If the patient develops an uncontrollable cough (eg, hemoptysis) during the procedure, the FNA is stopped and rescheduled.

Anticoagulant therapy or hemorrhagic diathesis are contraindications that may be remedied before FNA by cessation of the anticoagulant therapy, infusion of platelets, or other measures.

Advanced emphysema of the lung is a contraindication because of the increased risk of pneumothorax; however, we do not consider emphysema to be an absolute contraindication. With the small (22-gauge) needle used in our hospital, no serious FNA-related complications have occurred in patients with emphysema.

Severe pulmonary hypertension is also a contraindication to FNA because of the increased risk of postbiopsy bleeding. If the pulmonary hypertension is mild to moderate and the lesion is peripheral, then an FNA may be obtained if indicated. A central lesion should not be aspirated if the patient has pulmonary hypertension.[37]

Contralateral pneumonectomy is a significant but not an absolute contraindication.[41] Even a small pneumothorax may give rise to serious consequences. When FNA is attempted in these patients, a means of rapid suction should therefore be readily available.

Lung Fine Needle Aspiration Procedure Used at University of Virginia Medical Center

The general technique used for FNA was described in detail in chapter 2; therefore, this description is limited to the pulmonary FNA procedure followed at the University of Virginia Medical Center.[28,33,34,37,41] It is a modification of the Dahlgren and Nordenström technique.[28]

Equipment and Materials

A complete list of items required for FNA is listed in the "Equipment and Materials" section in chapter 2. The following equipment is additionally needed for the lung FNA procedure used at our institution: biplane or single-plane C-arm fluoroscopic control for guidance of a 3½-in., 6-in., or 8-in., 22-gauge needle or Rotex screw needle (Surgimed Inc, Summerville, SC), see Figure 26.

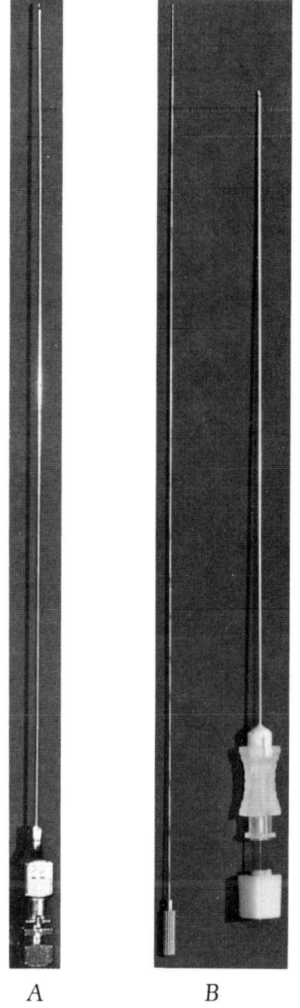

A B

Figure 26. *A:* Six-inch, 22-gauge needle used for lung FNA. *B:* Rotex screw needle used for lung biopsy.

Preaspiration Procedure

For a complete description of the preaspiration procedure, see the "Preaspiration Procedure" section in chapter 2. At the University of Virginia Medical Center, all lung FNAs are now performed by radiologists with special knowledge of thoracic lesions and experience with the FNA technique. The procedure is accomplished on an inpatient basis with careful explanation of the method to the patient. An informed consent for the FNA is obtained prior to the aspiration. Premedication is generally not required, however, if the patient is acutely apprehensive despite reassurance, mild sedation may be employed.

Aspiration

1. Review the chest roentgenogram for the general location of the lesion (Figure 27). Identify the lesion on the fluoroscope and sterilize the area for needle insertion.

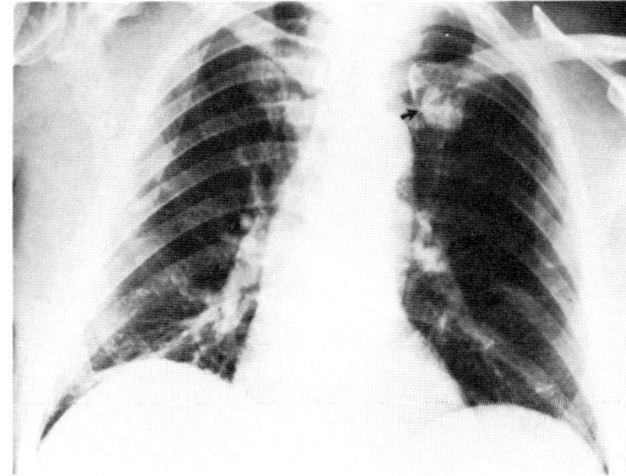

Figure 27. Typical chest roentgenogram.

2. Place the tip of a sterile hemostat or other radiopaque marker on the chest wall directly over the lesion and inject anesthesia (1% lidocaine [Xylocaine]) locally over the chosen entry site (Figure 28). The site chosen should enable the needle to traverse the lower half of the intercostal space and avoid injury to the intercostal vessels.

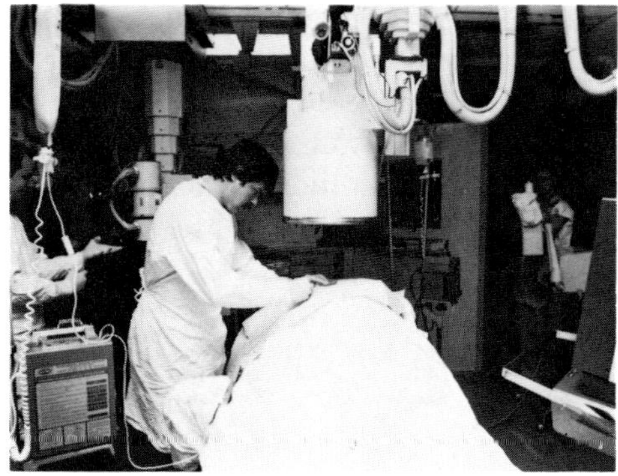

Figure 28. Radiopaque marker is placed on chest wall directly over lesion.

3. Make a small incision in the skin and subcutaneous tissue with a no. 11 scalpel blade (optional). This facilitates free passage of the needle through the skin and enables better appreciation of increased resistance when the needle tip encounters the lung lesion.

4. Insert a 22-gauge needle with the stylet in place through the chest wall (Figure 29). Position the needle exactly perpendicular to the patient. Allow the patient to breathe normally during the introduction of the needle, and instruct the patient to hold his or her breath momentarily while the needle is passed through the pleura.

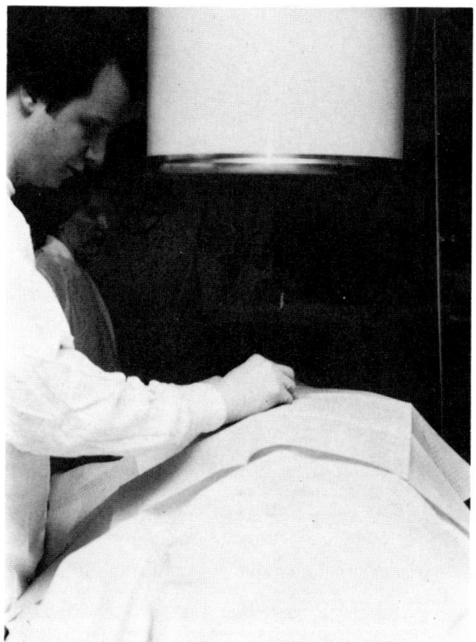

Figure 29. A 22-gauge needle with stylet in place is inserted through chest wall.

5. After the lung has been penetrated by the needle, ask the patient not to take deep breaths. Advance and guide the needle slowly towards the lesion with frequent monitoring under fluoroscopy (Figure 30). It is important to place the fluoroscope so that the needle is in the center of the image to avoid parallax problems.

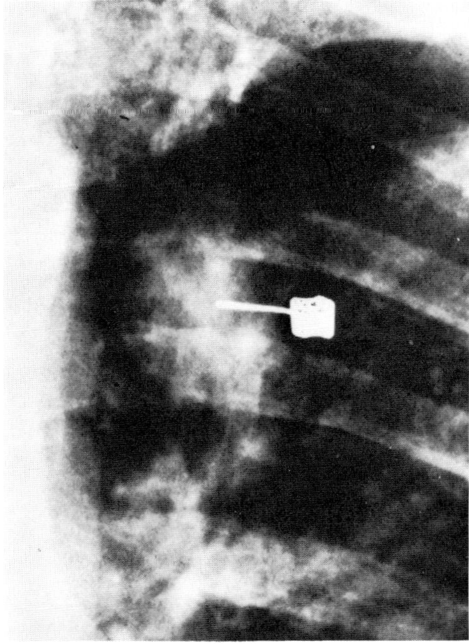

Figure 30. Needle is advanced slowly and guided towards lesion using frequent fluoroscopic monitoring.

6. When the needle tip reaches the lesion, an increased resistance is felt. Ask the patient to suspend respiration momentarily to avoid movement of the lesion while the mass is being penetrated. It is usually possible to feel the needle tip entering the lesion, and most operators feel this is the most useful sign. Verification of accurate needle placement can be documented by lateral fluoroscopy (Figure 31) or by synchronous movement of the needle tip and the lesion during shallow respiration when using either single-plane or biplane fluoroscopy. When the needle has entered the lesion, discontinue fluoroscopy and ask the patient to breath normally.

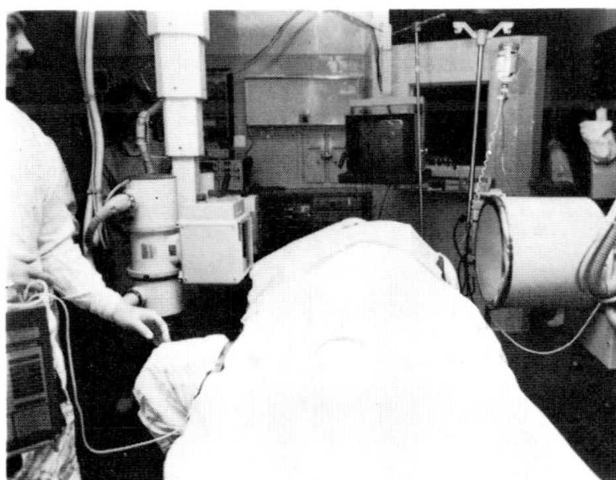

Figure 31. Accurate placement of needle is documented by lateral fluoroscopy.

7. When the tip of the needle is in its optimal position, instruct the patient to hold his or her breath. Remove the stylet from the needle and place the thumb over the open needle hub to avoid air embolism.

8. Attach a 20-mL disposable syringe to the needle. Instruct the patient to breathe normally. Retract the plunger of the syringe to create negative pressure in the syringe and needle lumen (Figure 32).

9. Rotate the needle with attached syringe clockwise and counterclockwise while moving it slightly forward and backward within the lesion (Figure 32).

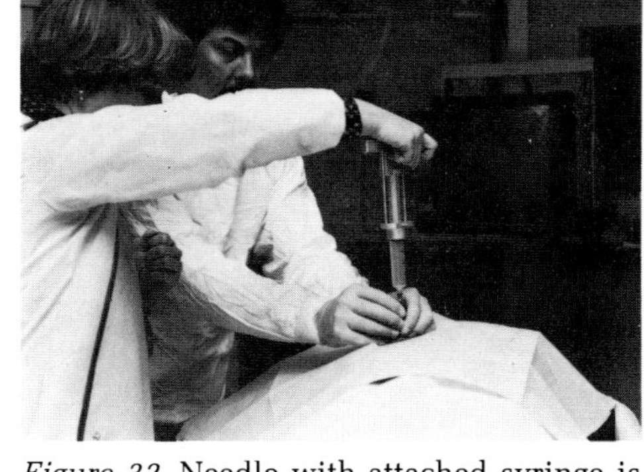

Figure 32. Needle with attached syringe is rotated clockwise and counterclockwise while being moved slightly backward and forward within lesion.

10. Maintain constant negative pressure throughout this manipulation by keeping the plunger of the syringe retracted. Unless negative pressure can be achieved, a successful aspiration is unlikely; therefore, the needle is advanced or retracted until negative pressure is obtained.

11. When the aspiration is completed, allow the pressure in the syringe to return to atmospheric pressure by gently releasing the plunger. Do not release the plunger quickly to prevent aspirated material from being blown out of the needle.

12. Withdraw the needle and syringe as a unit from the lesion and chest wall. Never remove the needle while any negative pressure is applied to the syringe. Such pressure would force aspirated material out of the needle and into the syringe making preparation of smears difficult.

13. *The aspirated material should remain within the needle and not the syringe.* Therefore, if material is seen entering the syringe, discontinue the negative pressure and withdraw the needle. Prepare and stain the smears in the same manner as previously described for palpable masses (chapter 2).

Screw Needle Biopsy

A biopsy done with a screw needle permits the collection of cellular material from the lung mass with minimal dilution of the material by fluid or blood. The apparatus is composed of a 205-mm, stainless steel needle in which the distal 17 mm has been designed in the form of a screw (Figure 33).

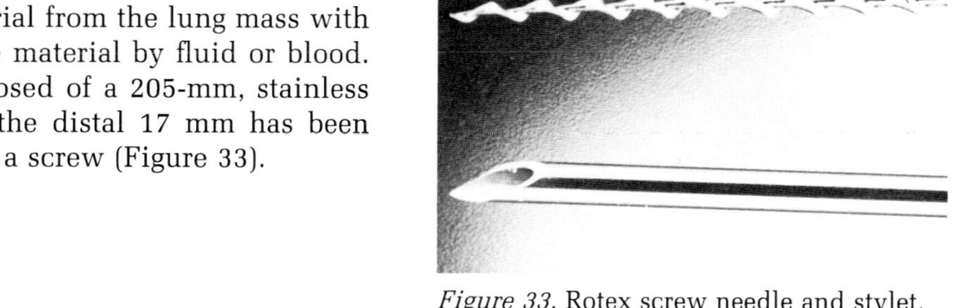

Figure 33. Rotex screw needle and stylet.

1. Under fluoroscopic guidance, place the biopsy needle with a central stylet at the edge of the mass (Figure 34).
2. Substitute the screw for the stylet and advance it beyond the tip of the outer needle (Figure 35). Rotate the screw clockwise into the lesion.
3. Push the biopsy needle downward into the lesion to cover the screw (Figure 36).
4. Withdraw the entire assembly.
5. Push the screw out of the needle and roll the material off the screw onto glass slides.
6. Immediately fix the slides in 95% ethyl alcohol and stain in the routine manner. If the material removed is in the form of a tissue fragment, place it in formalin for embedding and sectioning as a tissue biopsy specimen.

We have had limited experience with this type of needle because it is seldom used at our hospital. Conventional 22-gauge needles generally yield adequate material for diagnosis.

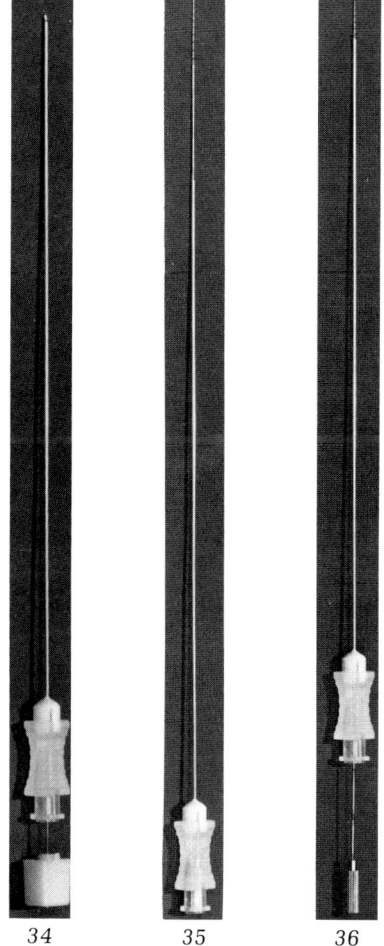

34 35 36

Figure 34. Biopsy needle with central stylet is placed at edge of lung mass.

Figure 35. Screw is substituted for stylet and advanced beyond tip of outer needle.

Figure 36. Needle is pushed downward into lesion to cover screw.

Postaspiration Procedure

An adhesive bandage is placed over the needle site, and fluoroscopy is performed immediately after the procedure to evaluate whether pneumothorax is present. Follow-up chest roentgenograms are obtained to check for the development of pneumothorax. The timing of these films is scheduled on a patient by patient basis, as needed. At the University of Virginia, a film is taken in the late afternoon, usually two to three hours after the procedure. Further films are then taken as indicated.

Complications

Complications of lung FNA include pneumothorax, hemoptysis, empyema, air embolism, hemothorax, subcutaneous or mediastinal emphysema, implantation of tumor cells along the needle tract, hematogenous spread of cancer, and death. Although this list appears ominous, the majority of complications are of no consequence and resolve spontaneously, eg, hemoptysis and pneumothorax. Nevertheless, fatal complications and tumor implants have occurred, but are very rare (Tables 8 and 9).

Pneumothorax

Pneumothorax is by far the most common and most important complication associated with needle aspiration of the lung.[33,37,40,41,46] Factors influencing the incidence of pneumothorax are as follows: the condition of the patient (eg, age, lung emphysema), the technique used, experience of the operator performing the FNA, characteristics of the lung lesion and the extent to which the patients were evaluated after the procedure. The incidence of pneumothorax in reported series ranged from 6% to 57% (see Table 8). The majority of pneumothoraces were small, asymptomatic, and resolved spontaneously; but active treatment by simple aspiration of air using a needle and syringe or intercostal tube was necessary in 5% to 57.0% of the patients (see Table 8).

The health and age of the patients undergoing lung FNA are dissimilar in different series. For example, in the Berquist et al series, the lung FNAs were performed primarily on elderly and inoperable patients.[38] The incidence of pneumothorax in that series was 49% (211 of 430). Similarly, other studies have shown an increased incidence of pneumothorax in elderly patients.[34,37,46] Sinner noted pneumothorax in 16.6% of patients younger than 20 years who had a lung aspiration and in 43.3% of patients older than 70 years.[46] However, Zornoza noted no significant difference in the incidence of pneumothorax with regard to the patient's age.[41] Advanced age itself is not an absolute contraindication to a lung aspiration. Cardiopulmonary function tests should be obtained in borderline cases.[46]

The presence of emphysema in patients having a lung aspiration is strongly correlated with the complication of pneumothorax. Sinner noted a significant difference in the incidence of pneumothorax when lung aspirates were obtained from patients with emphysema: no emphysema, 16.9% pneumothorax; moderate emphysema, 47% pneumothrax; and severe emphysema, 66.6% pneumothorax.[46]

Not only does the risk of pneumothorax increase according to the severity of emphysema, but the necessity for chest tube drainage, sometimes for prolonged periods, is also more frequent. For example, in the Sagel et al series of lung aspirations "five patients with severe bullous emphysema needed sustained drainage for seven to ten days before the leak closed."[34] Because of the potential risk of developing pneumothorax, emphysema is considered one of the relative contraindications to lung aspirations. However, in each patient the advantage of having an established diagnosis has to be weighed against the risk of the procedure.

The depth, size, and diffuse or discrete nature of the lung lesion also influence the incidence of pneumothorax with FNA. Pneumothorax is more frequent with increasing depth of the lesion.[34,37,41,46] For example, in Sinner's series he noted 9.1% pneumothorax with lesions at a depth of 0.1 to 1.9 cm, 35.7% pneumothorax with lesions at 4.0 to 4.9 cm, and 48.4% pneumothorax with lesions at 11.9 cm in depth.[46]

Although Zornoza noted no significant difference in the rate of pneumothorax relative to the size of the lung lesion, others experienced significant differences.[37,41,46] Stitik observed a higher incidence of pneumothorax in patients with smaller lesions.[37] Sinner found the incidence of pneumothorax comparatively low in the groups of patients with lesions having a diameter of 2.6 to 3.5 cm.[46] He felt this was due to the fact that it was easier to obtain cytologic material from these lesions. Like Stitik, he noted a much higher incidence of pneumothorax in patients with lesions less than 2 cm or greater than 3.5 cm.[37,46] Fine needle aspirations of the large lesions may be more difficult because of central necrosis and surrounding inflammation. This necessitates several punctures to obtain representative material, and thereby increases the risk of pneumothorax.

TABLE 9. Fatalities from Transthoracic Needle Biopsies of the Lung

Author	Year	Needle Size*	Total Needle Biopsies	No., Cause of Death
Rosemond et al[18]	1949	18.0†	271	1, PTX;‡ 1, unknown
Woolf[63]	1954	18.0	94	1, unknown (? air embolus)
Smith[73]	1964	14.0§	96	1, pulmonary hemorrhage
Lauby et al[29]	1965	18.0	626	1, tension PTX;‡ 1, unknown cause
Adamson & Bates[74]	1967	14.0§	71	1, pulmonary hemorrhage
Meyer et al[55]	1970	14.0§	1	1, pulmonary hemorrhage and oversedation‡
Jones[67]	1970	14.0§	45	1, PTX
Weg[75]‖	1970	14.0§	ID	1, air embolus; 1, endobronchial hemorrhage; 1, unknown
Youmans et al[75]	1970	14.0§	220	1, endobronchial hemorrhage
Westcott[62]	1973	18.0	1	1, air embolus
Boylen et al[76]	1973	Drill§	75	1, pulmonary hemorrhage
Pearce & Patt[80]	1974	18.0	1	1, pulmonary hemorrhage
McCartney[78]	1974	14.0§ Drill	1 1	1, pulmonary hemorrhage 1, pulmonary hemorrhage
Norenberg et al[79]	1974	14.0§	5	2, endobronchial hemorrhage
Sargent et al[32]	1974	16.0 & 18.0	410	1, PTX and pulmonary hemorrhage (same patient)
Chaudhary et al[53]	1977	20.0	228	1, pulmonary hemorrhage
Lalli et al[33]	1978	18.0	1,296	1, unknown cause
Sinner[36]	1979	0.9–1.1 mm	5,300	0‡,¶
Milner et al[81]	1979	20.0	1	1, hemothorax and intraparenchymal hemorrhage
Berquist et al[38]	1980	18.0	430	2, pulmonary hemorrhages

Abbreviations: ID = insufficient data; PTX = pneumothorax.

*Size of needles used for the fine needle aspiration procedures is given in gauge, unless the unit "mm" appears. The measurements in millimeters indicate the outside diameter of the needle.

†Modified Franzen needle.

‡Potentially preventable deaths.

§Cutting or drill biopsies.

‖This material appeared in Youmans et al.[75]

¶There were no deaths in the series reported by Sinner,[36] but he mentioned a fatality that occurred at another hospital, after the same aspiration biopsy technique was used. The death was caused by unrecognized tension pneumothorax.

Similarly, FNA of small lesions may necessitate several punctures to obtain representative material and thus increase the risk for pneumothorax.[46,59]

No significant differences in the incidence of pneumothorax have been observed with lesions located in different lobes of the lung.[46]

However, the incidence of pneumothorax is greater in patients with diffuse rather than discrete pulmonary lesions. Zornoza noted 35% pneumothorax in patients with diffuse versus 26% in patients with discrete lesions.[41]

The technique used plays a significant role in the incidence of pneumothorax associated with FNA. The experience of the radiologist performing the FNA is directly related to the frequency of pneumothorax. For example, in Sinner's series, if the radiologist had performed less than 20 FNAs, the frequency of pneumothorax was 44.5%; if 21 to 80 FNAs, the frequency of pneumothorax was 20%; and if more than 80 FNAs, the frequency of pneumothorax was 15%.[46] Similarly, Zornoza[41] and Stitik[37] noted an increased frequency of pneumothorax when the FNA was done by a less experienced radiologist.

The size of the needle used for the aspiration is also directly related to the incidence of pneumothorax. Sinner noted that the relative frequency of pneumothorax increased as the outer diameter of the needle increased.[46] For example, there was a 20.6% incidence of pneumothorax with the 0.9-mm (outside diameter) needle and 25% pneumothorax with the 1.4-mm (outside diameter) needle.[46] Not only is the incidence of pneumothorax higher when larger needles are used, but the necessity of chest tube drainage is also increased (see Table 8).[32,33,38,44,46]

The incidence of pneumothorax increases sharply if the needle puncture is repeated. Sinner noted 20% pneumothorax with one puncture (using a 0.9-mm needle), 35.2% pneumothorax with two punctures, and 42.9% pneumothorax with three punctures.[46] Similarly, Zornoza observed a rise in the incidence of pneumothorax in patients if more than one puncture was required: 27% pneumothorax with one puncture, 35% pneumothorax with two punctures, and 45% pneumothorax with three or four punctures.[41]

Hemoptysis

The reported incidence of hemoptysis is variable (1% to 19%). This is not surprising in view of the different size needles used for biopsy. Stitik used a 16- to 18-gauge needle, which obtained a core of tissue for histologic examination and cells for cytologic evaluation with a 17% to 19% incidence of hemoptysis.[37] Sinner[46] and Zornoza[41] used a smaller needle (21- to 22-gauge) with a 2% to 7% incidence of hemoptysis. In general, the large needle is associated with a higher incidence of hemoptysis (see Table 8). In most patients, hemoptysis is mild, self-limited, and does not necessitate treatment by transfusion or surgery.[32–34,37,41]

Empyema

An objection to FNA is that infection will spread as the needle is withdrawn from the lung; however, this complication is rare. No evidence of spread of infection occurred in the Dahlgren and Nordenström series.[28]

Air Embolus

Although air embolus is a well recognized complication of thoracentesis and therapeutic pneumothorax, only one well-documented case of air embolus following needle biopsy of the lung has been reported.[60–62] Westcott described a fatal case of air embolus following needle biopsy of the lung using an 18-gauge needle.[62] Roentgenograms of the skull taken immediately after death showed air in the basilar artery and in branches of the middle cerebral arteries. In addition, roentgenograms of the heart showed numerous air bubbles in the coronary arteries and cardiac chambers. Gross examination of the lung demonstrated a puncture wound 3-cm deep in the superior segment of the lower lobe of the left lung with a communication between the puncture wound, a peripheral bronchus, and a peripheral pulmonary vein.

There are other reported cases with only circumstantial clinical evidence rather than pathologic and radiographic proof of air emboli. Woolf reported a fatality after needle (18-gauge) biopsy of the lung and questioned air embolus as the cause of death.[63] Ten seconds after the biopsy, the patient became unconscious and pulseless. At autopsy no air emboli were found in the cerebral vessels; but the needle had traversed a cavity in the lung with large vessels on its inner surface. Rosemond et al also reported a fatality after needle (18-gauge) biopsy of the lung.[18] In this case, shortly after the biopsy was begun, the patient developed shock and convulsions and then died. The autopsy showed no definite cause of death. However, the brain was not examined and therefore cerebral air embolus could not be ruled out. Blady noted two possible instances of cerebral air emboli during needle (18-gauge) biopsy of lung tumors.[16] Both patients became unconscious and subsequently developed transient partial hemiplegia necessitating brief hospitalization.

Although death from air embolus is uncommon, certain precautions may further reduce its incidence. It is essential to avoid atmosphere-to-pulmonary-vein communication.[62] This can be accomplished by making certain that when the needle is inserted into the lung, the needle is *closed with a stylet,* and that after the needle has reached the target, the stylet is removed and the syringe is connected to the needle *without delay.* The patient should be thoroughly instructed to avoid coughing or straining; and the procedure should be discontinued if coughing persists.[62]

Implants

The danger of implanting tumor cells in the needle tract has fostered considerable controversy about the safety of the continued use of FNA. However, this risk is more theoretical than real. There have only been eight reported cases of implants resulting from needle biopsies of the lung. All the implants, except one, occurred when large-caliber cutting needles (Vim-Silverman or Franklin-Silverman) were used for the needle biopsies.[20,23,24–27]

Sinner and Zajicek reviewed the case histories of 1,264 patients who had a malignant tumor diagnosed by FNA of the lung using 0.9- to 1.1-mm outside diameter needles. They were able to show a tumor implant at the biopsy site in only one of the 1,264 cases.[27] A search of the literature has shown no additional reports of implants from FNA of the lung. Therefore, the risk of implanting tumor cells with this technique is minimal.

Another source of concern to some physicians is the risk of disseminating tumor cells into the pleural cavity as a result of pulmonary FNA. This is an important consideration because the presence of pleural involvement has a direct bearing on the operability and prognosis of lung tumors. The combination of a pulmonary malignancy and a malignant effusion is regarded as evidence of inoperability and incurability. Thus, a needle biopsy would convert an operable and potentially curable lesion into a fatal disease. Fortunately, the risk of pleural dissemination of tumor cells by lung FNA is minimal. Sinner and Zajicek noted an increase in the pleural fluid in only four of the 1,264 patients in whom FNA of the lung was diagnostic of malignancy.[27] Cytologic evaluation of the pleural fluid in these four cases was negative for malignancy and no tumor growth developed during the follow-up period. This suggests that FNA of the lung does not cause tumor cell dissemination into the pleural cavity. A search of the literature reveals no reported cases documenting such a complication.

Berger et al reported two cases in which a hydropneumothorax followed lung biopsies with a 14-gauge needle.[64] Reported results of the cytologic examination showed that the fluid in both cases contained cancer cells. However, Naylor reviewed the cytologic preparations from these cases and disagreed with the cytologic interpretation.[65] He could not confirm the diagnosis of carcinoma in either of these cases. There has been no bonafide documentation of dissemination of tumor cells in the pleural fluid after needle biopsy of the lung.

Subcutaneous implantation of tumor cells has rarely been reported following needle biopsy of parietal pleura; and in all reported cases, a cutting needle (14-gauge) was used.[66–68]

Despite the absence of reported cases of dissemination of tumor cells into the pleural cavity by FNA of the lung, this does not mean that it does not happen. It probably does occur rarely, but apparently the number and viability of tumor cells is insufficient to permit implantation. Spjut et al searched for carcinoma cells in pleural cavity washings obtained during thoracotomy.[69] Cancer cells were identified in the washings from 10 of 17 patients (59%) who had either a pneumonectomy or lobectomy for cancer. The significance of their findings was not apparent when their paper was published, but their findings illustrate the potential danger of cancer implantation in a pleural cavity during thoracic surgery.

Moreover, the presence of malignant cells in the pleural fluid need not necessarily be attributed to a needle biopsy because the appearance of tumor cells in the fluid could arise ab initio from the lung cancer.

Hematogenous spread of cancer with resultant shortening of survival is another conceivable complication of needle aspirations. However, studies on survival rates showed no significant difference between those patients who had FNA before surgery for kidney cancer,[70] breast cancer,[71] and lung cancer[27] and those patients who did not have FNA before surgery for these tumors.

Fatalities

Needle biopsy of the lung is not an innocuous procedure, and review of the literature since 1935 revealed 27 reported deaths due to transthoracic needle biopsies of the lung (Table 9).[72–81] It is important to separate a cutting (14-gauge) needle biopsy that obtains a tissue core for histologic study from an FNA (22-gauge needle) that obtains cellular material for cytologic study. The majority of deaths from lung needle biopsies have resulted from cutting needle biopsies.[73–79] A search of the literature disclosed only one fatality resulting from a fine-gauge needle (0.9 to 1.1 mm, outside diameter) used for a lung aspiration.[35] In Sinner's series of 5,300 FNAs, there were no fatalities. However, he refers to a death in another hospital where the same technique was used.[36] The patient developed an unrecognized tension pneumothorax and died untreated. This was a preventable death. Reported fatalities in studies of transthoracic needle biopsy cases have resulted from pulmonary hemorrhage (fifteen), pneumothorax (five), air embolism (three), hemothorax (one), and unknown causes (four). Undoubtedly, other deaths have occurred but the case reports have not been published.

Any of the previously discussed complications of FNA can result in a fatality; therefore, it is important that complications be recognized and treated without delay. The two complications of lung FNA most frequently reported as the cause of death are pulmonary hemorrhage and pneumothorax.

Pulmonary Hemorrhage

Approximately two months before the introduction of the FNA procedure for evaluation of lung lesions at the University of Virginia Medical Center, a fatality occurred as a result of a biopsy with a large bore (14-gauge) cutting needle.

A 68-year-old man had a right upper lobectomy for a large-cell undifferentiated carcinoma, but the hilum was considered unresectable. He received radiation therapy, postoperatively. He was lost to follow-up, but seven years later he noticed pain along the left sternal border. A chest roentgenogram revealed a mass in the upper lobe of the left lung, approximately 2 × 3 cm, and he was referred to the University of Virginia Medical Center.

The physical examination showed a right thoracotomy scar, and examination of his lung showed decreased breath sounds in the region of the upper lobe of the left lung. Results of sputum cytologic evaluations and bronchoscopy were negative. A needle biopsy (14-gauge) of the lung mass was performed. The biopsy went well, but four hours after the procedure the patient suddenly died. At autopsy there was a left hemothorax (900 mL), and examination of the left lung showed a hemorrhagic area at the biopsy site. On opening the lung, there was a tear in the pulmonary artery (Figure 37) and a 3-cm carcinoma with hemorrhage in the adjacent parenchyma. This region corresponded to the biopsy site. The specimen from the cutting needle biopsy consisted of three cores of lung parenchyma (Figure 38) that contained a moderately well-differentiated squamous cell carcinoma. The cause of death was pulmonary hemorrhage and hemothorax secondary to the needle biopsy.

This case illustrates the major complication that may result from a cutting needle biopsy—pulmonary, endobronchial, or intraparenchymal hemorrhage. Ten of the thirteen reported deaths with a cutting needle or drill biopsy have resulted from pulmonary, endobronchial, or intraparenchymal hemorrhage (see Table 9). This hemorrhage occurs because this type of needle may lacerate a major pulmonary vessel in the process of obtaining a core biopsy, as observed in our case. Similarly, in the fatal cases reported by Adamson and Bates (1 of 71)[74] and Youmans et al (1 of 220),[75] the biopsy specimens contained portions of pulmonary vessels, and the patients died from pulmonary hemorrhage. The incidence of hemoptysis and hemor-

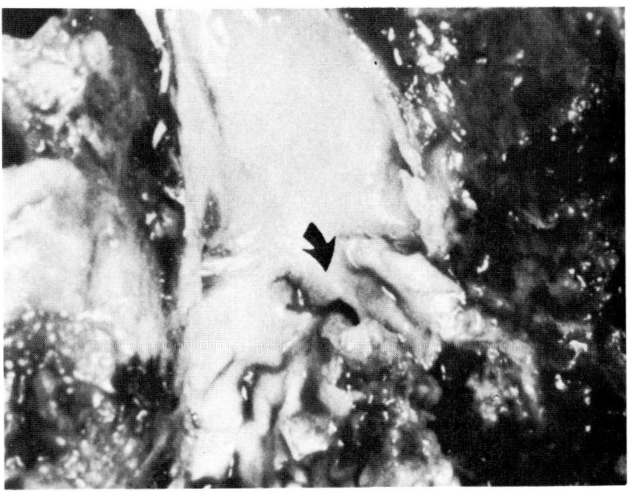

Figure 37. Tear in pulmonary artery with hemorrhage in adjacent parenchyma and carcinoma shown at autopsy (see arrow).

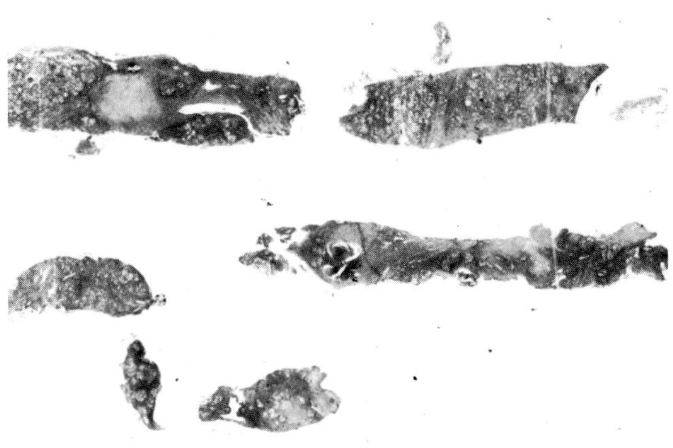

Figure 38. Three cores of lung parenchyma containing squamous carcinoma from cutting needle biopsies.

rhage is much higher with the cutting needle (5% to 30%) than with FNA biopsies (average hemoptysis incidence is 4.8% and pulmonary hemorrhage is uncommon).[46]

Pneumothorax

The second most frequently reported cause of death related to lung needle biopsy is pneumothorax. Three of the five fatal cases indicated in Table 9 had potentially preventable deaths (eg, unrecognized tension pneumothorax and inadequate treatment). It is therefore essential to closely monitor patients after needle sampling of the lung to detect any pneumothorax that may develop several hours after the procedure. It is also helpful to inform patients of the symptoms of pneumothorax so that they can seek treatment if the symptoms should occur. Our experience demonstrates that the majority of the patients who develop pneumothorax show no evidence of pneumothorax on chest roentgenograms immediately following the FNA procedure, but develop changes within 3 to 24 hours. Similarly, Berquist et al noted that most patients in whom pneumothorax developed did not experience pneumothorax immediately; the pneumothorax was detected either 24 hours later on follow-up chest roentgenograms or the day after the procedure because respiratory symptoms were noticed.[38]

Accuracy

A review of the literature shows excellent FNA results for the diagnosis of lung malignancies, with accuracy rates ranging from 72% to 97% (Table 7). Similarly, our experience with lung FNAs done at the University of Virginia Medical Center showed an accuracy rate of 87%. The variations in these percentages may result from differences in technique, size and type of needle, patient population, experience of the radiologist and pathologist, and the other previously discussed factors. These accuracy rates are most impressive considering that conventional cytology (sputum and bronchial cytology) in most of these series was nondiagnostic before FNA.

Dahlgren and Lind compared FNA and sputum cytology diagnoses for benign and malignant lesions and concluded that FNA was more accurate in the diagnosis and typing of both kinds of lesions, regardless of location.[82] They also reported that the accuracy rates for FNA and sputum cytology did not vary with the size of the tumor. Landman et al compared the accuracy of FNA and bronchial washings, and reported that FNA diagnostic accuracy was better for lesions less than 2 cm, lesions not originating in the bronchial epithelium, and peripherally located lesions.[83] Similarly, Francis and Borgeskov noted improved accuracy using FNA results as opposed to fiberoptic bronchoscopy.[84] However, they did find that the rate of diagnostic accuracy for centrally located lesions was similar with either FNA or bronchial brushings. In 1978, Mark et al confirmed results that FNA was an improved method for diagnosing peripherally located lesions.[85] Statistical comparison between FNA and conventional cytologic methods is difficult because FNA is usually performed either in lieu of sputum or bronchial cytology or when these methods have failed to yield a definitive diagnosis.

Typing Tumors by Fine Needle Aspiration

Numerous authors have reported on the accuracy of typing lung tumors by FNA.[82,86–89] These studies demonstrate a wide range in interpretive results for all major categories of lung malignancies with the exception of small-cell undifferentiated carcinoma. Fine needle aspiration showed consistently high diagnostic accuracy for this tumor type (82% to 100%).[82,86–89] Accuracy ranges for the other major lung cancers are as follows: squamous cell carcinoma, 48% to 49%; adenocarcinoma, 47% to 80%; and large-cell undifferentiated carcinoma, 20% to 100%. The variations in these results may be due to several factors, the most significant of which are the quality of the cytologic preparations and the skill and experience of the person evaluating the smears. Similar discrepancies in typing accuracy have also been noted for sputum and bronchial cytology.[82,90–94]

False-Negative Diagnoses

The FNA diagnosis was negative in 3% to 28% of patients with malignancies in the lung (see Table 7). The false-negative rate in our series was 13%. There are several reasons for failure of the FNA. The most frequent reason is the failure to obtain adequate material, and not from incorrect interpretation of the aspirate. Incomplete sampling of the lesion may result from several causes. The most common problem is faulty technique. For example, initially, our lung aspirations were obtained with needle guidance by single-plane fluoroscopy, and frequently the tumor depth was miscalculated. Another problem that resulted from using single-plane fluoroscopy was improper positioning of the needle. Although biplane fluoroscopy is not essential, it enables more accurate guidance of the needle. The greatest single reason for not obtaining sufficient material is the failure to maintain adequate negative pressure during the manipulation of the needle after it is inserted into the tumor.[95]

Often, the tumor is partially necrotic, which causes the aspirate to contain necrotic debris. This is especially true of squamous cell carcinoma. This type of lesion frequently cavitates, and if the needle is inserted into the center of the mass, mainly necrotic material will be obtained. This problem may be resolved by inserting the needle into the periphery of the lesion. At the University of Virginia Medical Center, the patient remains in the fluoroscopy suite until adequate material is obtained. Adequacy is determined by examining material from the FNA with the rapid Papanicolaou stain. If the sample is insufficient, the FNA is repeated. Just as multiple sputum cytology specimens improve the rate of positive diagnoses, so multiple FNAs increase the chance of a correct diagnosis.[32,34]

Another source of false-negative results is the placement of the needle into the inflammatory area distal to a tumor that has obstructed the bronchus. The roentgenogram in such a case gives a false impression of the size of the malignancy.

Difficulties in visualizing a lesion due to its size and location (eg, near the cardiac silhouette) are also contributory factors in a false-negative diagnosis.

The composition of the tumor may also result in a poor sample. Marked cohesion between tumor cells, especially in mesenchymal tumors, may impede adequate penetration with the fine needle.[41] And some lesions may be very firm, defy insertion of the needle, and elude the needle tip.

A negative diagnosis of FNA should *not* be accepted as proof against a malignant lesion or in favor of a benign process. However, Sagel et al reported that in their experience, two negative aspiration biopsies sufficed to exclude cancer with greater than 98% accuracy.[34] This figure corresponds to other recent reports of approximately 95% accuracy in the diagnosis of malignant lesions by aspiration biopsy of the lung.[36]

False-Positive Diagnoses

False-positive diagnoses of malignancy are reported in less than 1% to 4% of cases in most series (see Table 7). There were no false-positive diagnoses made in our series of lung aspirations. One of the most notable diagnostic pitfalls is atypical alveolar lining cells, which may be associated with various benign disease processes. These processes include tuberculosis, fungal infections,[28,30,35,40,46] organizing pneumonia,[40] silicosis,[96] fibrotic lung disease,[33,35,40,46] and pulmonary infarct.[40]

Therapeutic procedures such as radiation and chemotherapy may also elicit cytologic changes that may be confused with malignancy. It is therefore essential for the pathologist to be well acquainted with the clinical history of the patient and to be aware of previous therapy. Close collaboration between the radiologist and pathologist is imperative in decreasing the risk of diagnostic error. To facilitate such teamwork at the University of Virginia, a cytotechnologist always assists the radiologist in the preparation of the cell smears, and the pathologist will usually attend the FNA. Both the pathologist and the radiologist review the rapid Papanicolaou-stained slides to determine the adequacy of the sample and discuss the cytologic interpretation of the aspirated material.

Interpretation of Lung Fine Needle Aspirations

The accuracy of lung FNA depends not only on the quality of the cellular material obtained by the radiologist, but also on the skill of the pathologist in interpreting the FNA sample. Fortunately, pathologists familiar with sputum and bronchial cytology will find that the morphologic criteria used in those methods will apply to FNA smears with equally good results. The cytologic features for diagnosing various lung diseases by respiratory cytology are well documented in the literature and are familiar to most physicians who evaluate cytologic specimens (Table 10). They are described in detail in the illustrated case studies and will not be discussed here. However, there are a few areas of diagnostic difficulty that deserve special emphasis.

Atypical alveolar lining cells are perhaps the most common source of false-positive diagnoses. These cells may be associated with many benign lung diseases and may show significant nuclear atypia that mimic carcinoma (lung Color Plates 28 and 29). Another difficulty is that alveolar cells tend to be scant in sputum and bronchial cytologic specimens but may be abundant in FNA, giving a low-power impression of malignancy. Differential diagnosis from bronchioloalveolar carcinoma is possible, however, upon careful examination of the cellular material and adequate clinical information. The benign alveolar cells tend to show distinct cell

TABLE 10. Cytologic Features of Primary Lung Carcinomas

Feature	Carcinoma Type				
	Squamous Cell (Well-Differentiated)	Squamous Cell (Poorly Differentiated)	Adenocarcinoma	Large-Cell (Undifferentiated)	Small-Cell (Undifferentiated)
Slide Background	Often contains necrotic debris	Necrotic debris frequent	Clean or tumor diathesis	Frequently contains necrotic debris	Necrotic debris
Cellular Arrangement	Usually single cells; occasional aggregates and sheets	Single cells and syncytial arrangements	Single cells, clusters, balls, acinar groupings; nuclear molding within groups	Single cells and syncytial arrangements	Single cells and syncytial groupings with nuclear molding
Cytoplasm	Strikingly pleomorphic; orangophilic, acidophilic, basophilic staining; moderate or scant	Dense granular appearance; basophilic staining; moderate or scant amount; indistinct cell borders	Basophilic staining; usually vacuolated (lacy appearance to large, distended vacuoles); moderate or scant; some cylindrically shaped cells	Basophilic staining; dense; granular; moderate or scant; may show some vacuolization	Basophilic staining; very scant; indistinct cell borders
Nuclear Configuration	Irregular shapes; size variation	Round, oval, irregular shapes; size variation	Round or oval shape with occasional nuclear membrane irregularities; size variation	Round or oval shape with occasional nuclear membrane irregularities; size variation	Round, oval, irregular shapes; size variation, some molding
Nuclear:Cytoplasmic Ratio	Moderately increased	Increased	Increased	Increased	Very high
Chromatin Pattern	Coarsely granular; irregularly distributed; hyperchromatic, opaque forms frequent	Finely granular; irregularly distributed; hyperchromatic	Finely granular; irregularly distributed	Finely granular; irregularly distributed	Granular, irregularly distributed with clumping and parachromatin clearing
Nucleolus	Usually not evident	Large, single, round to irregular shapes	Prominent, present in almost every cell; may be multiple, irregularly shaped	Large, present in almost every cell; may be multiple; may be irregular	Small but visible

borders and well-organized cell groups. Their nuclear outlines are smooth and even. The chromatin pattern is finely granular and evenly distributed despite the prominent, sometimes multiple nucleoli. Another helpful hint is the presence of a spectrum of cell changes from obviously benign alveolar cells to the more pleomorphic forms. The absence of two distinct populations, one benign and one malignant, aids in the recognition of benign disease.

The diagnosis of malignancy is usually a fairly clear-cut interpretation in lung FNA; however, typing the lesions may be difficult. Poorly differentiated squamous carcinoma, poorly differentiated adenocarcinoma, and large-cell undifferentiated carcinoma may present a similar cytologic picture. In these cases, the FNA report generally reads "poorly differentiated carcinoma, not small-cell type." No further typing is made. In those patients having a previous malignant diagnosis, the FNA smears can be compared with the primary lesion for typing.

The differential diagnoses among the small-cell tumors may also cause some interpretation problems. Oat cell carcinomas tend to yield cells in FNA smears that are twice as large as those seen in sputum and bronchial washings. The cell pattern more closely resembles that seen in bronchial brushings. This difference is probably an artifact of sampling method (ie, direct sampling versus natural exfoliation). The malignant cells, however, retain the characteristic features of prominent nuclear molding, granular chromatin, and scant cytoplasm. In contrast, carcinoid tumors shed a more uniform cell population with finely granular chromatin and nuclear overlapping rather than molding.

Lymphomas and leukemias are frequently recognized in cytologic specimens by the preponderance of individual cells and the absence of cell groups and sheets. We have seen several cases in which the FNA smears from lymphoma or leukemia have contained cell aggregates or groups similar to the epithelial fragments of carcinoma, especially at low-power magnification. Examination of these groups at high power shows that the cells lack the granular, dense cytoplasm or the vacuolization characteristic of carcinomas. This cytoplasm tends to be scant and indistinct. The nuclei within these aggregates may occasionally show flattened, opposing nuclear surfaces that mimic the molding of oat cell carcinoma. However, this finding is usually widespread and lacks the sharp definition seen in the oat cell pattern.

Normal Cytology

The normal cytology seen in lung FNAs is identical to that described in detail in the literature for sputum and bronchial cytology. For this reason, these cells will not be discussed here. Normal respiratory cells are seen in Color Plates 30 and 36, and pulmonary macrophages are noted in the background of Color Plate 33. Normal alveolar lining cells (pneumocytes) are found admixed with atypical forms in Color Plate 28. Mesothelial cells, which are not seen in sputum or bronchial cytologic specimens, may be identified in lung aspirates. These cells are described more fully in Color Plate 28.

Summary

Fine needle aspiration of the lung is a diagnostic tool complementary to the conventional methods of sputum and bronchial cytology. Cytologic evaluation of sputum samples is a screening procedure particularly useful for small lesions not visible on chest roentgenograms, whereas cytologic evaluation of bronchoscopy samples is the method of choice for centrally located lesions of the tracheobronchial tree. The FNA enables the radiologist to sample small, radiographically demonstrated lesions and more peripheral lesions not accessible by bronchoscopy. It is also effective for lung lesions in which sputum and bronchial cytology have failed to yield a diagnosis. Together, these three diagnostic techniques provide clinicians with effective and highly accurate methods for the detection and evaluation of lung masses without the risks and complications of thoracotomy.

References

1. Leyden H: Uber infectiose pneumonie. *Deutsch Med Wochnschr* 1883;9:52–54.

2. Krönig G: Diagnostischer Beitrag Zur Herz-und Lungen pathologie *Berl Klin Wochnschr* 1887;24(51):961–967.

3. Ménétrier P: Cancer primitif du Poumon. *Bull Soc Anat Paris* 1886;4:643.

4. Russell AE: Lung puncture. *Lancet* 1909;2:1539–1540.

5. Netter A: L' épidémie d'influenza de 1918. *Bull Acad Med* 1918;80:275–286.

6. Lyon AB: Bacteriologic studies of 165 cases of pneumonia and postpneumonic empyema in infants and children. *Am J Dis Child* 1922;23:72–87.

7. Stewart D: Lung puncture in acute lobar pneumonia. *Lancet* 1930;2:520–521.

8. Ellison JB: Pneumonia in measles. *Arch Dis Child* 1931;6:37–52.

9. Sappington SW, Favorite GO: Lung puncture in lobar pneumonia. *Am J Med Sci* 1936;191:225–234.

10. Waldvogel H: Zwischenfalle bei der Thorakozentose, speziell uber das Wesen der albuminosen Expektoration. *Deutsch Arch Klin Med* 1907;89:322–341.

11. Stahelin F: Uber todliche Blutungen bei Probepunktionen der Lunge. *Berl Klin Wochnschr* 1919;56:562–564.

12. Martin HE, Ellis EB: Biopsy by needle puncture and aspiration. *Ann Surg* 1930;92:169–181.

13. Martin HE, Ellis EB: Aspiration biopsy. *Surg Gynecol Obstet* 1934;59:578–589.

14. Stewart FW: The diagnosis of tumors by aspiration. *Am J Pathol* 1933;9:801–812.

15. Craver LF, Binkley JS: Aspiration biopsy of tumors of the lung. *J Thorac Cardiovasc Surg* 1939;8:436–463.

16. Blady JV: Aspiration biopsy of tumors in obscure or different locations under roentgenoscopic guidance. *Am J Roentgenol Rad Ther* 1939;42:515–524.

17. Gledhill EY, Spriggs JB, Binford CH: Needle aspiration in the diagnosis of lung carcinoma: Report of experience with 75 aspirations. *Am J Clin Pathol* 1949;19:235–242.

18. Rosemond BP, Burnett WE, Hall JH: Value and limitations of aspiration biopsy of lung lesions. *Radiology* 1949;52:506–510.

19. Ochsner A, DeBakey M: Primary pulmonary malignancy: Treatment by total pneumonectomy. *Surg Gynecol Obstet* 1939;58:435–451.

20. Ochsner A, De Bakey M, Dixon JL: Primary cancer of the lung. *JAMA* 1947;135:321–327.

21. Overholt RH: Curability of primary carcinoma of the lung. Early recognition and management. *Surg Gynecol Obstet* 1940;70:479–490.

22. Storey CF, Reynolds BM: Biopsy techniques in the diagnosis of intrathoracic lesions. *Dis Chest* 1953;23:357–382.

23. Allbritten FF Jr, Neadon T, Gibbon JH Jr, et al: The diagnosis of lung cancer. *Surg Clin North Am* 1952;32:1657.

24. Dutra FR, Geraci C: Needle biopsy of the lung. *JAMA* 1954;155:21–24.

25. Meakins JF, Groszman M: Needle biopsy as an aid to the precise diagnosis of intrathoracic disease. *Can Med Assoc J* 1963;88:120–127.

26. Wolinsky H, Lischner MW: Needle track implantation of tumor after percutaneous lung biopsy. *Ann Intern Med* 1969;71(2):359–362.

27. Sinner WN, Zajicek J: Implantation metastasis after percutaneous transthoracic needle aspiration biopsy. *Acta Radiol Diagn* 1976;17:473–480.

28. Dahlgren S, Nordenström B: *Transthoracic Needle Biopsy.* Chicago, Yearbook Medical Publishers, Inc, 1966.

29. Lauby VW, Burnett WE, Rosemond GP, et al: Value and risk of biopsy of pulmonary lesions by needle aspiration: Twenty-one years' experience. *J Thorac Cardiovas Surg* 1965;49:159–172.

30. Stevens GM, Weigen JF, Lillington GA: Needle aspiration biopsy of localized pulmonary lesions with amplified fluoroscopic guidance. *Am J Roentgenol Rad Ther Nucl Med* 1968;103:561–571.

31. Fontana RS, Miller WE, Beabout JW, et al: Transthoracic needle aspiration of discrete pulmonary lesions: experience in 100 cases. *Med Clin North Am* 1970;54:961–971.

32. Sargent EN, Turner AF, Gordonson J, et al: Percutaneous pulmonary needle biopsy report of 350 patients. *Am J Roentgenol Rad Ther Nucl Med* 1974;122:758–758.

33. Lalli AF, McCormack LJ, Zelch M, et al: Aspiration biopsies of chest lesions. *Radiology* 1978;127:35–40.

34. Sagel SS, Ferguson TB, Forrest JV, et al: Percutaneous transthoracic aspiration needle biopsy. *Ann Thorac Surg* 1978;26:399–405.

35. Flower CDR, Verney GI: Percutaneous needle biopsy of thoracic lesions—an evaluation of 300 biopsies. *Clin Radiol* 1979;30:215–218.

36. Sinner WN: Pulmonary neoplasms diagnosed with transthoracic needle biopsy. *Cancer* 1979;43:1533–1540.

37. Stitik F: Percutaneous lung biopsy, in Siegelman SS, et al (eds): *Pulmonary System.* New York, Grune & Stratton, 1979, vol I: *Multiple Imaging Procedures,* pp 181–219.

38. Berquist TH, Bailey PB, Cortese DA, et al: Transthoracic needle biopsy. Accuracy and complications in relation to location and type of lesion. *Mayo Clin Proc* 1980;55:475–481.

39. Jackson R, Coffin L, DeMeules J, et al: Percutaneous needle biopsy of pulmonary lesions. *Am J Surg* 1980;139:586–590.

40. Westcott JL: Direct percutaneous needle aspiration of localized pulmonary lesions: Results in 422 patients. *Radiology* 1980;137:31–35.

41. Zornoza J (ed): *Percutaneous Needle Biopsy.* Baltimore, Williams & Wilkins Co, 1981.

42. Cardozo L, DeGraaf SP, DeBoer MJ, et al: The results of cytology in 1,000 patients with pulmonary malignancy. *Acta Cytol* 1967;11:120–130.

43. Sanders DE, Thompson DW, Pudden BJE: Percutaneous aspiration lung biopsy. *Can Med Assoc J* 1971;104:139–142.

44. Dick R, Heard BE, Hinson KFW, et al: Aspiration needle biopsy of thoracic lesions: An assessment of 227 biopsies. *Br J Dis Chest* 1974;68:86–94.

45. Poe RH, Tobin RE: Sensitivity and specificity of needle biopsy in lung malignancy. *Am Rev Resp Dis* 1980;122:725–729.

46. Sinner WN: Complications of percutaneous transthoracic needle aspiration biopsy. *Acta Radiol Diagn* 1976;17:813–828.

47. Weiss W: Operative mortality and five-year survival rates in men with bronchogenic carcinoma. *Chest* 1974;66:483–487.

48. Cahan WG, Castro EB, Hajdu SI: The significance of a solitary lung shadow in patients with colon carcinoma. *Cancer* 1974;33:414–421.

49. Moertel CG, Hagedorn AB: Leukemia or lymphoma and coexistent primary malignant lesions—A review of the literature and a study of 120 cases. *Blood* 1957;12:788–803.

50. Cahan WG, Shah J: Benign solitary lung lesions found with an extrathoracic cancer: A report of 12 cases. *Chest* 1972;62:360.

51. Castellino RA, Blank N: Etiologic diagnosis of focal pulmonary infection in immunocompromised patients by fluoroscopically guided percutaneous needle aspiration. *Radiology* 1979;132:563–567.

52. Castellino RA: Percutaneous pulmonary needle diagnosis of pneumocystic carinii pneumonitis. *Nat Cancer Inst Monogr* 1976;43:137–140.

53. Chaudhary S, Hughes WT, Feldman S, et al: Percutaneous transthoracic needle aspiration of the lung. *Am J Dis Child* 1977;131:902–907.

54. Walls WJ, Thornbury JR, Naylor B: Pulmonary needle aspiration biopsy in the diagnosis of pancoast tumors. *Radiology* 1974;111:99–102.

55. Meyer JE, Ferrucci JT Jr, Janower ML: Fatal complications of percutaneous lung biopsy. *Radiology* 1970;96:47–48.

56. Lalli AF: Roentgen-guided aspiration biopsies of thoracic, renal and skeletal lesions, in Meaney T, Lalli AF, Altidi RJ (eds): *Complications and Legal Implications of Radiologic Special Procedures.* St. Louis, CV Mosby Co, 1973; chapter 8, pp 83–91.

57. Allen AR, Fullmer CD: Primary diagnosis of pulmonary echinococcosis by the cytologic technique. *Acta Cytol* 1972;16:212–216.

58. Jacobson ES: A case of secondary echinococcosis diagnosed by cytologic examination of pleural fluid and needle biopsy of pleura. *Acta Cytol* 1973;17:76–79.

59. Sinner WN: Transthoracic needle biopsy of small peripheral malignant lung lesions. *Invest Radiol* 1973;8:305–314.

60. Chattenberg HJ, Ziskind J: Air embolism as a complication of artificial pneumothorax. *Am J Clin Pathol* 1939;9:477–482.

61. Taylor JD: Postmortem diagnosis of air embolism by radiography. *Br Med J* 1952;1:890–892.

62. Westcott JL: Air embolism complicating percutaneous needle biopsy of the lung. *Chest* 1973;63:108–110.

63. Woolf CR: Applications of aspiration lung biopsy with a review of the literature. *Dis Chest* 1954;25:286–301.

64. Berger RL, Dargan EL, Huang BL: Dissemination of cancer cells by needle biopsy of the lung. *J Thorac Cardiovasc Surg* 1972;63:430–432.

65. Naylor B: Dissemination of cancer cells after needle biopsy of lung. *J Thorac Cardiovasc Surg* 1972;64:324.

66. Mestitz P, Purves MJ, Pollard AC: Pleural biopsy in the diagnosis of pleural effusion: A report of 200 cases. *Lancet* 1958;275:1349–1353.

67. Jones FL, Jr: Subcutaneous implantation of cancer: A rare complication of pleural biopsy. *Chest* 1970;57:189–190.

68. Schachter EN, Basta W: Subcutaneous metastasis of an adenocarcinoma following a percutaneous pleural biopsy. *Am Rev Resp Dis* 1973;107:283–285.

69. Spjut HJ, Hendrix VJ, Ramirez GA, et al: Carcinoma cells in pleural cavity washings. *Cancer* 1958;11:1222–1225.

70. Von Schreeb T, Arner O, Skousted G, et al: Renal adenocarcinoma. Is there a risk of spreading tumor cells in diagnostic puncture? *Scand J Urol Nephrol* 1967;1:270–276.

71. Berg JW, Robbins G: A late look at the safety of aspiration biopsy. *Cancer* 1962;15:826–827.

72. Smith WG: Needle biopsy of the lung. *Thorax* 1964;19:68–78.

73. Smith WB: Needle biopsy of lung. *Lancet* 1964;2:318.

74. Adamson JS, Jr, Bates JH: Percutaneous needle biopsy of the lung. *Arch Intern Med* 1967;119:164–169.

75. Youmans CR, Jr, DeGroot WJ, Marshall R, et al.: Needle biopsy of the lung in diffuse parenchymal disease: An analysis of 151 cases. *Am J Surg* 1970;120:637–643.

76. Boylen CT, Johnson NR, Richters V, et al: High speed trephine lung biopsy: Method and results. *Chest* 1973;63:59–62.

77. Jones FL Jr: A comparison of trephine and Franklin-Silverman needles for percutaneous lung biopsy. *Am Rev Resp Dis* 1974;109:625–629.

78. McCartney R: Hemorrhage following percutaneous lung biopsy. *Radiology* 1974;112:305–307.

79. Norenberg R, Claxton CP, Takaro T: Percutaneous needle biopsy of the lung: report of two fatal complications. *Chest* 1974;66:216–218.

80. Pearce JG, Patt NL: Fatal pulmonary hemorrhage after percutaneous aspiration lung biopsy. *Am Rev Resp Dis* 1974;110:346–349.

81. Milner LD, Ryan K, Gullo J: Fatal intrathoracic hemorrhage after percutaneous aspiration lung biopsy. *Am J Radiol* 1979;132:280–281.

82. Dahlgren SE, Lind B: Comparison between diagnostic results obtained by transthoracic needle biopsy and by sputum cytology. *Acta Cytol* 1972;16:53–58.

83. Landman S, Burgener FA, Kim GHK: Comparison of bronchial brushing and percutaneous needle aspiration biopsy in the diagnosis of malignant lung lesions. *Radiology* 1975;115:275–278.

84. Francis D, Borgeskov S: Progress in preoperative diagnosis of pulmonary lesions. *Acta Cytol* 1975; 19(3):231–234.

85. Mark JBD, Marglin SI, Castellino RA: The role of

bronchoscopy and needle aspiration in the diagnosis of peripheral lung masses. *J Thorac Cardiovasc Surg* 1978;76:266–268.

86. Nasiell M: Diagnosis of lung cancer by aspiration biopsy and a comparison between this method and exfoliative cytology. *Acta Cytol* 1967;11:114–119.

87. Hastrup J: Cytologic-histologic correlation in the diagnosis of carcinoma of the lung. Presented at Third International Congress of Cytology, Rio de Janiero, Brazil, 1968.

88. Francis D: Transthoracic aspiration biopsy. Cytological classification of aspirated malignant tumour cells. *Acta Pathol Microbiol Immunol Scand* 1977;85:535–538.

89. Taft PD, Szyfelbein W, Greene R: A study of variability in cytologic diagnoses based on pulmonary aspiration specimens. *Am J Clin Pathol* 1980;73:36–40.

90. Suprun H, Pedio G, Ruttner JR: The diagnostic reliability of cytologic typing in primary lung cancer with a review of the literature. *Acta Cytol* 1980;24:494–500.

91. Lange E, Heg K: Cytologic typing of lung cancer. *Acta Cytol* 1972;16:327–330.

92. Kanhouwa SB, Matthews MJ: Reliability of cytologic typing of lung cancer. *Acta Cytol* 1976;20:229–232.

93. Foot NC: The identification of types of pulmonary cancer in cytologic smears. *Am J Path* 1952;28:963–977.

94. Kirsch MM, Orvald T, Naylor B, et al: Diagnostic accuracy of exfoliative pulmonary cytology. *Ann Thorac Surg* 1970;9:335–358.

95. Dahlgren SE: Aspiration biopsy of intrathoracic tumours. *Acta Pathol Microbiol Immunol Scand* 1967;70:566–576.

96. Grunze H: Cytologic diagnosis of tumors of the chest. *Acta Cytol* 1973;17:148–159.

97. Dahlgren SE: Aspiration biopsy of intrathoracic tumours. *Acta Pathol Microbiol Immunol Scand* 1967;70:566–576.

6

Illustrated Case Studies of Lung Diseases

PLATE 27

Lipid Pneumonia

Note. Most of the patients whose conditions are described in chapter 6 were seen at the University of Virginia Medical Center.

Clinical History. A 60-year-old male smoker was in his usual state of good health until four days before admission to another hospital, when he noted the spontaneous onset of sharp, severe constant pain in the left shoulder and left side of the chest. A chest roentgenogram showed a lesion in the left lung that was suspected of being malignant (Figure A). The patient was unaware of other symptoms except for chronic dyspnea on exertion without any recent change. He was referred to the University of Virginia Medical Center for further evaluation.

Auscultation and palpation of his chest revealed that the lung was clear, and the remainder of his examination results, within normal limits. Results from the patient's pulmonary function tests were very poor. His blood gases in room air showed a Po_2 of 59 mm Hg, pco_2 of 50 mm Hg, and pH 7.4. A percutaneous FNA of his lung lesion was performed under fluoroscopic guidance.

Cytologic Findings. The FNA smears contained inflammatory cells and numerous macrophages with abundant, vacuolated basophilic cytoplasm and vesicular nuclei (Plate 27–1). When stained with the Sudan IV stain, these macrophages were positive for lipid material (Plate 27–2). A diagnosis of lipid pneumonia was made.

Pathologic Findings. Because the FNA indicated benign disease, an open lung biopsy was performed to confirm the absence of malignancy. Microscopic sections confirmed the presence of lipid pneumonia with no evidence of malignancy (Plate 27–3, 27–4).

Refer to Slide 51 in Optional Slide Set.

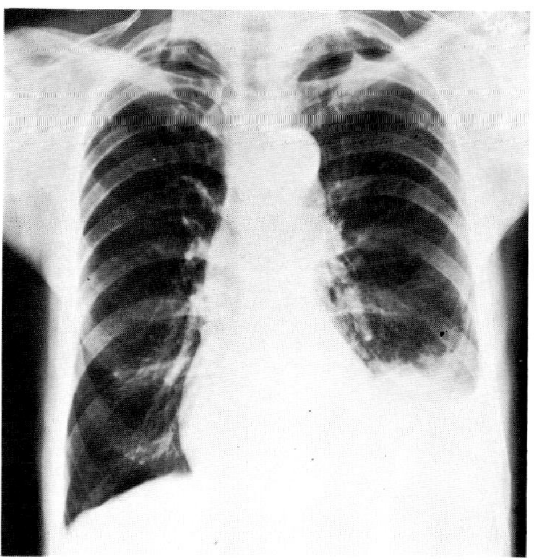

Figure A. Chest roentgenogram showing infiltrate in lower lobe of left lung.

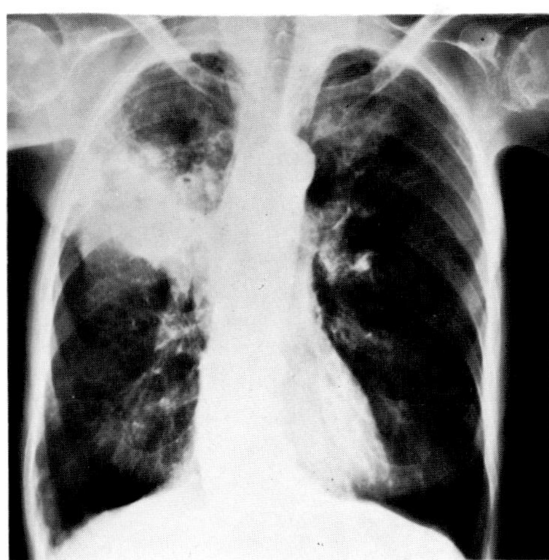

Figure B. Chest roentgenogram showing infiltrate in upper lobe of right lung and right hilar mass.

PLATE 27

Aspiration Pneumonia (Phytopneumonitis)

Clinical History. A generally healthy 80-year-old female nonsmoker with a ten-year history of chronic bronchitis first noticed exacerbation of her mild chronic cough with production of white, nonfoul smelling sputum three months before admission to the University of Virginia Medical Center. The sputum production was accompanied by chest pain. The patient also noticed a low-grade fever but was unaware of other symptoms.

A chest roentgenogram revealed upper lobe pneumonia and a hilar mass in the right lung (Figure B). Subsequent tomograms showed a 5 × 5.5-cm mass felt to be carcinoma with postobstructive pneumonia beyond it. Findings from sputum cytologic evaluations were negative. Bronchoscopy was performed, but the brushings and washings showed no evidence of malignancy. A transbronchial biopsy specimen contained chronic inflammation but no evidence of tumor. The sputum culture grew mixed oropharyngeal flora with *Pseudomonas* species, *Streptococcus* species, and *Staphylococcus aureus.* Results of fungal serologic evaluations were all negative. The patient underwent FNA of the right hilar mass.

Cytologic Findings. The aspirate consisted of an inflammatory exudate with numerous histiocytes, plasma cells, and angular structures with thick, refractile, green-staining cell walls (Plate 27–5 to 27–7). The cytoplasm of the structures contained numerous dark-blue-staining bodies about 5 to 7 μm in diameter, which were probably some kind of storage vacuole. The structures were often surrounded by active histiocytes with mildly atypical nuclei (Plate 27–6). The foreign material was felt to be of vegetable origin, and a diagnosis of aspiration pneumonia (phytopneumonitis) was made. It was suggested that the right hilar enlargement seen on the chest roentgenogram was a hyperplastic lymph node in reaction to the inflammatory process in the right lung.

Pathologic Findings. The patient underwent an upper gastrointestinal (GI) series, and she was found to have esophageal dismotility with some degree of esophageal reflux of gastric contents. Her previous transbronchial biopsy specimen was reviewed and recuts were made. One slide showed refractile, nonstaining structures within the lung tissue that closely resembled those seen in the aspiration smears (Plate 27–8). Chronic inflammation was also noted (Plate 27–9, 27–10). The patient was treated with antibiotics and instructed to elevate the head of her bed at night. Within four months, her chest roentgenograms were clear.

Refer to Slide 52 in Optional Slide Set.

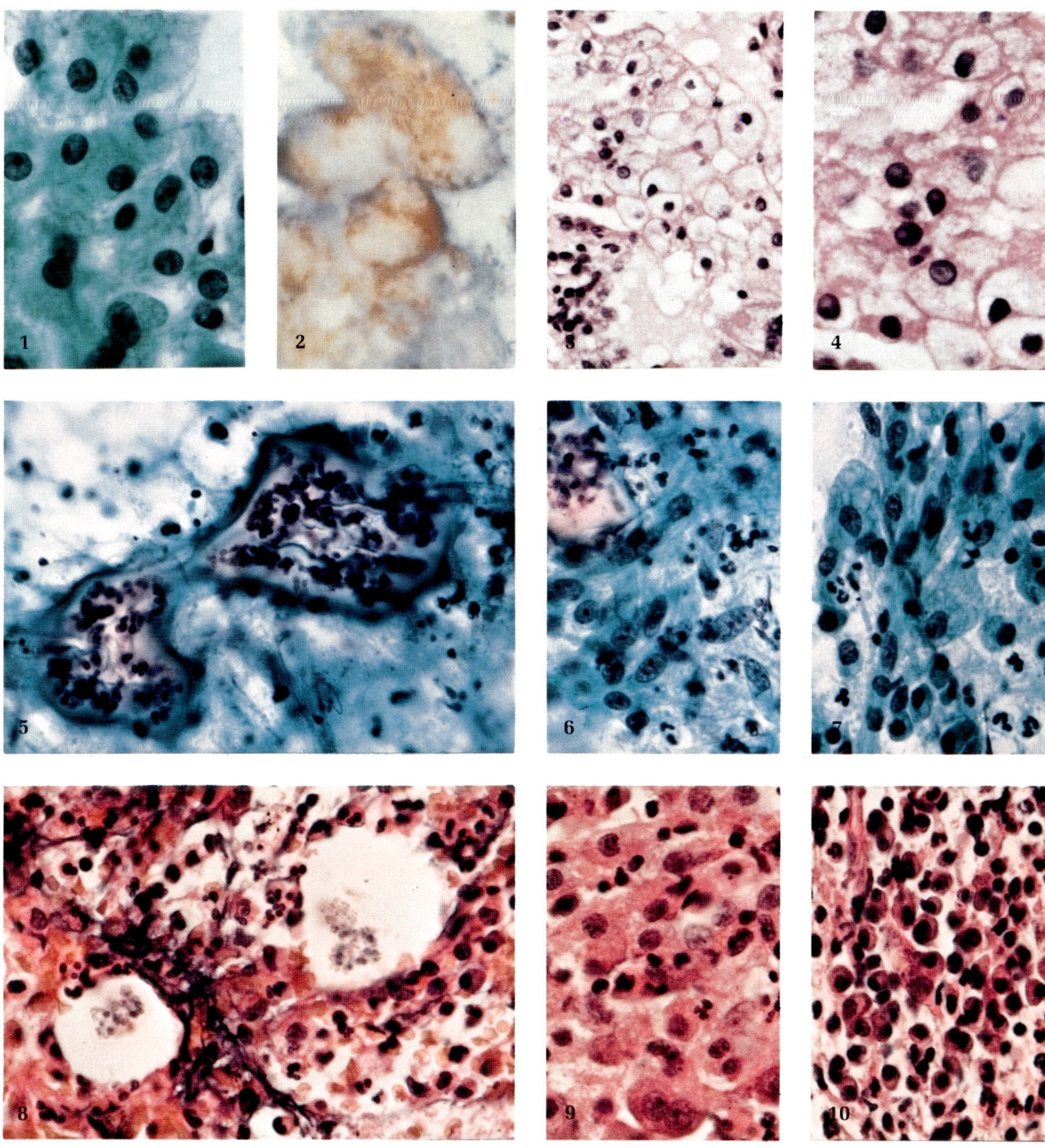

PLATE 27

Lipid Pneumonia

Plate 27–1. Lipid-laden macrophages from lipid pneumonia in FNA smear of the lung (Papanicolaou stain, ×400).

Plate 27–2. Fat-positive material in macrophages (Sudan IV stain, × 400).

Plate 27–3, 27–4. Lipid pneumonia in open lung biopsy specimen (H & E; 27–3, × 200; 27–4, × 400).

Aspiration Pneumonia (Phytopneumonitis)

Plate 27–5, 27–6. Vegetable material and inflammatory exudate from aspiration pneumonia in FNA smears of the lung (Papanicolaou stain, × 400).

Plate 27–7. Macrophages, plasma cells, and leukocytes from aspiration pneumonia in FNA smear of the lung (Papanicolaou stain, × 400).

Plate 27–8. Chronic inflammation and vegetable material in transbronchial biopsy specimen (H & E, × 400).

Plate 27–9, 27–10. Macrophages and plasma cells in lung tissue (H & E, × 400).

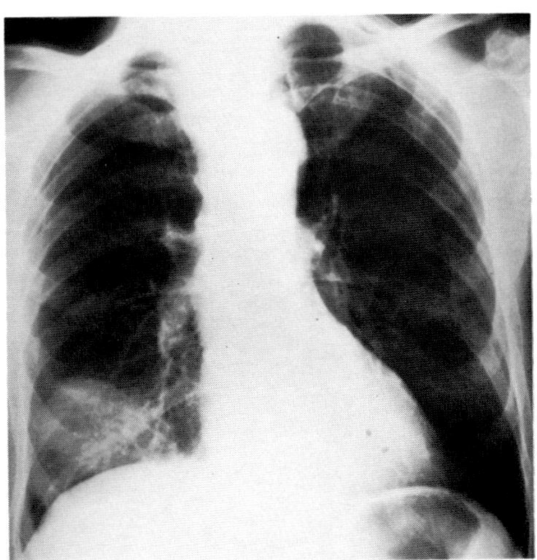

Figure A. Chest roentgenogram showing density in posteroinferior region of right lung.

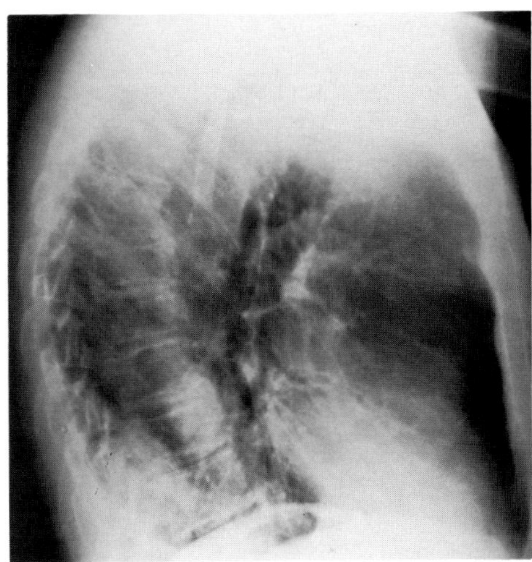

Figure B. Lateral view of same patient shown in Figure A.

PLATE 28

Pulmonary Infarct

Clinical History. A 73-year-old man was admitted to his local hospital for laboratory tests because he had been experiencing repeated falls and hemoptysis. He had a long-standing history of Parkinson's disease. He recently had pain in the right posterior part of the chest, at least one associated episode of hemoptysis, and had lost 15 to 20 lb during the previous 6 to 12 months, despite a continued good appetite. Chest roentgenograms showed a density in the right posteroinferior lung field (Figures A, B), which apparently originated from the pleural cavity. Differential diagnoses included old pleural thickening, loculated fluid, or neoplasm.

Cytologic Findings. An FNA of the lung was performed, and the smears contained numerous markedly atypical cells in a bloody background (Plate 28–1 to 28–4). These cells had enlarged, round or oval nuclei with a moderate or scant amount of dense granular cytoplasm (Plate 28–2, 28–3). The chromatin pattern was finely granular and evenly distributed with occasional chromocenters. The nuclear membranes were smooth and regular (Plate 28–3). Prominent nucleoli were seen in almost every cell. The cells were arranged singly and in sheets with well-defined cell borders (Plate 28–2). Occasional mitotic figures were visible (Plate 28–4).

At first glance, these cells were suspected of being malignant. However, upon careful examination, the nuclei, although definitely atypical, were not strikingly pleomorphic. The nucleoli were prominent, but the chromatin and nuclear membranes appeared normal. The cell borders were distinct and cellular adhesion was preserved within the sheets. For these reasons, the cells were identified as atypical benign alveolar lining cells (pneumocytes). This cell pattern was felt to be consistent with the reactive cells seen with a pulmonary infarct. Sheets of mesothelial cells were identified by their cuboidal shape, uniform vesicular nuclei, prominent nucleoli, distinct cell borders, and orderly arrangement (Plate 28–5).

Pathologic Findings. Two weeks after FNA, mediastinoscopy revealed normal lymph nodes. A right lower lobectomy showed a resolving pulmonary infarct and no evidence of malignancy. Microscopic sections showed a pulmonary infarct with adjacent atypical alveolar lining cells (Plate 28–6 to 28–9). These cells were probably the source of cytologic atypia seen in the aspirate. The patient's postoperative course was uncomplicated, and he was discharged in satisfactory condition.

Refer to Slides 53 and 54 in Optional Slide Set.

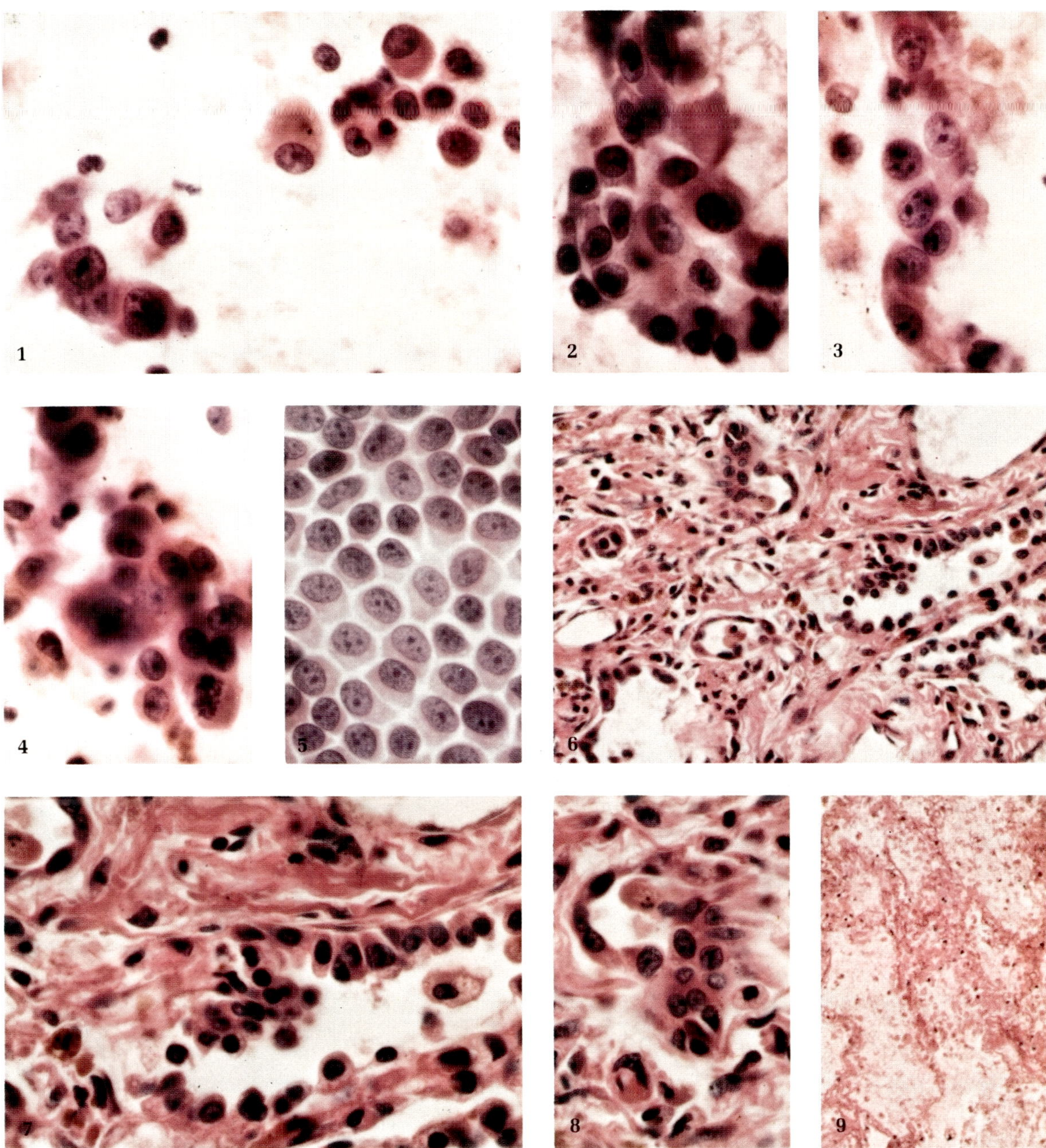

PLATE 28

Pulmonary Infarct

Plate 28–1 to 28–4. Benign histiocytes and atypical alveolar lining cells associated with pulmonary infarct in FNA smears of lung (H & E, × 400).

Plate 28–5. Benign mesothelial cells in FNA smear of lung (H & E, × 400).

Plate 28–6 to 28–8. Atypical alveolar lining cells adjacent to pulmonary infarct in microscopic section of lung (H & E; 28–6, × 200; 28–7, 28–8, × 400).

Plate 28–9. Pulmonary infarct in microscopic section of the lung (H & E, × 100).

PLATE 29

Diffuse Alveolar Damage Due to Radiation and Chemotherapy

Clinical History. The lungs of a 10-year-old boy with acute myelogenous leukemia developed infiltrates that were presumed to be leukemic in origin. The boy was treated with chemotherapy and radiation at another hospital, and the pulmonary infiltrates initially regressed and then reappeared. He developed respiratory insufficiency and was referred to the University of Virginia Medical Center for further evaluation and treatment. An FNA of his lung was performed under fluoroscopic guidance.

Cytologic Findings. The FNA smears contained numerous pleomorphic cells arranged singly and in sheets (Plate 29–1). These cells varied widely in size and shape. Their cytoplasm was basophilic, finely granular with occasional degenerative vacuoles, and scant to abundant in amount. Cell borders were generally distinct. The nuclei were enlarged, usually round or oval, and varied greatly in size. The chromatin pattern was finely granular with some chromocenters and showed some mild hyperchromatism. Prominent nucleoli were present in almost every cell. The characteristics of these cells were not compatible with a diagnosis of leukemia; and despite their pleomorphism in size, the nuclear abnormalities were similar from cell to cell. In view of the patient's history of radiation and chemotherapy, the cells were interpreted as severely atypical, but benign and consistent with the effects of therapy.

Pathologic Findings. The patient could not be weaned from a ventilator. His lungs developed progressive pulmonary infiltrates; he then suffered respiratory failure and died. At autopsy, his lungs were heavy; and microscopic sections showed diffuse alveolar damage. There was fibrosis with marked nuclear atypia of the alveolar lining cells. Their nuclei were enlarged and hyperchromatic with prominent nucleoli (Plate 29–2, 29–3). These changes were consistent with the effects of radiation and chemotherapy.

Refer to Slide 55 in Optional Slide Set.

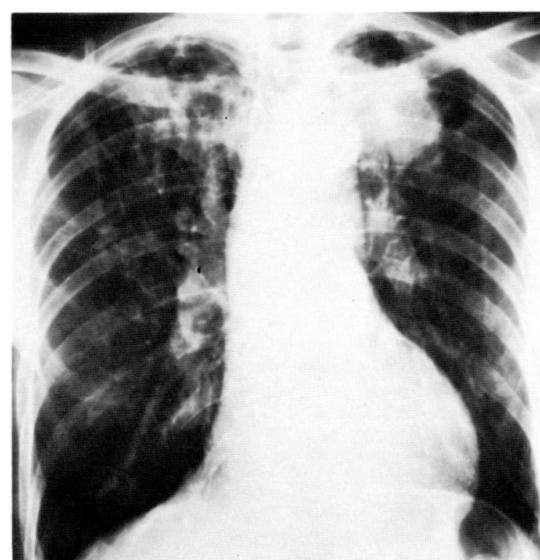

Figure A. Chest roentgenogram depicting irregular mass in apex of left lung.

PLATE 29

Tuberculosis with Coexisting Squamous Cell Carcinoma

Clinical History. A 73-year-old man had been experiencing fever, chills, night sweats, cough, anorexia, weight loss, and hemoptysis when admitted to the University of Virginia Medical Center. Findings from sputum cultures were positive for *Mycobacterium tuberculosis,* and he was treated with preparations of isoniazid (INH) and rifampin, administered orally. His chest roentgenogram showed an irregular mass in the apex of the left lung (Figure A) and an infiltrate with multiple lucent areas in the upper lobe of the right lung. Results of sputum cytologic evaluations and bronchoscopy with biopsy, washings, and brushings were negative. An FNA of the left lung mass was performed under fluoroscopic guidance.

Cytologic Findings. The FNA smears contained acute and chronic inflammatory cells and scattered multinucleated giant cells (Plate 29–4). The giant cells had abundant, finely granular, basophilic cytoplasm and 10 to 30 uniform, vesicular nuclei. Special stains were done to determine the presence of microorganisms; acid-fast stain demonstrated a few aggregates of acid-fast organisms averaging about 4 μm in length and less than 1 μm in diameter (Plate 29–5). A diagnosis of tuberculosis was made. A repeat aspiration of the mass was performed because the clinical findings suggested the presence of a malignant lesion. These smears contained scattered, abnormal keratinizing squamous cells characteristic of a well-differentiated squamous cell carcinoma (Plate 29–6, 29–7). The two aspirations from this same lung mass indicated a squamous cell carcinoma coexisting with tuberculosis.

Pathologic Findings. The patient discontinued his medication because he was feeling well, but then developed recurrent respiratory symptoms, a tender abdomen, and bone tenderness. The patient subsequently died. Autopsy revealed tuberculosis in both upper pulmonary lobes, a 6 × 5 × 3-cm squamous carcinoma in the upper lobe of the left lung, and metastatic disease in the liver, adrenal glands, and vertebrae.

Refer to Slide 56 in Optional Slide Set.

PLATE 29

Nocardiosis

Clinical History. A 67-year-old woman had bilateral supraclavicular lymphadenopathy; and a lymph node biopsy specimen was diagnosed as malignant lymphoma of possible Hodgkin's type. She was treated with chemotherapy and administration of prednisone orally for one year, which resulted in moderate resolution of the lymphadenopathy.

She was then transferred to the University of Virginia Medical Center for further evaluation and treatment. The slides prepared at the other hospital were reviewed and interpreted as atypical hyperplasia, not lymphoma. The chemotherapy was discontinued and the quantity of steroids administered was gradually decreased. Computerized axial tomography showed extensive lymphadenopathy in the retroperitoneum, posterior mediastinum, and left paratracheal region. She had experienced night sweats for two months before admission to the University of Virginia Medical Center and developed shortness of breath, dyspnea, and progressive left-sided pleuritic chest pain. She had no weight loss and had never smoked. A chest roentgenogram taken at the time of admission showed a 4-cm density in the lower lobe of her left lung, which was not present one month before admission (Figure B). The physical examination showed that she had generalized lymphadenopathy, and auscultation and palpation revealed that her lungs were normal. An FNA of the lung mass was performed under fluoroscopic guidance.

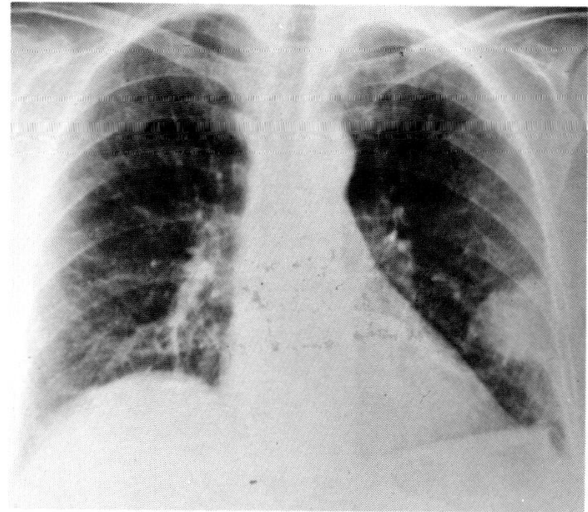

Figure B. Chest roentgenogram showing density in lower lobe of left lung.

Cytologic Findings. The FNA smears contained a severe acute inflammatory exudate and necrotic debris (Plate 29–8). Special stains were done on some slides for the identification of microorganisms. The Brown-Hopps gram stain and the Fite's method for acid-fast organisms showed delicate, branching filamentous hyphae 0.5 to 1.0 μm in diameter and 10 to 20 μm in length (Plate 29–9, 29–10). The branching was more or less at right angles. No sulfur granules were seen. The hyphae did not stain with either the Papanicolaou or hematoxylin and eosin methods. A diagnosis of nocardiosis was made.

Follow-up. A culture from the lung aspiration grew *Nocardia,* and the patient was treated with administration of erythromyocin and ampicillin because she was allergic to sulfur.

Refer to Slide 57 in Optional Slide Set.

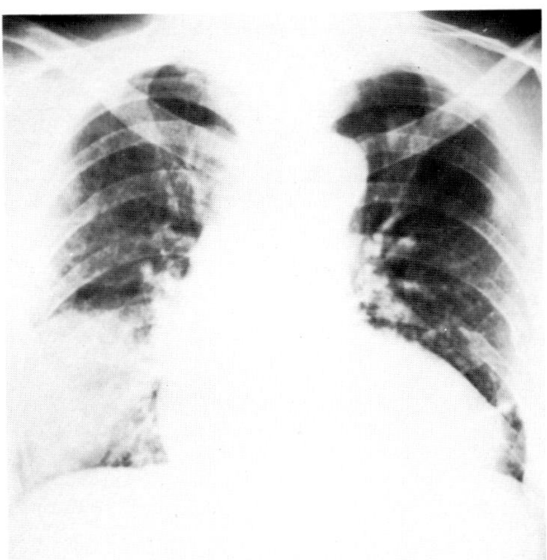

Figure C. Chest roentgenogram showing infiltrate in middle lobe of right lung.

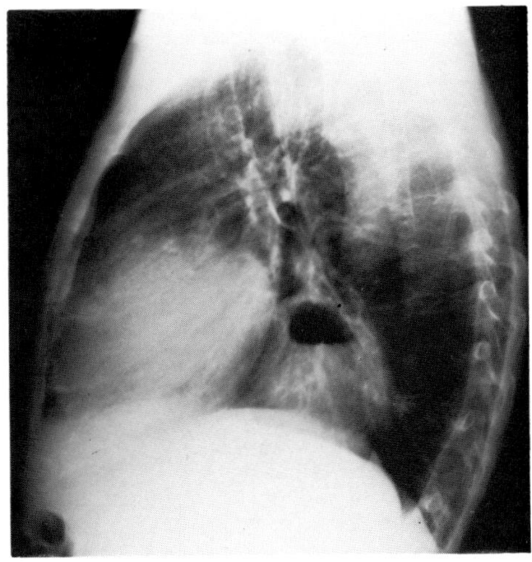

Figure D. Chest roentgenogram showing lateral view of same patient whose roentgenogram was seen in Figure C, infiltrate in middle lobe of right lung.

PLATE 29

Legionella micdadei Pneumonia

Clinical History. A 42-year-old man had end-stage renal disease diagnosed by the presence of obstructive uropathy and was treated with hemodialysis. He responded poorly to the dialysis and was referred to the University of Virginia Medical Center for a renal transplant. He underwent a cadaveric renal transplant but shortly after surgery had a decrement in urine output, which remained persistently low. He received radiation therapy (4 doses of 150 rads) to the transplanted kidney and a bolus of methylprednisolone sodium succinate (Solu-Medrol) treatment for three days, as well as immunosuppression therapy with high-dose prednisone and azathioprine (Immuran). This treatment resulted in a gradual improvement of renal function. During the third week postoperatively, he became febrile and developed an infiltrate in the middle lobe of the right lung (Figures C & D). An FNA of the infiltrate was performed under fluoroscopic guidance.

Cytologic Findings. The FNA smears contained a mixed inflammatory exudate of polymorphonuclear leukocytes and macrophages. Fite's method for acid-fast organisms revealed intracytoplasmic, short (2 to 3 μm) acid-fast bacilli within the cytoplasm of the neutrophils (Plate 29–11, 29–12). Extracellular acid-fast bacilli were also seen (Plate 29–12, 29–13). A direct fluorescent antibody stain for *Legionella micdadei* on an aspiration smear was positive (Plate 29–14).

Pathologic Findings. Despite therapy with intravenously administered erythromycin and tapering of the immunosuppression therapy, the lung infiltrate persisted. There was marked deterioration of the patient's renal function during the period of severe pneumonia, and the renal allograft became nonfunctioning. He received dialysis, but died.

Autopsy demonstrated the lungs to be heavy (right, 620 g; left, 685 g), congested, and focally consolidated. Microscopic sections showed extensive pneumonia with alveolar spaces packed with polymorphonuclear leukocytes (Plate 29–15, 29–16). Special stains revealed numerous intracellular and extracellular acid-fast bacteria. Results of lung cultures were positive for *L micdadei.*

Refer to Slide 58 in Optional Slide Set.

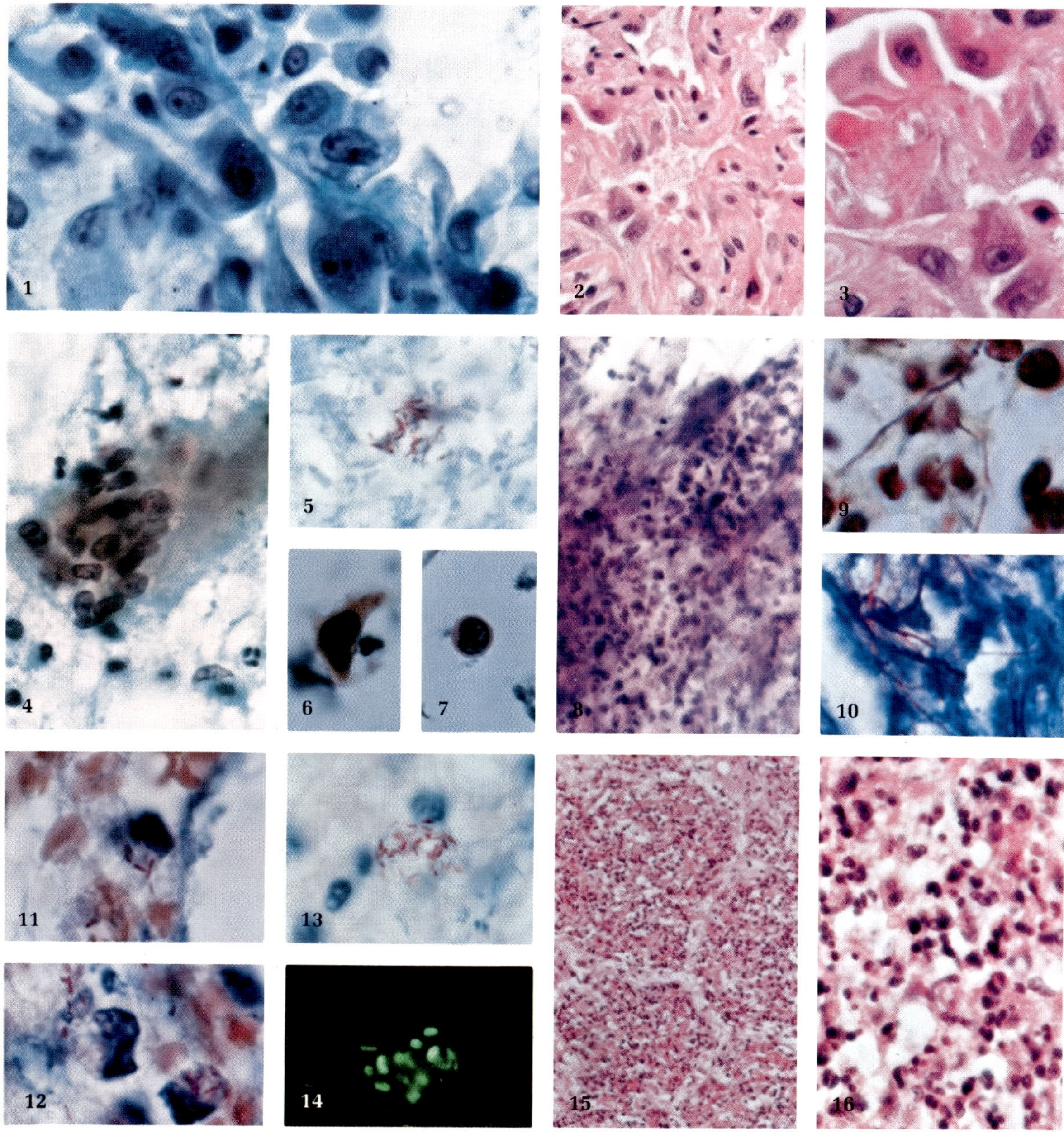

PLATE 29

Diffuse Alveolar Damage Due to Radiation and Chemotherapy

Plate 29–1. Highly atypical alveolar lining cells associated with radiation and chemotherapy effect in FNA smear of the lung (Papanicolaou stain, × 400).

Plate 29–2, 29–3. Diffuse alveolar damage due to radiation and chemotherapy in microscopic sections of the lung at autopsy (H & E; 29–2, × 200; 29–3, × 400).

Tuberculosis with Coexisting Squamous Cell Carcinoma

Plate 29–4. Multinucleated giant cell associated with tuberculosis in FNA smear of the lung (Papanicolaou stain, × 400).

Plate 29–5. Acid-fast bacilli of tuberculosis in FNA smear of the lung (acid-fast stain, × 1,000).

Plate 29–6, 29–7. Keratinizing squamous cell carcinoma in FNA smears of the lung. Filter preparation (Papanicolaou stain, × 400).

Nocardiosis

Plate 29–8. Marked, acute inflammation and necrosis associated with nocardiosis in FNA smear of the lung (Papanicolaou stain, × 200).

Plate 29–9. Nocardia asteroides in FNA smear of the lung (Brown-Hopps gram stain, × 1,000).

Plate 29–10. N asteroides in FNA smear of the lung (Fite's method for acid-fast organisms, × 1,000).

Legionella micdadei Pneumonia

Plate 29–11 to 29–13. Intracytoplasmic and extracellular acid-fast bacilli of *Legionella micdadei* in FNA smear of the lung (Fite's method for acid-fast organisms, × 1,000).

Plate 29–14. Direct fluorescent antibody stain for *L micdadei* (× 1,000).

Plate 29–15, 29–16. Extensive pneumonia with polymorphonuclear leukocytes packed in alveolar spaces in microscopic sections of the lung at autopsy (H & E; 29–15, × 100; 29–16, × 400).

PLATE 30

Histoplasmosis

Clinical History. A 17-year-old female student complained of increasing fatigue and shortness of breath that had been occurring for approximately two months. During the month prior to her visit, she had lost 8 lb voluntarily and had not experienced any cough or fever.

During the physical examination, her lungs were clear and there were no abdominal abnormalities. A chest roentgenogram taken at her college disclosed a right hilar lesion (Figure A), and she was referred to the University of Virginia Medical Center for evaluation.

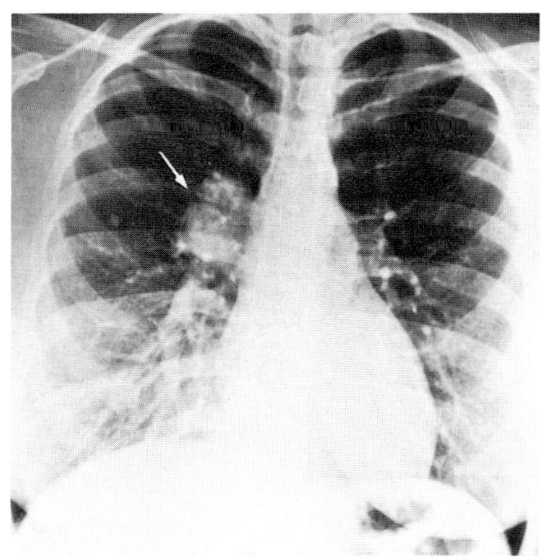

Figure A. Chest roentgenogram showing hilar lesion in right lung *(see arrow).*

Cytologic Findings. Fluoroscopically directed FNA of the right lung produced smears containing abundant macrophages of varying sizes with vesicular nuclei and abundant "bubbly" cytoplasm (Plate 30–1 to 30–4). High-power examination of the cytoplasm revealed innumerable small, round or oval structures measuring 1 to 5 μm in diameter and surrounded by a rigid cell wall. The protoplasm appeared to have pulled away from the cell wall, resulting in a clear space (Plate 30–2, 30–4). This was felt to be an artifact of fixation. A Gomori methenamine silver stain confirmed the presence of the fungal organisms, *Histoplasma capsulatum* (Plate 30–5).

Follow-up. Cultures from the aspirate were positive for *Histoplasma capsulatum.*

Refer to Slide 59 in Optional Slide Set.

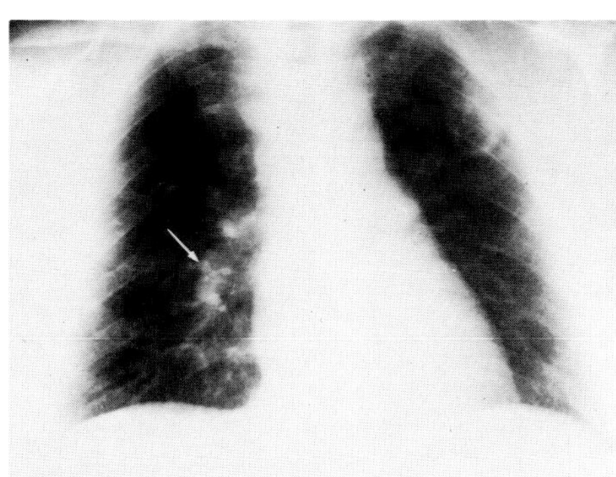

Figure B. Chest roentgenogram demonstrating cystic lesion in left lung *(see arrow).*

PLATE 30

Cryptococcosis

Clinical History. A 20-year-old man with fever, shortness of breath, and productive cough was admitted to the University of Virginia for evaluation of his pulmonary problem. A chest roentgenogram showed a cystic lesion in the left lung (Figure B). A transtracheal aspirate, material from bronchoscopy, and sputum contained no organisms. Fluoroscopically directed FNA of the lung lesion was performed.

Cytologic Findings. Filter preparations from the aspiration material demonstrated numerous round or oval bodies about 5 to 8 μm surrounded by a clear capsule 3 to 5 μm in thickness (Plate 30–6 to 30–8). They did not stain with the Papanicolaou stain, but were made clearly visible by the background staining of the filter. Budding forms were also noted. These buds were single and attached by a thin wall and narrow pore forming a "teardrop" appearance (Plate 30–7). No true hyphae were seen. These organisms were interpreted as *Cryptococcus neoformans.*

Follow-up. The patient was treated with amphotericin B, intravenously, and his condition progressively improved. The presence of *Cryptococcus* organisms was confirmed by culture of FNA material.

Refer to Slide 60 in Optional Slide Set.

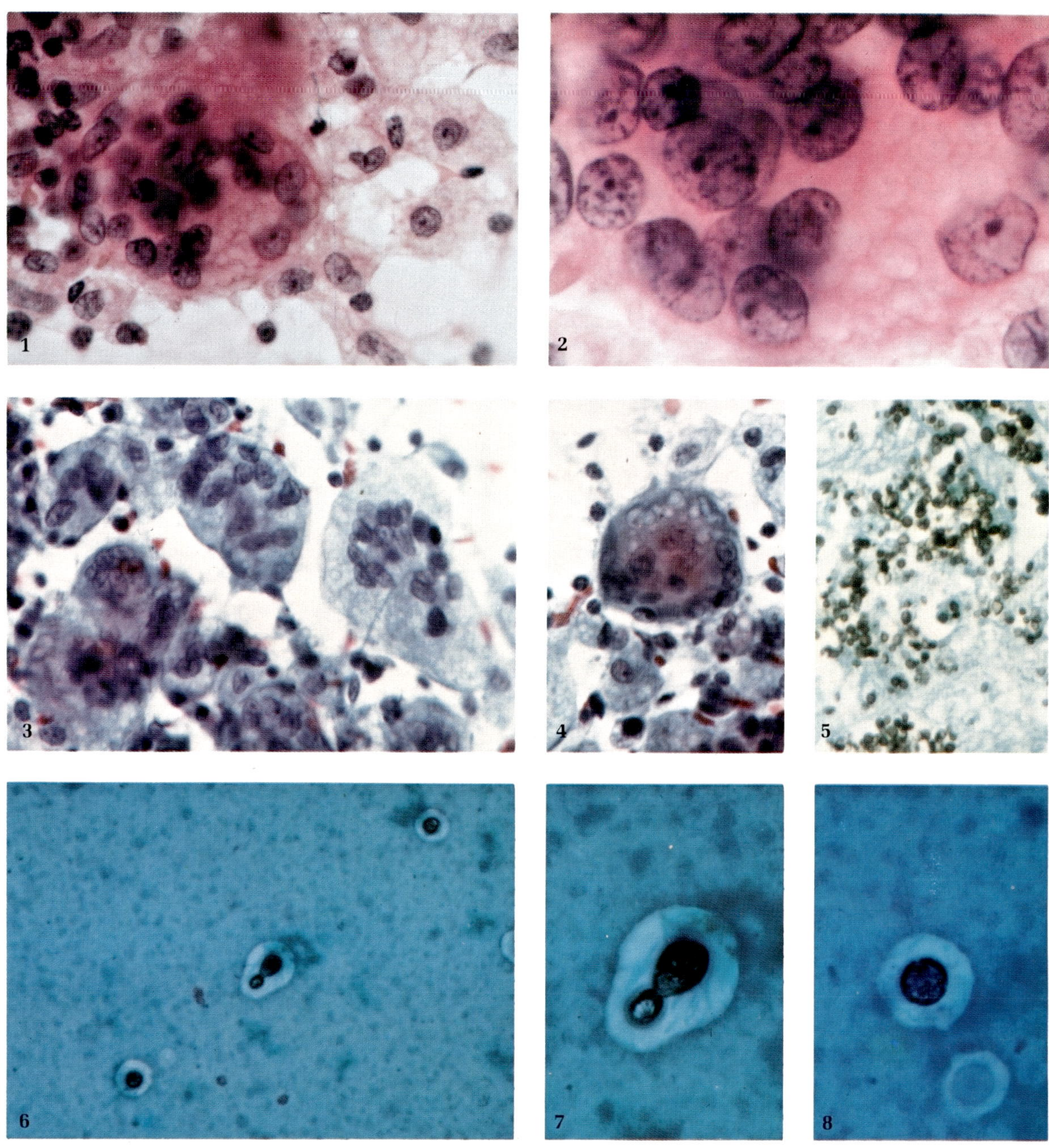

PLATE 30

Histoplasmosis

Plate 30–1, 30–2. Macrophages containing *Histoplasma capsulatum* in lung FNA smear (H & E; 30–1, × 400; 30–2, × 1,000).

Plate 30–3, 30–4. Macrophages containing *H capsulatum* in lung FNA smears. (Papanicolaou stain, × 400).

Plate 30–5. H capsulatum (Gomori methenamine silver stain, × 400).

Cryptococcosis

Plate 30–6 to 30–8. Cryptococcus neoformans in filter preparation of needle washings of lung FNA (Papanicolaou stain; 30–6, × 400; 30–7, 30–8, × 1,000).

PLATE 31

Blastomycosis

Clinical History. A 28-year-old male smoker was referred to the University of Virginia Medical Center for evaluation of an infiltrate at the apex of the left lung shown on chest roentgenogram (Figure A). He was in excellent health until three to four months before admission when he developed left-sided pleuritic chest pain and a nonproductive cough.

Results of sputum cultures were negative for acid-fast bacilli and fungi. Results of skin tests for histoplasmosis, coccidiomycosis, and tuberculosis were negative. Results of serologic tests were negative for cryptococci. Bronchoscopy revealed inflammation of the upper lobe of the left lung and a white exudate in the apical segment of the upper lobe of the left lung. Washings showed no evidence of malignancy, and the findings from a culture of this material were negative for acid-fast bacilli and fungi.

He had explored caves approximately 12 times in the past year and had been exposed to significant levels of asbestos at his workplace for one to two years. An FNA of the lung infiltrate was performed under fluoroscopic guidance.

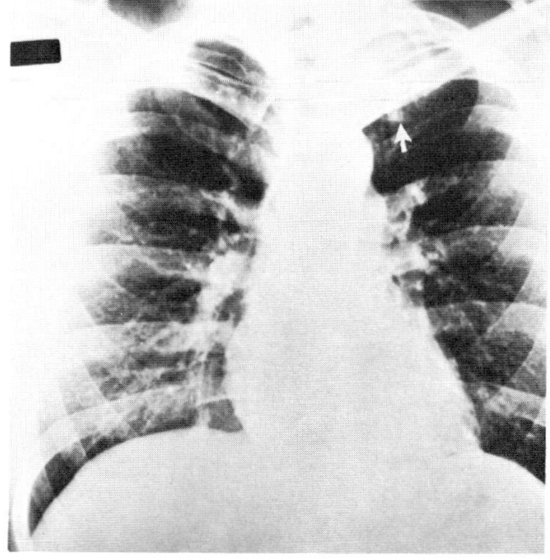

Figure A. Chest roentgenogram showing infiltrate in apex of left lung *(see arrow).*

Cytologic Findings. The FNA smears contain numerous inflammatory cells, multinucleated giant cells, epithelioid cells, and lipid-laden macrophages (Plate 31–1 to 31–5). The multinucleated giant cells ranged from 30 to 90 μm, and some contained more than 100 nuclei per cell (Plate 31–6). These nuclei frequently contained nucleoli. The epithelioid cells were in sheetlike or syncytial arrangements with abundant basophilic cytoplasm and elongated shapes (Plate 31–1, 31–3). The nuclei of these cells were round or oval with finely granular chromatin and frequent prominent nucleoli. Many of the macrophages had abundant cytoplasm that appeared "foamy" or "lacy"; such cytoplasm suggested the presence of lipid material (Plate 31–4). Small individual or budding spherical organisms about 8 to 15 μm in diameter were visible within the giant cells and associated with the epithelioid cells (Plate 31–1 to 31–5). The organisms had sharply defined, relatively thick, refractile cell walls that stained bluish green. The prominent protoplasm appeared brownish and was often retracted from the cell wall, leaving a clear space (Plate 31–5) The budding forms showed a single bud with a broad-based attachment characterized by a broad, flat wall segment between the bud and the parent cell. The organisms were mucin-negative (Plate 31–7). This cell pattern was interpreted as granulomatous inflammation with fungal forms consistent with the presence of *Blastomyces dermatitidis.*

Follow-up. A culture of the aspirated material confirmed the presence of *Blastomyces* organisms.

Refer to Slide 61 in Optional Slide Set.

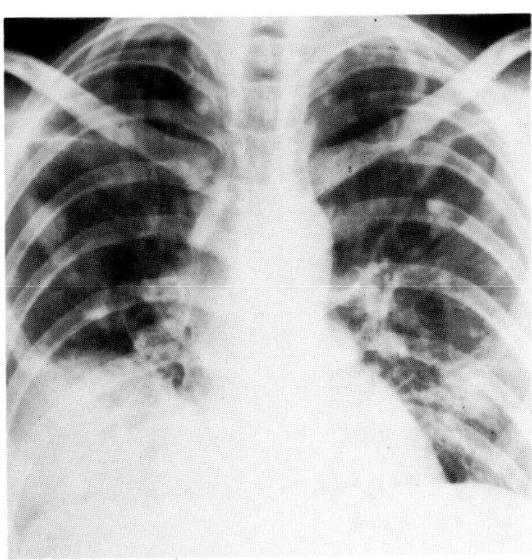

Figure B. Chest roentgenogram showing multiple areas of patchy infiltrate throughout both lungs.

PLATE 31

Aspergillosis

Clinical History. Three weeks before admission, a 71-year-old male smoker had finished receiving locally administered radiation therapy and one course of chemotherapy for treatment of chronic lymphocytic leukemia. On admission, he complained of increased lethargy, anorexia, fever, and a rattling cough. Chest roentgenograms revealed extensive consolidation in the lower lobe of the right lung and an ill-defined area of consolidation in the upper lobe of the right lung. There were multiple areas of patchy infiltrate throughout both lungs (Figure B).

Cytologic Findings. The FNA smears contained scattered hyphae approximately 3 to 4 μm in diameter with uniform dichotomous branching (Plate 31–8, 31–9). The angle of branching was acute (about 45°) resulting in terminal branching that resembled a forked stick. Staining with Gomori methenamine silver stain showed the fungal forms with clearly visible septae (Plate 31–10). These hyphae were interpreted as *Aspergillus fumigatus.* The background of the smear contained scattered benign respiratory cells and acute and chronic inflammatory cells.

Pathologic Findings. The patient died six days later of progressive respiratory failure. Examination of the lungs at autopsy revealed multiple light yellow nodules scattered throughout the pulmonary parenchyma. Microscopic sections showed a severe hemorrhagic pneumonia, and postmortem cultures confirmed the presence of *A fumigatus.* Special stains of lung tissue showed massive quantities of fungal hyphae. Evidence of disseminated aspergillosis was found in the colon, brain, and left ethmoid sinus.

Refer to Slide 62 in Optional Slide Set.

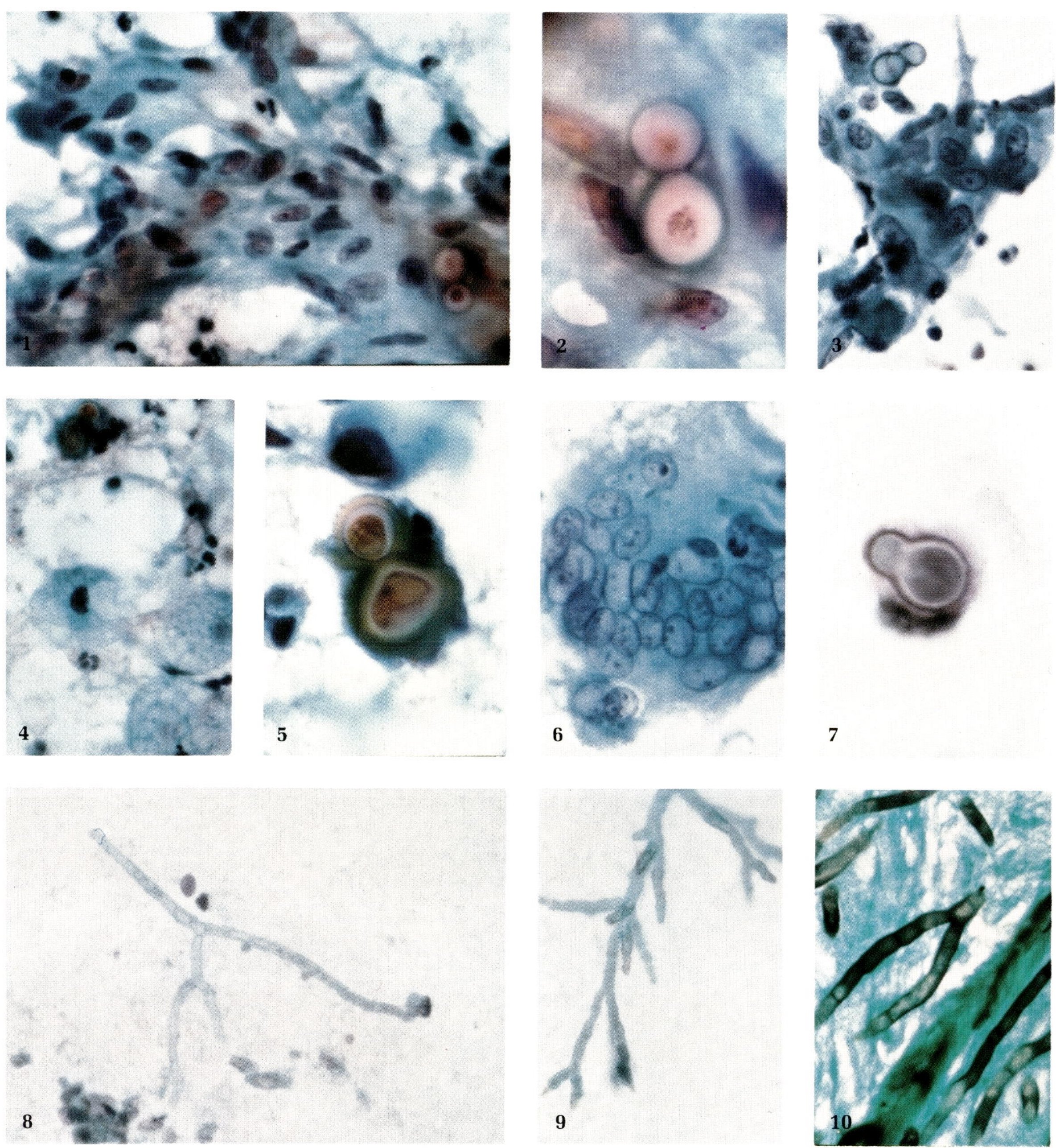

PLATE 31

Blastomycosis

Plate 31–1 to 31–3. Epithelioid cells with *Blastomyces dermatitidis* in lung FNA smears (Papanicolaou stain; 31–1, 31–3, × 400; 31–2, × 1,000).

Plate 31–4. Lipid-laden macrophages in lung FNA smear (Papanicolaou stain, × 400).

Plate 31–5. Blastomyces organisms in lung FNA smear (Papanicolaou stain, × 1,000).

Plate 31–6. Multinucleated giant cell in lung FNA smear (Papanicolaou stain, × 400).

Plate 31–7. Budding yeast form of *B dermatitidis* (mucicarmine stain, × 1,000).

Aspergillosis

Plate 31–8, 31–9. Hyphae of *Aspergillus fumigatus* in lung FNA smear. Filter preparation of needle washings of lung FNA (Papanicolaou stain, × 400).

Plate 31–10. Hyphae of *A fumigatus* in lung FNA smear (Gomori methenamine silver stain, × 400).

PLATE 32

Coccidioidomycosis

Clinical History. A 25-year-old female student at the University of Arizona was admitted to a local hospital for removal of a ganglion cyst of the wrist. A routine chest roentgenogram done during her admission examination showed a mass in the left lung (Figure A). The patient claimed to be asymptomatic; however, careful questioning disclosed that she had a history of a cough that produced yellowish sputum. Two months before her symptoms appeared, she had visited Mexico. An FNA of the lung mass was performed.

Cytologic Findings. The FNA smears contained scattered, large, spherical structures lying singly or within macrophages (Plate 32–1 to 32–4). Some of these spherules contained smaller structures or endospores, which were clearly shown by the Gomori methenamine silver stain (Plate 32–4). A diagnosis of fungal forms compatible with *Coccidioides immitis* was made.

Pathologic Findings. Although it is not the usual policy at our hospital, a needle-core biopsy was performed along with the FNA. Tissue sections showed granulomatous inflammation with giant cells containing spherules of *C immitis* (Plate 32–5). Her chest roentgenogram showed spontaneous improvement, and no further surgery was required.

Refer to Slide 63 in Optional Slide Set.

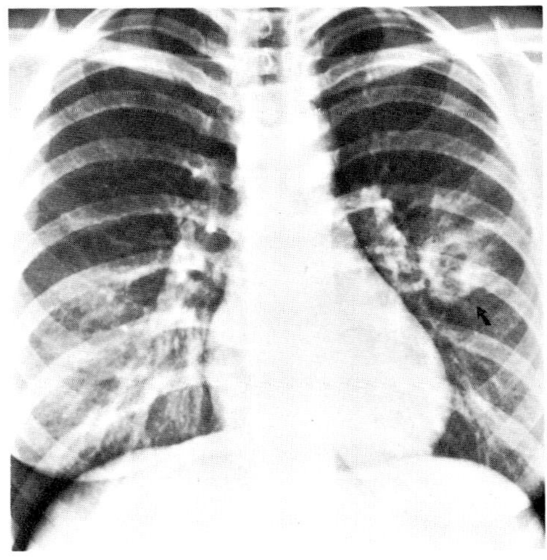

Figure A. Chest roentgenogram showing mass in left lung *(see arrow)*.

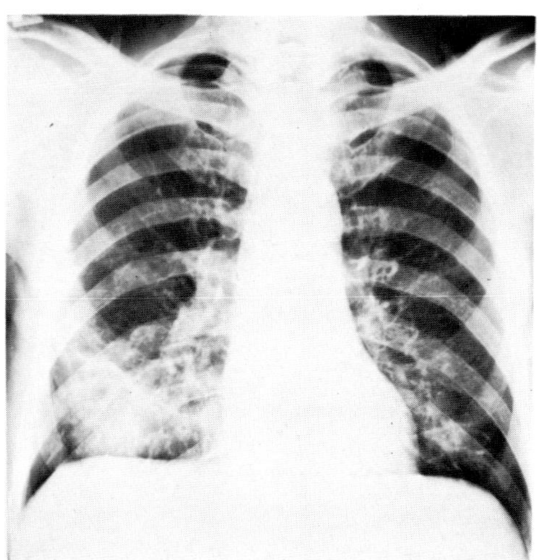

Figure B. Chest roentgenogram demonstrating infiltrate in lower lobe of right lung.

PLATE 32

Mucormycosis

Clinical History. A 64-year-old man with adult-onset diabetes mellitis was admitted to the University of Virginia Medical Center with a history of dyspnea, pleuritic chest pain, 20-lb weight loss, and temperature to 38.8 °C. A chest roentgenogram showed an infiltrate in the lower lobe of the right lung (Figure B). Results of blood cultures and purified protein derivative were negative. He was treated with intravenously administered ampicillin for 14 days, and he responded to therapy. Following discharge, he gradually developed worsening pleuritic chest pain and dyspnea and was readmitted for further evaluation of the infiltrate and his symptoms.

The physical examination showed that he was thin and had mild tachypnea. Percussion revealed dullness with decreased breath sounds at the right base. The remainder of the physical examination and results of laboratory tests were normal, except for an elevated white blood cell count.

Oral administration of penicillin was initiated for treatment of possible postobstructive pneumonia. Multiple sputum samples tested for fungi, tuberculosis, and malignancy showed negative results. No evidence of bronchial obstruction appeared on tomograms or bronchoscopy.

Cytologic Findings. An FNA of the lower lobe of the right lung showed numerous very broad, rarely septate, tubelike hyphae that varied greatly in thickness and shape (Plate 32–6, 32–7). The hyphae stained orange-brown with the Papanicolaou stain. Branching was common although the angle and spacing of the branches was very irregular. Partially collapsed and distorted hyphae were also visible. These organisms showed poor sensitivity to fungal stains. The diagnosis was fungal forms consistent with the presence of mucormycosis. The smears also contained acute and chronic inflammatory cells and benign respiratory cells.

Pathologic Findings. Cultures of the aspirated material failed to confirm the presence of fungus. A repeat bronchoscopy with transbronchial biopsy revealed no evidence of fungal infection. On open lung biopsy, a large fibrotic abscess cavity was discovered and drained copious amounts of yellow, purulent debris. Nonbranching hyphae consistent with mucormycosis were present on the potassium hydroxide preparation of this material. Microscopic examination of the lung tissue from the edges of the cavity showed vascular invasion by hyphae with necrosis (Plate 32–8). Results of cultures were again negative.

Refer to Slide 64 in Optional Slide Set.

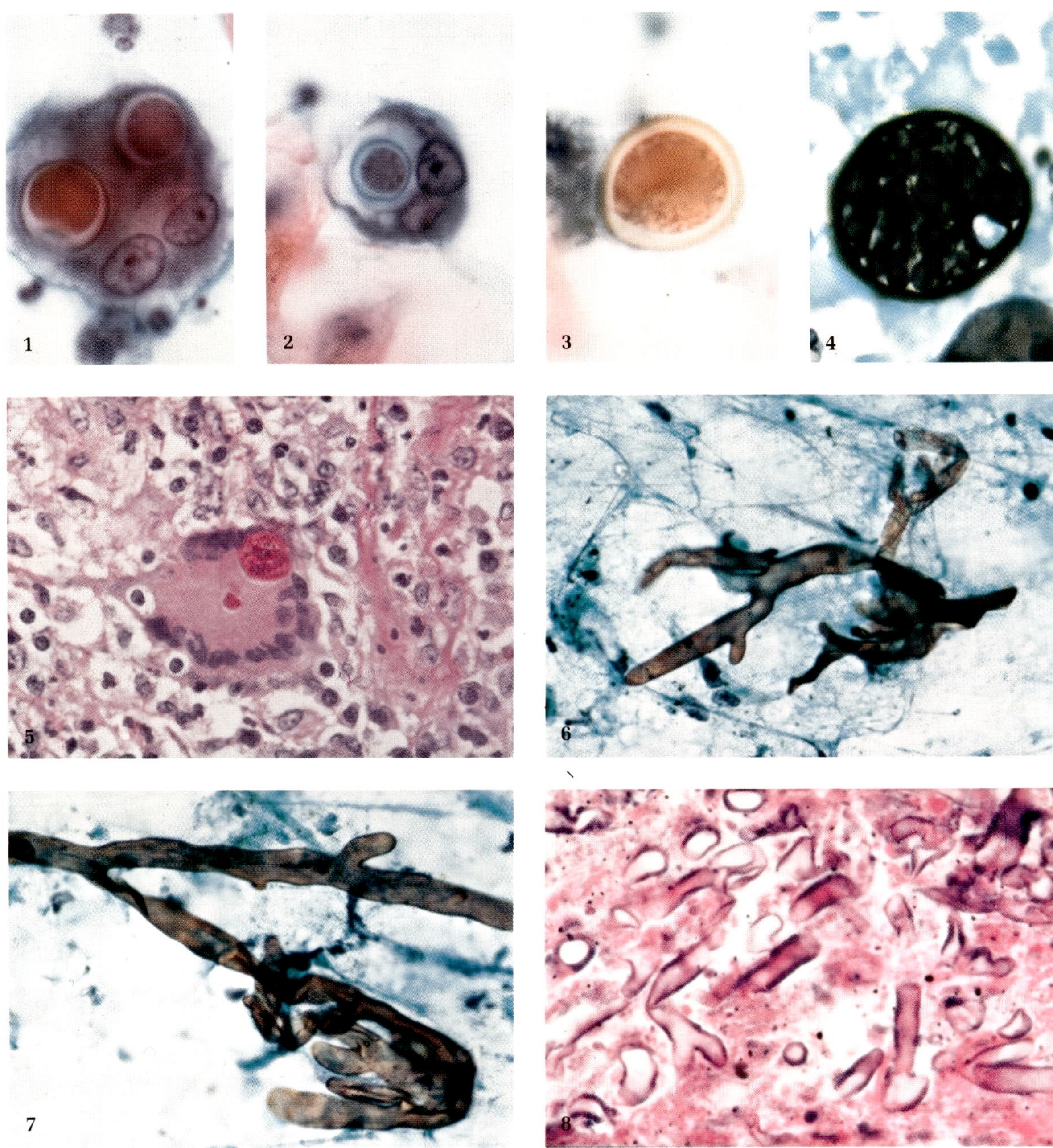

PLATE 32

Coccidioidomycosis

Plate 32–1, 32–2. Macrophages containing *Coccidioides immitis* in lung FNA smear (Papanicolaou stain; 32–1, × 400; 32–2, × 1,000).

Plate 32–3. C immitis spherule in lung FNA smear (Papanicolaou stain, × 1,000).

Plate 32–4. C immitis spherule in lung FNA smear (Gomori methenamine silver stain, × 1,000).

Plate 32–5. Granulomatous inflammation with *C immitis* spherules in microscopic section of the lung (H & E, × 200).

Mucormycosis

Plate 32–6, 32–7. Fungal hyphae of mucormycosis in lung FNA smear (Papanicolaou stain, × 400).

Plate 32–8. Fungal hyphae of mucormycosis in microscopic section of the lung (H & E, × 400).

PLATE 33

Cytomegalic Inclusion Disease

Clinical History. A 17-year-old girl was diagnosed as having acute myelomonocytic leukemia two months before her current admission to the University of Virginia Hospital. She had been treated with chemotherapy and had remission of her leukemia. Upon admission she was febrile. No organisms could be identified, and she was treated with multiple antibiotics. A chest roentgenogram showed diffuse mixed alveolar interstitial pulmonary infiltrates (Figure A). An FNA of the lung infiltrate was done under fluoroscopic guidance.

Cytologic Findings. The FNA smears contained scattered enlarged epithelial cells with large, single basophilic inclusions within their nuclei (Plate 33–1 to 33–3). These inclusions were surrounded by a large, clear halo and a sharply defined nuclear membrane lined by residual condensed chromatin (Plate 33–2). This produced the classic "owl's eye" appearance of the nuclei. Most affected cells were mononucleated; however, occasional binucleated forms were seen (Plate 33–2 to 33–3). Rare cells showed cytoplasmic inclusions (Plate 33–3). Benign respiratory cells and pulmonary macrophages composed the other cellular components of the smear. A diagnosis of cytomegalic inclusion disease was made.

Pathologic Findings. The patient was treated with a broad spectrum of antibiotics, but she showed no response. Chest roentgenograms showed progression of the infiltrates. After a few episodes of hypotension, she had a fatal cardiopulmonary arrest. Examination of the lung at autopsy showed numerous small lesions with the appearance of abscesses scattered throughout the lung parenchyma. Microscopic sections of the lung contained numerous cytomegalovirus inclusions (Plate 33–4, 33–5). The presence of cytomegalovirus was confirmed by culture.

Refer to Slide 65 in Optional Slide Set.

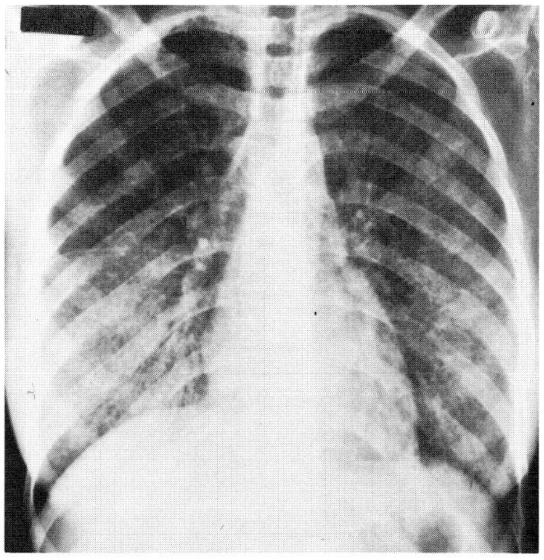

Figure A. Chest roentgenogram showing mixed alveolar-interstitial pulmonary infiltrates.

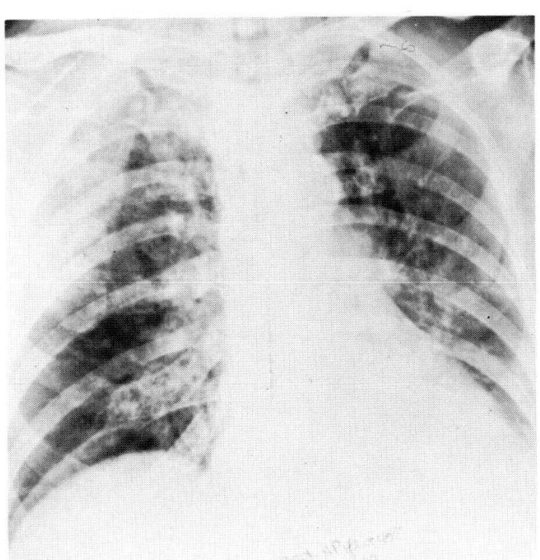

Figure B. Chest roentgenogram demonstrating bilateral, diffuse, fluffy alveolar infiltrates.

PLATE 33

Herpes Simplex Pneumonia

Clinical History. A 78-year-old woman, who was previously treated for myasthenia gravis with high dosages of steroids at the University of Virginia Medical Center, experienced what her physician suspected to be a large pulmonary embolus, one month before her current admission. She came to the hospital because of difficulty in breathing and was admitted. A chest roentgenogram showed bilateral, diffuse, fluffy alveolar infiltrates (Figure B). Results of bronchoscopy with transbronchial biopsy and multiple cultures of sputum and blood were normal. A high fever developed, and chest roentgenograms showed progressive pulmonary infiltrates. An FNA of the lung was performed under fluoroscopic guidance.

Cytologic Findings. The FNA smears contained single cells and multinucleated cells. Both had enlarged nuclei and scant, dense, basophilic cytoplasm. The nuclear chromatin was clumped along the inner nuclear membrane, leaving a bland, refractile center; this gave the nuclei a characteristic "ground glass" appearance (Plate 33–6 to 33–8). Other multinucleated cells had large, eosinophilic intranuclear inclusion bodies surrounded by more or less prominent, clear halos (Plate 33–9). No cytoplasmic inclusions were seen. The cells with multiple nuclei showed nuclear molding without overlapping (Plate 33–7, 33–8). A diagnosis of herpes simplex pneumonia was made.

Pathologic Findings. The patient became progressively hypoxic with progressive diffuse lung infiltrates and died. Microscopic sections of the lung at autopsy demonstrated histologic changes compatible with herpes simplex pneumonia (Plate 33–10 to 33–12). A culture of this specimen grew herpes simplex virus.

Refer to Slide 66 in Optional Slide Set.

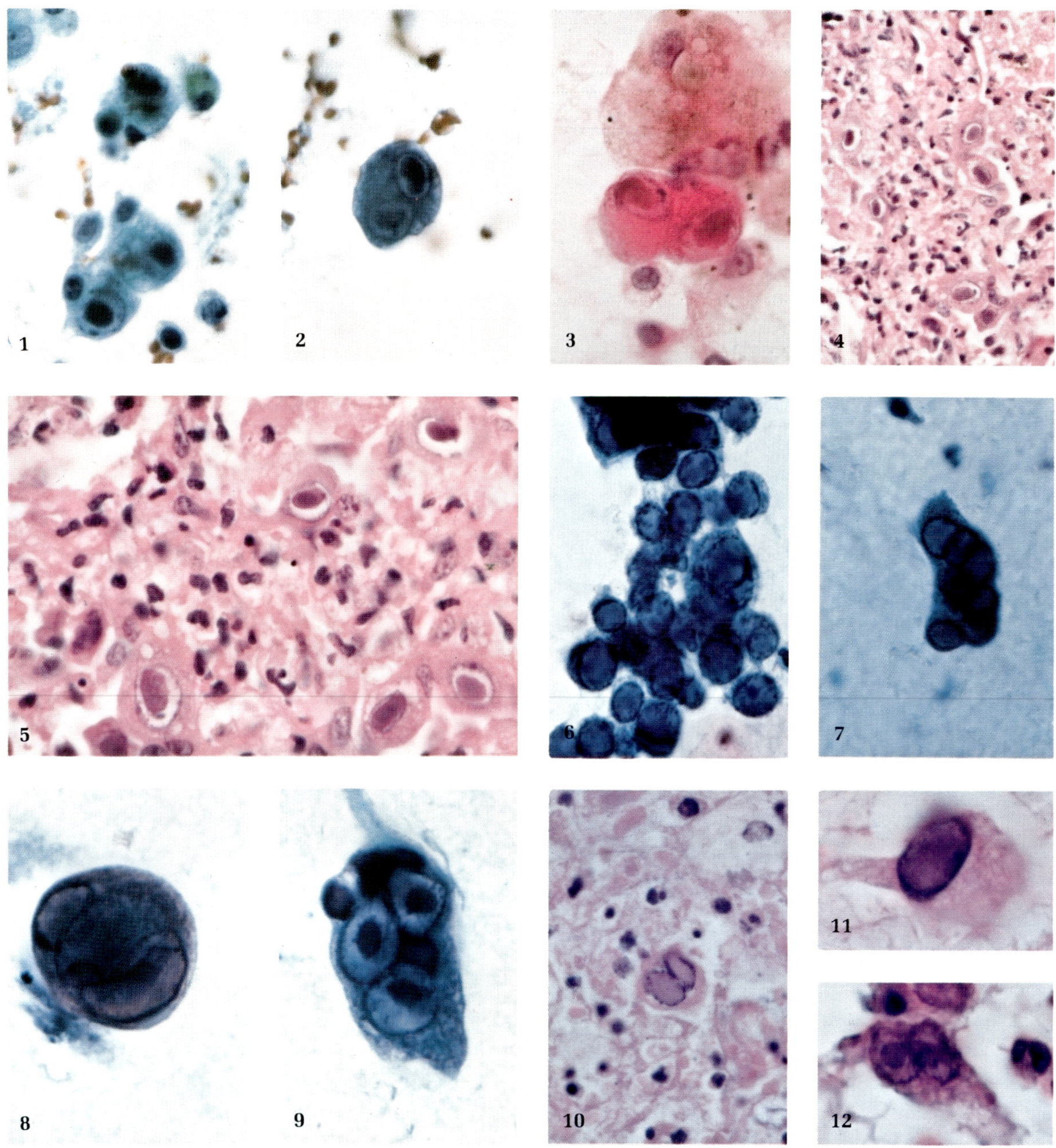

PLATE 33

Cytomegalic Inclusion Disease

Plate 33–1, 33–2. Viral changes consistent with cytomegalovirus (CMV) in lung FNA smear (Papanicolaou stain, × 1,000).

Plate 33–3. Viral changes consistent with CMV in lung FNA smear (H & E, × 1,000).

Plate 33–4, 33–5. Microscopic sections of the lung at autopsy demonstrating CMV inclusions (H & E; 33–4, × 400; 33–5, × 1,000).

Herpes Simplex Pneumonia

Plate 33–6. Single cells showing viral changes of herpes infection in lung FNA smear (Papanicolaou stain, × 400).

Plate 33–7 to 33–9. Multinucleated giant cells showing viral changes of herpes infection. Millipore filter preparation of needle washings of lung FNA (Papanicolaou stain, 33–7, × 400; 33–8, 33–9, × 1,000).

Plate 33–10 to 33–12. Herpes simplex changes in microscopic sections of lung tissue at autopsy (H & E; 33–10, × 400; 33–11, 33–12, × 1,000).

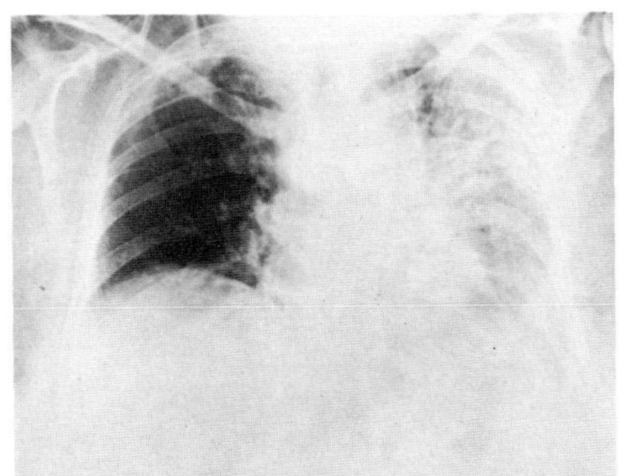

Figure A. Chest roentgenogram showing diffuse infiltrates in left lung.

PLATE 34

Pneumocystis carinii Pneumonia

Clinical History. A 56-year-old woman with chronic glomerulonephritis and previous rejection of a renal transplant was readmitted to the University of Virginia Medical Center because of fever and difficulty in breathing. A chest roentgenogram showed diffuse infiltrates in her left lung (Figure A). Because she had a history of immunosuppression (prednisone, azathioprine), the most likely causative agent of the pneumonia was an opportunistic agent. Studies of sputum and a transtracheal aspirate and of cultures from these materials did not reveal any organisms. An FNA of the left lung was performed.

Cytologic Findings. The FNA slides stained with Gomori methenamine silver stain contained groups of rounded, cup-shaped, and comma-shaped organisms 4 to 5 μm in diameter (Plate 34–1). Modified Wright-Giemsa–stained slides demonstrated doubly refractile cyst walls containing one to eight pleomorphic intracystic structures (Plate 34–2). These organisms were interpreted as being *Pneumocystis carinii.*

Pathologic Findings. Despite pentamidine therapy, the lung infiltrates progressed to both lungs; and the patient died from respiratory failure. At autopsy, both lungs were firm and heavy with massive consolidation. The cut surfaces of the lung were pink and consolidated. Microscopically, the alveoli contained a foamy, pink intra-alveolar exudate (Plate 33–3). At higher magnification, the alveolar contents consisted of a honeycomblike material with very fine-walled cystic spaces (Plate 33–4). The Gram-Weigert stain showed innumerable *Pneumocystis* organisms (Plate 33–5). The organisms stained purple-blue and measured 4 to 5 μm in diameter (Plate 33–6).

Refer to Slides 67 and 68 in Optional Slide Set.

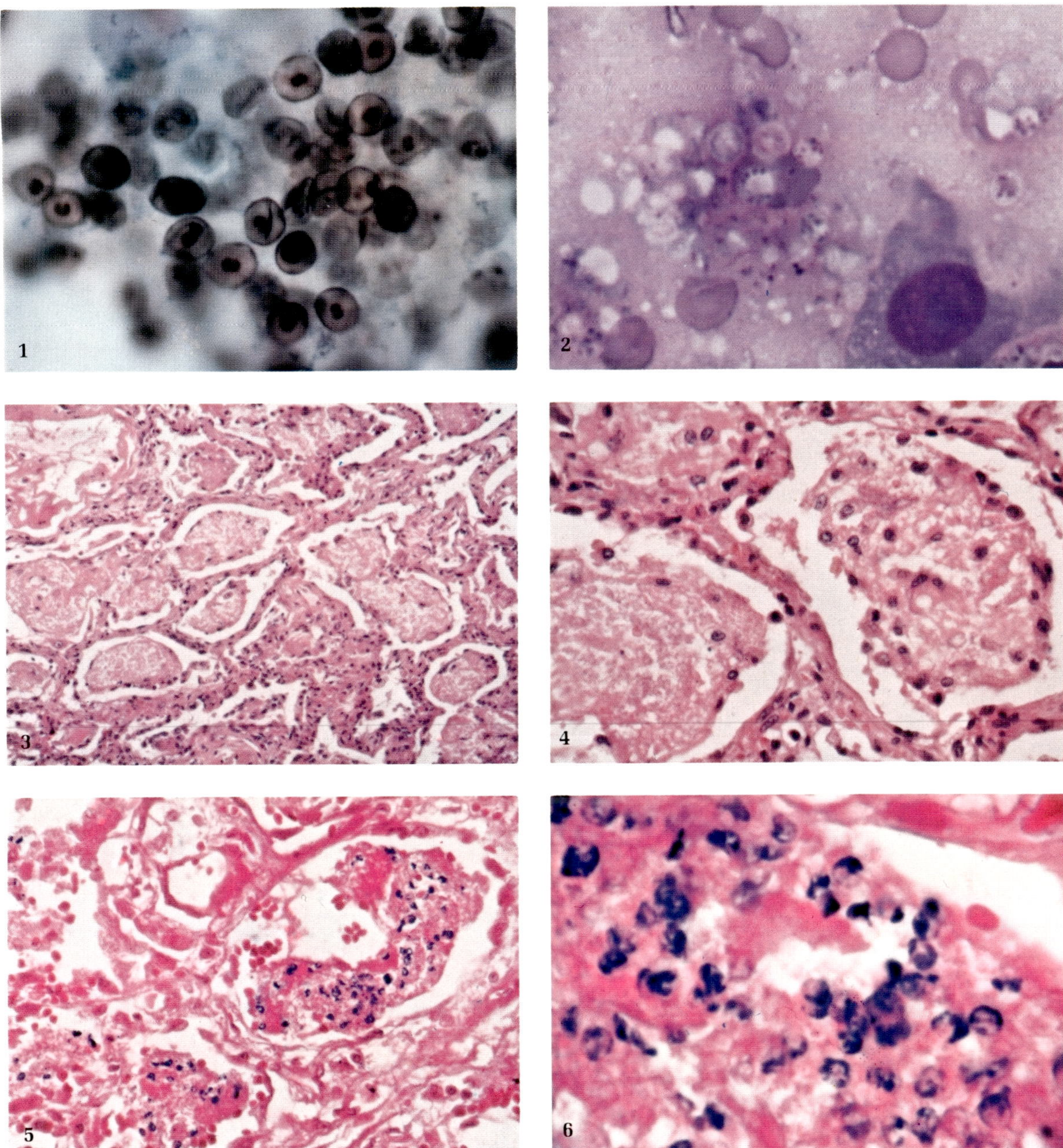

PLATE 34

Pneumocystis carinii Pneumonia

Plate 34–1. Pneumocystis carinii in lung FNA smear (Gomori methenamine silver stain, × 1,000).

Plate 34–2. P carinii cyst wall with intracystic structures in lung FNA smear (modified Wright-Giemsa stain, × 1,000).

Plate 34–3, 34–4. Pneumocystis infection in microscopic section of the lung at autopsy (H & E; 34–3, × 100; 34–4, × 400).

Plate 34–5, 34–6. P carinii in microscopic section of the lung at autopsy (Gram-Weigert stain; 34–5, × 200; 34–6, × 1,000).

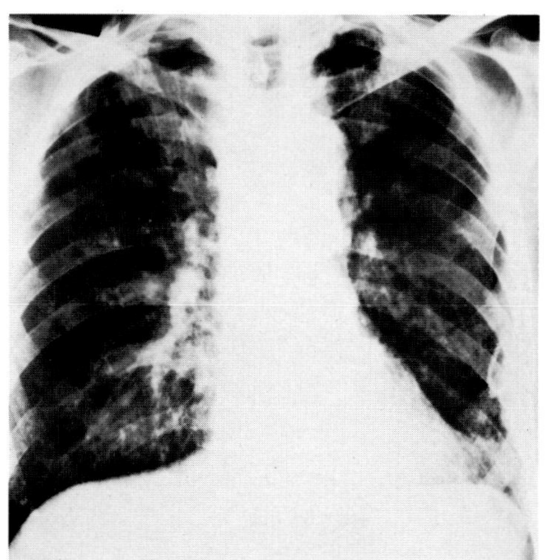

Figure A. Chest roentgenogram showing nodule in lower lobe of right lung.

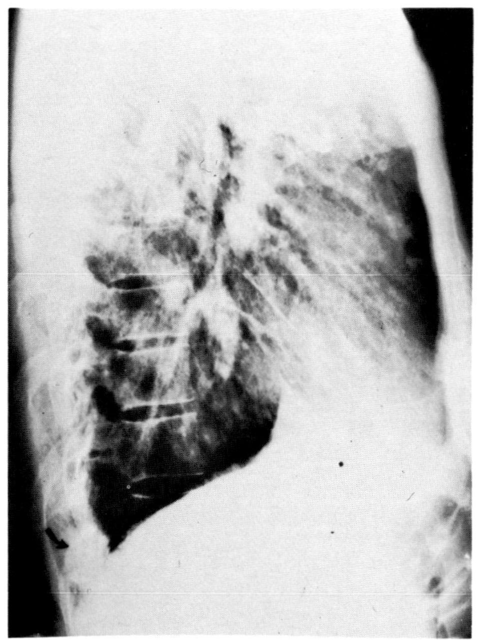

Figure B. Chest roentgenogram showing lateral view of patient shown in Figure A. A nodule in lower lobe of right lung is visible *(see arrow).*

PLATE 35

Pulmonary Nodular Amyloidosis

Clinical History. A 78-year-old man was referred to the University of Virginia Medical Center for evaluation of chronic diarrhea and weight loss. Examination of his stools showed *Entamoeba histolytica,* and he was treated with metronidazole (Flagyl) for amebiasis. A chest roentgenogram taken at admission showed an approximately 3-cm nodule in the lower lobe of his right lung (Figures A, B). Auscultation and percussion revealed that the lungs were normal. His past medical history included resection of an amyloid nodule in his left lung seven years previously. Serum electrophoresis showed an IgM monoclonal spike. Findings from rectal and bone marrow biopsies were normal.

Cytologic Findings. The FNA smears contained abundant waxy, amorphous, acellular material that was bluish green with the Papanicolaou stain (Plate 35–1, 35–2). Congo red stain identified this material as amyloid (Plate 35–3). Scattered lymphocytes were mixed with the amyloid. Occasional groups of benign ciliated respiratory cells were seen (Plate 35–4).

Pathologic Findings. A wedge resection of the lower lobe of the right lung was performed. The excised material contained a subpleural mass measuring 2.0 × 1.0 × 1.5 cm. The mass was difficult to cut, rather gritty, and translucent to grey (Plate 35–5). Microscopic sections showed the nodule to be largely composed of amorphous eosinophilic material (Plate 35–6). When stained with the Congo red, this material was red-orange (Plate 35–7). Polarized light of the Congo red–stained sections showed the apple green birefringence characteristic of amyloid (Plate 35–8).

Refer to Slides 69 and 70 in Optional Slide Set.

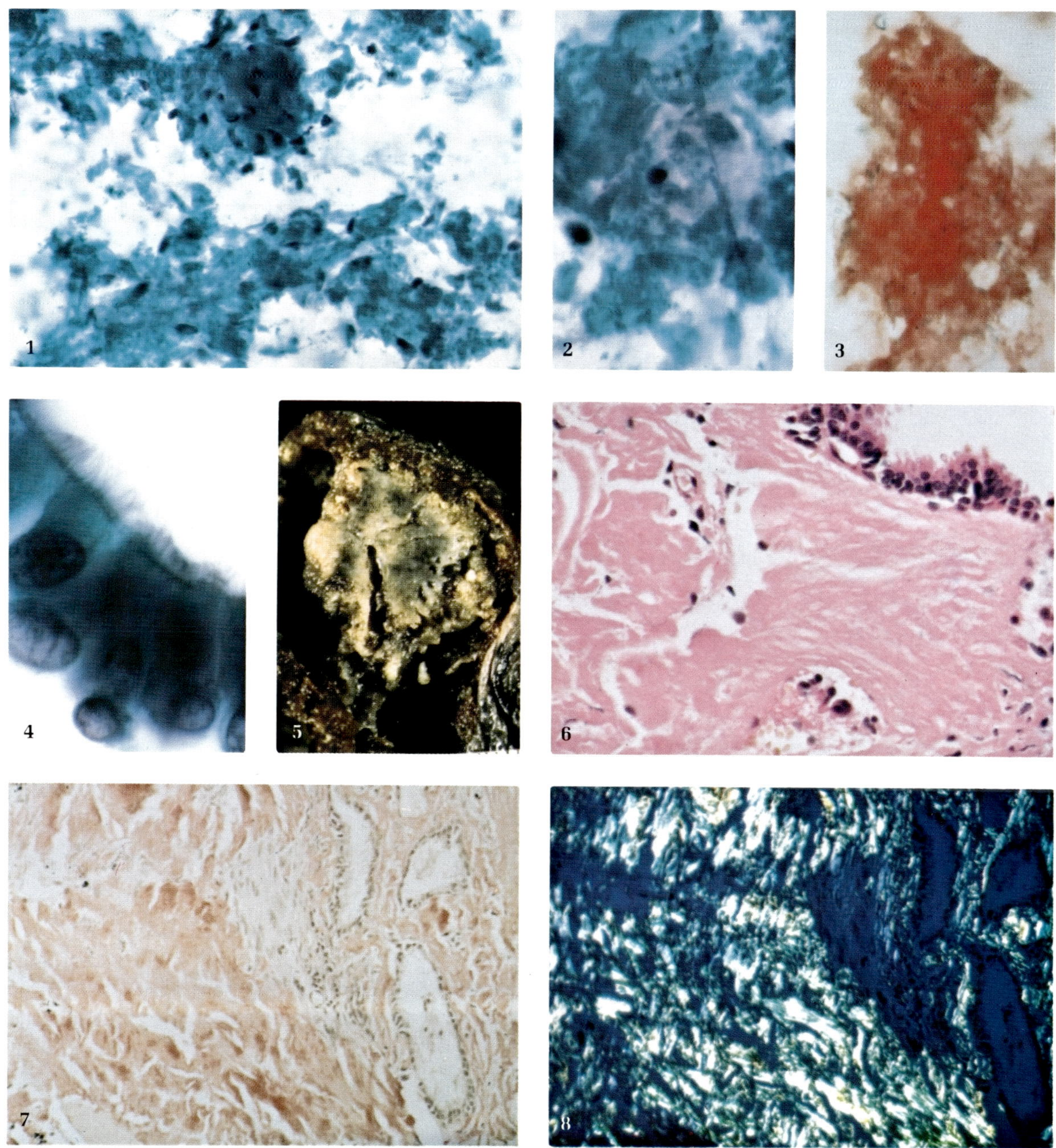

PLATE 35

Pulmonary Nodular Amyloidosis

Plate 35–1, 35–2. Amyloid in lung FNA smear (Papanicolaou stain; 35–1, × 200; 35–2, × 400).

Plate 35–3. Amyloid in lung FNA smear (Congo red stain, × 200).

Plate 35–4. Normal bronchial epithelial cells from amyloidosis in lung FNA smear (Papanicolaou stain, × 1,000).

Plate 35–5. Gross specimen of nodule in lung wedge resection.

Plate 35–6. Amyloidosis in microscopic section of the lung (H & E, × 200).

Plate 35–7. Amyloidosis in microscopic section of the lung (Congo red stain, × 100).

Plate 35–8. Same section as in 35–7, under polarized light (× 100).

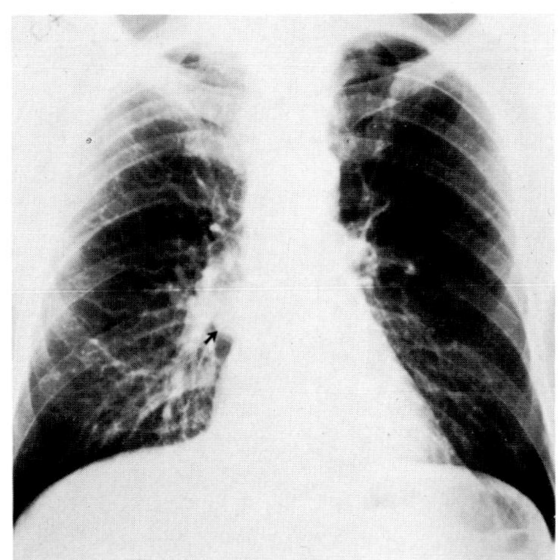

Figure A. Chest roentgenogram showing mass in lower lobe of right lung *(see arrow)*.

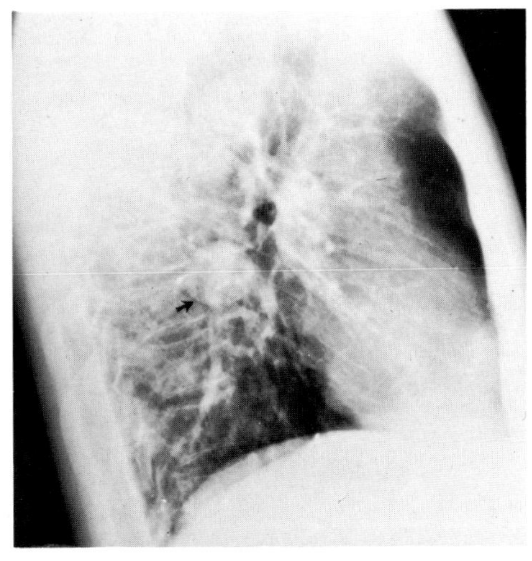

Figure B. Chest roentgenogram showing lateral view of patient shown in Figure A. A mass in lower lobe of right lung is visible (see arrow).

PLATE 36

Pulmonary Hamartoma

Clinical History. A 52-year-old man had routine chest roentgenography. On the roentgenogram, a mass was visible in the lower lobe of his right lung (Figures A, B), but he had no respiratory symptoms. He was referred to the University of Virginia Medical Center for evaluation of the lung mass. Auscultation and percussion revealed that the lungs were normal. The remainder of the examination showed no abnormalities. Bronchoscopy also showed no abnormalities, and evaluation of washings, brushings, and sputum yielded negative results. Under fluoroscopic guidance, an FNA of the lung was performed.

Cytologic Findings. The FNA smears contained scattered fragments of benign ciliated respiratory epithelium (Plate 36–1) and numerous irregularly shaped fragments of cartilaginous matrix. This matrix stained purplish with the Papanicolaou and the hematoxylin and eosin stains, and it contained scattered, oval-to-elongated vesicular nuclei (Plate 36–2, 36–3). This cytologic pattern was interpreted as a pulmonary hamartoma.

Pathologic Findings. The patient underwent a thoracotomy with excision of the mass. The specimen consisted of a sharply circumscribed, spherical tumor with a diameter of 3.1 cm. On cut section, the tumor was lobulated, grey-white, and cartilaginous in appearance (Plate 36–4). Tissue sections showed a hamartoma that contained islands of benign cartilage mixed with cleftlike spaces lined by ciliated respiratory epithelium (Plate 36–5 to 36–8). The gross and histologic features were diagnostic of a hamartoma.

Refer to Slides 71 and 72 in Optional Slide Set.

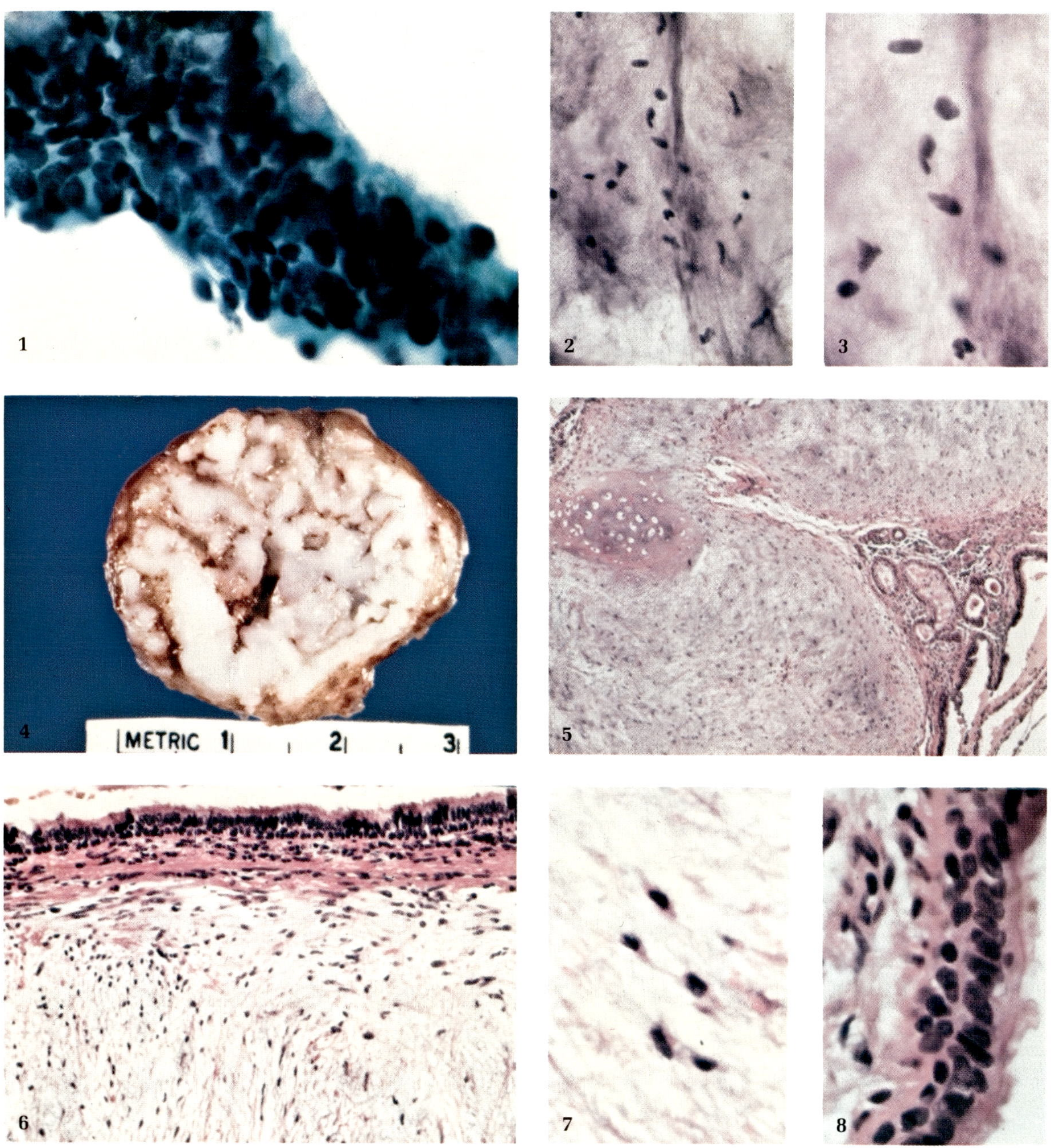

PLATE 36

Pulmonary Hamartoma

Plate 36–1. Fragment of ciliated respiratory epithelium from hamartoma in lung FNA smear (Papanicolaou stain, × 400).

Plate 36–2, 36–3. Cartilaginous matrix from hamartoma in lung FNA smear (H & E; 36–2, × 200; 36–3, × 400).

Plate 36–4. Gross appearance of hamartoma.

Plate 36–5 to 36–8. Benign cartilage mixed with cleftlike spaces lined by ciliated respiratory epithelium of hamartoma in microscopic sections of the lung, (H & E; 36–5, × 40; 36–7, × 100; 36–8, × 400).

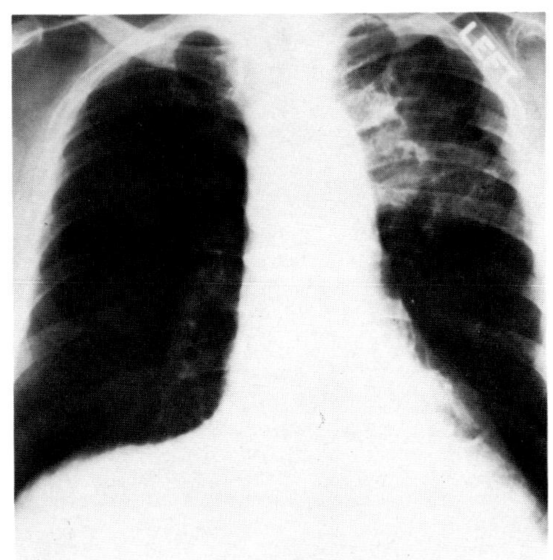

Figure A. Chest roentgenogram showing large mass in upper lobe of left lung.

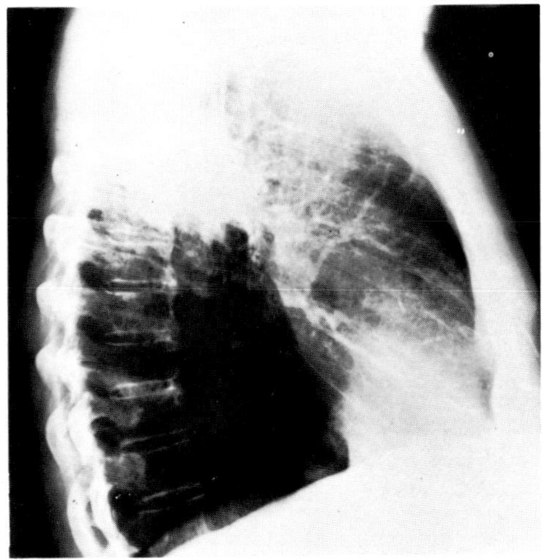

Figure B. Chest roentgenogram showing lateral view of patient shown in Figure A.

PLATE 37

Well-Differentiated Squamous Cell Carcinoma

Clinical History. A 71-year-old male smoker was admitted for evaluation of a large mass in the upper lobe of the left lung. The mass had been detected in a chest roentgenogram (Figures A, B). The patient had also been experiencing shortness of breath, increasing fatigue, and chronic cough with sputum production. A fluoroscopically guided FNA of the lung mass was performed.

Cytologic Findings. The FNA smears contained innumerable pleomorphic tumor cells lying singly or occasionally in aggregates in a background of inflammatory cells and cellular debris (Plate 37–1 to 37–5). The cells varied widely in size and shape with frequent bizarre, elongated forms (Plate 37–2, 37–4, 37–5). The cytoplasm was scant to abundant, and its responses to staining were basophilic, acidophilic, or orangophilic. Cell borders were distinct. The nuclei were hyperchromatic and varied in size and shape. The chromatin was granular and irregularly distributed. Nucleoli were absent. Cellular degeneration was common with many anucleated keratinized cells. The cell-in-cell arrangement was occasionally seen (Plate 37–3). Some of the squamous-type cells showed atypia but lacked obvious nuclear criteria of malignancy. These cells resembled dysplastic squamous cells seen in the uterine cervix (Plate 37–4, 37–5). A diagnosis of well-differentiated (keratinizing) squamous cell carcinoma was made.

Pathologic Findings. Six months following the FNA, the patient died. Microscopic sections of the lung at autopsy demonstrated a well-differentiated squamous cell carcinoma with foci of necrosis (Plate 37–6). Keratinized fiberlike cells and squamous pearls were abundant (Plate 37–7, 37–8).

Refer to Slides 73 and 74 in Optional Slide Set.

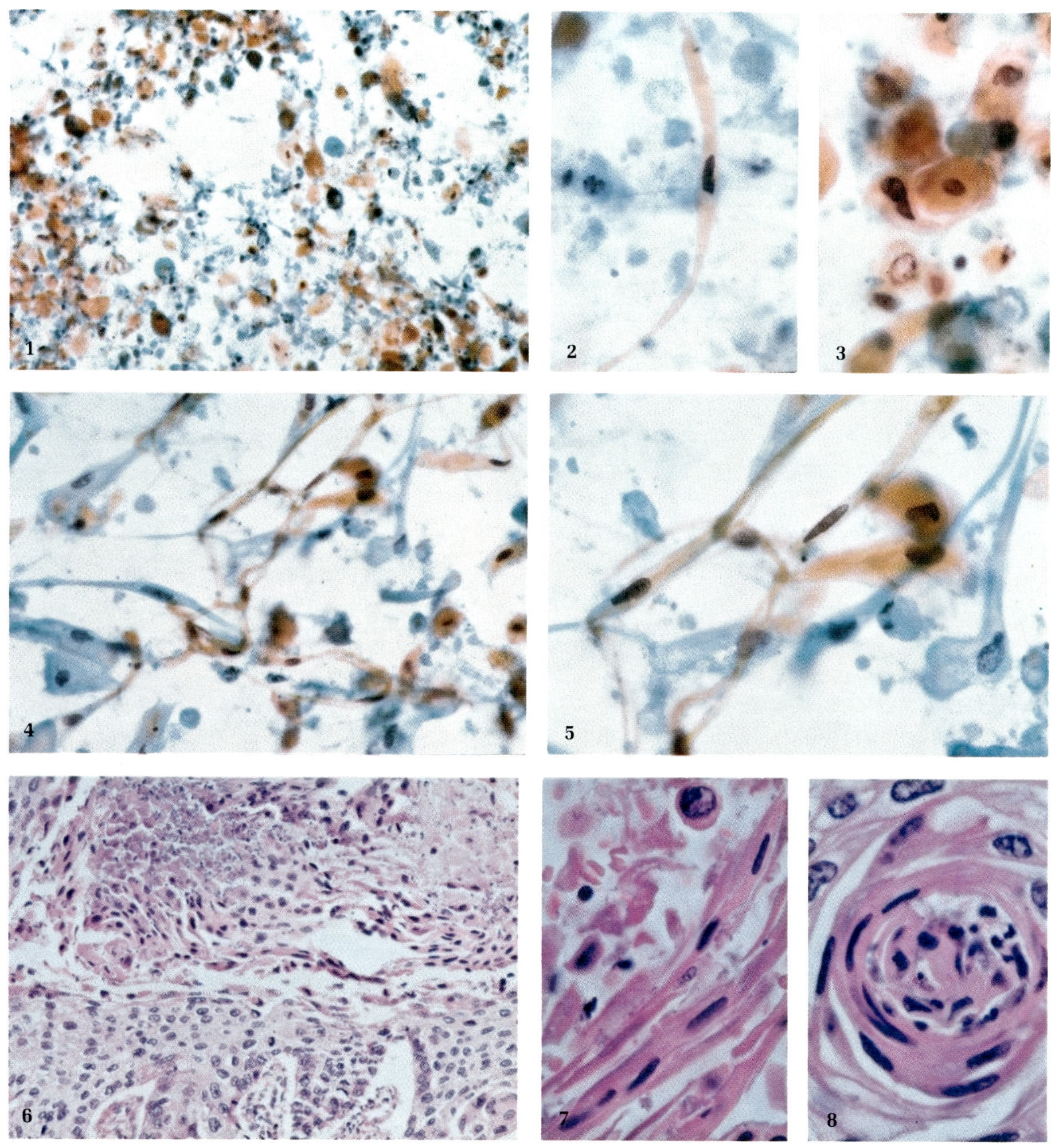

PLATE 37

Well-Differentiated Squamous Cell Carcinoma

Plate 37–1. Low-power view of well-differentiated squamous cell carcinoma in lung FNA smear (Papanicolaou stain, × 100).

Plate 37–2. Fiberlike cell from well-differentiated squamous carcinoma in lung FNA smear (Papanicolaou stain, × 400).

Plate 37–3. Cell-in-cell arrangement of keratinized cells from well-differentiated squamous cell carcinoma in lung FNA smear (Papanicolaou stain, × 400).

Plate 37–4, 37–5. Dysplastic squamous cells and fiberlike cells in squamous carcinoma in lung FNA smear (Papanicolaou stain; 37–4, × 200; 37–5, × 400).

Plate 37–6. Well-differentiated squamous cell carcinoma with focal necrosis in microscopic section of the lung at autopsy (H & E, × 200).

Plate 37–7. Keratinized fiberlike cells in microscopic section of well-differentiated squamous carcinoma of the lung at autopsy (H & E, × 400).

Plate 37–8. Abnormal squamous pearl in microscopic section of well-differentiated squamous carcinoma of the lung at autopsy (H & E, × 400).

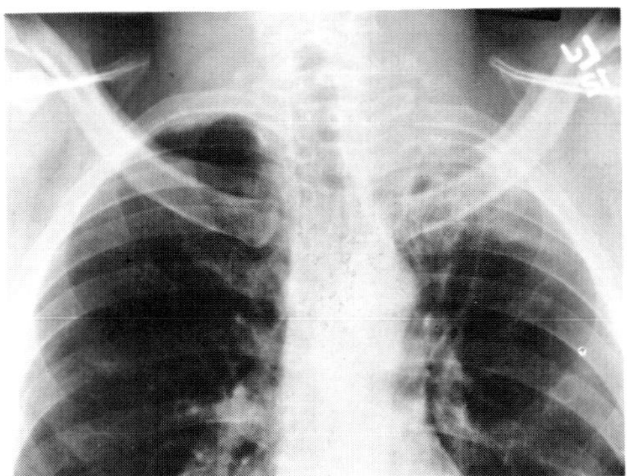

Figure A. Chest roentgenogram showing mass in apex of left lung with erosion of posterior aspect of first rib.

PLATE 38

Poorly Differentiated Squamous Cell Carcinoma with Pancoast's Syndrome

Clinical History. A 50-year-old man noticed progressive left hand and arm weakness associated with left chest and shoulder pain. He was seen in the medicine clinic at the University of Virginia Medical Center several times, and it was believed he had a degenerative joint disease or carpal tunnel syndrome. Because Horner's syndrome on the left side was noted during his latest clinic visit, apical tomograms were done and showed a lesion in the apex of the left lung eroding the posterior aspect of the first rib. He was admitted to the University of Virginia Medical Center and diagnosed as having a Pancoast's tumor with involvement of the brachial plexus.

His medical history showed a 32-pack year history of cigarette smoking and a 5-lb weight loss during the month before admission. He denied hemoptysis or coughing.

The physical examination showed ptosis of the left eyelid, anhidrosis, and moderate atrophy of the muscles of the left upper extremity. Auscultation of the lungs revealed a friction rub with decreased breath sounds at the apex of the left lung.

A chest roentgenogram showed a mass in the apex of the left lung, approximately 3 × 3 cm, which was eroding the posterior aspect of the first rib (Figure A).

Cytologic Findings. An FNA of the lung mass contained a moderate number of abnormal cells primarily in syncytial arrangements (Plate 38–1 to 38–3). The cytoplasm was scant, dense, and stained basophilic with the Papanicolaou stain or acidophilic with H & E stain. The nuclei varied in size and shape and showed some hyperchromatism. The chromatin pattern was finely granular and irregularly distributed with chromocenters present (Plate 38–2 to 38–4). Many of the cells showed single, rounded macronucleoli (Plate 38–2). These morphologic features were interpreted as consistent with poorly differentiated squamous cell carcinoma.

Pathologic Findings. The cancer was determined to be unresectable, and the patient was treated with radiation therapy. Ten months later, he died and autopsy confirmed the diagnosis of poorly differentiated squamous cell carcinoma (Plate 38–5 to 38–7).

Refer to Slides 75 and 76 in Optional Slide Set.

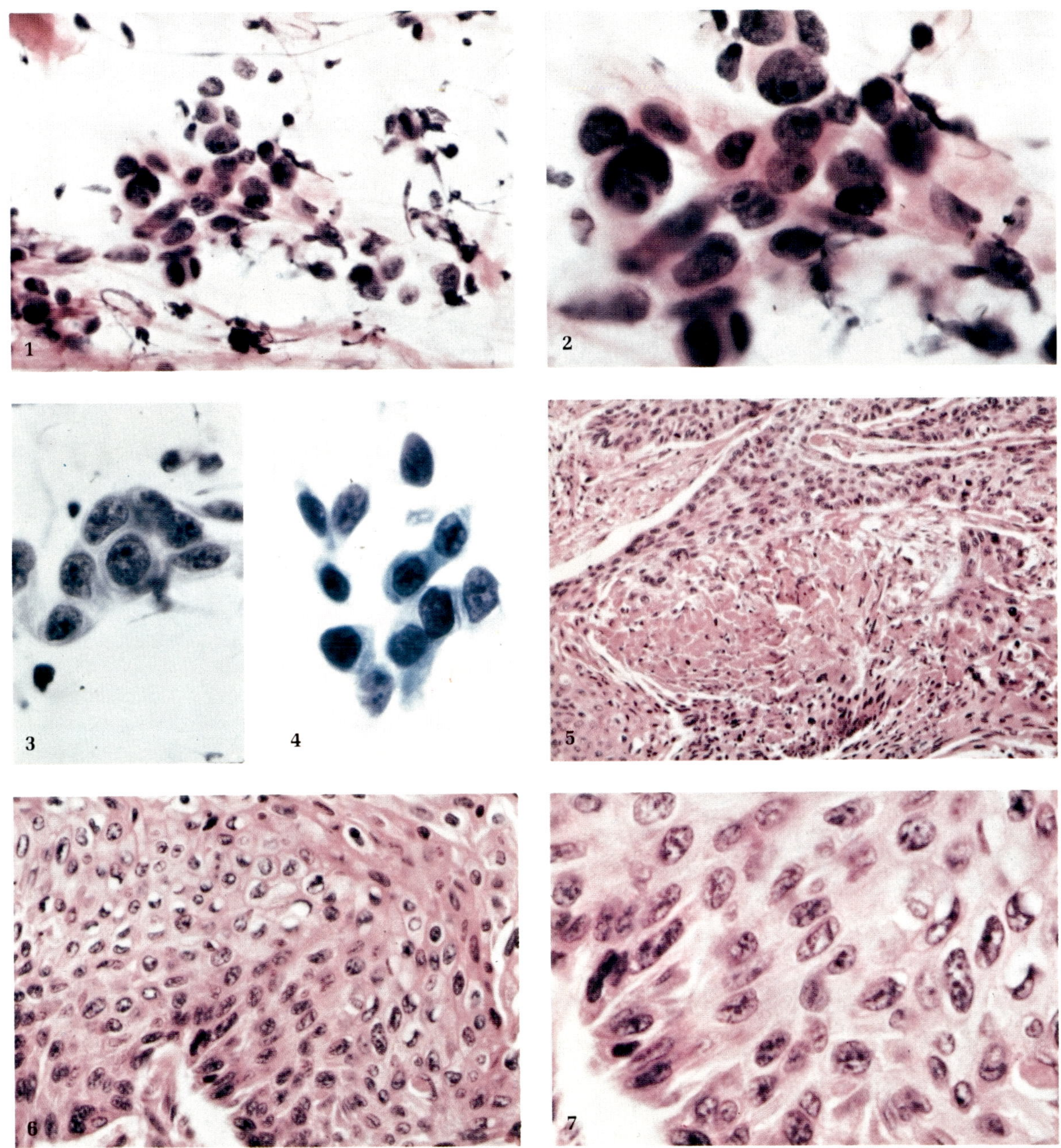

PLATE 38

Poorly Differentiated Squamous Cell Carcinoma with Pancoast's Syndrome

Plate 38–1, 38–2. Poorly differentiated squamous cell carcinoma in lung FNA smear (H & E; 38–1, × 200; 38–2, × 400).

Plate 38–3, 38–4. Poorly differentiated squamous cell carcinoma in lung FNA smear (Papanicolaou stain, × 400).

Plate 38–5 to 38–7. Poorly differentiated squamous cell carcinoma in microscopic section of the lung at autopsy (H & E; 38–5, × 100; 38–6, × 200; 38–7, × 400).

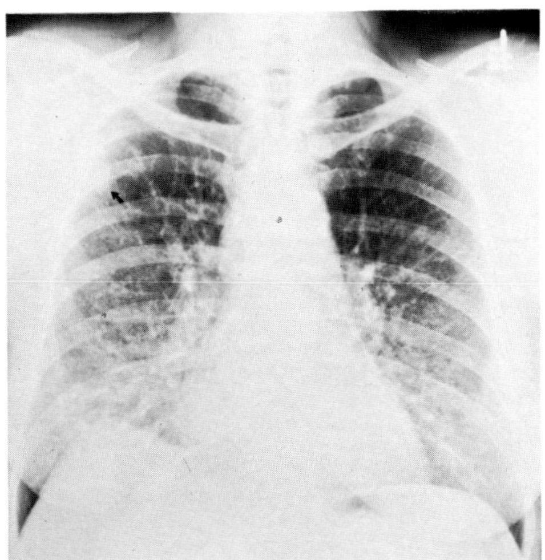

Figure A. Chest roentgenogram showing density in upper lobe of right lung *(see arrow).*

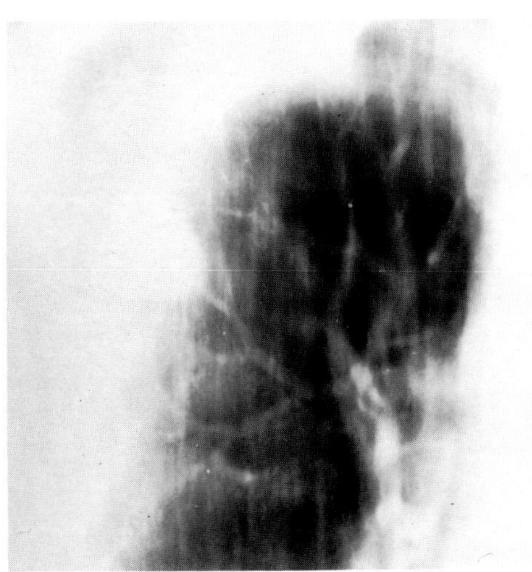

Figure B. Tomogram of same patient as shown in Figure A. A mass in upper lobe of right lung is shown at higher magnification.

PLATE 39

Adenocarcinoma

Clinical History. A 53-year-old woman was asymptomatic; however, 2 × 2-cm density was noted in the upper lobe of her right lung on a routine chest roentgenogram and a tomogram (Figures A, B). She was referred to the University of Virginia Medical Center for further evaluation. She had a 75-pack year smoking history. Auscultation and percussion revealed that her lungs were normal. The remainder of the physical examination was also normal. Fluoroscopically directed FNA of the lung was performed.

Cytologic Findings. The FNA smears were bloody and contained numerous large malignant cells arranged singly or in clusters with moderate or scant, basophilic, finely vacuolated cytoplasm (Plate 39–1 to 39–5). Although these cells varied in shape, some cells suggested glandular origin by the eccentrically placed nuclei in cylindrical cells (Plate 39–2) and cellular molding within the groups (Plate 39–6). The nuclei were round or oval and many nuclear membrane irregularities were visible (Plate 39–1). The chromatin was finely granular but irregularly distributed. The nucleoli were prominent, multiple, and sometimes irregular in shape (Plate 39–1 to 39–5). Some cells contained hypochromatic nuclei; however, this probably represented cellular degeneration (Plate 39–1). These cells were interpreted as adenocarcinoma.

Pathologic Findings. An upper lobectomy of the right lung was performed, and the excised tissue contained a nodular gray-black mass that was 2 cm at its maximum diameter. Microscopic sections showed a moderately to well differentiated adenocarcinoma (Plate 39–7, 39–8). A mass of matted lymph nodes from the hilum of the lung contained metastatic adenocarcinoma.

The patient was treated with radiation therapy administered postoperatively.

Refer to Slides 77 and 78 in Optional Slide Set.

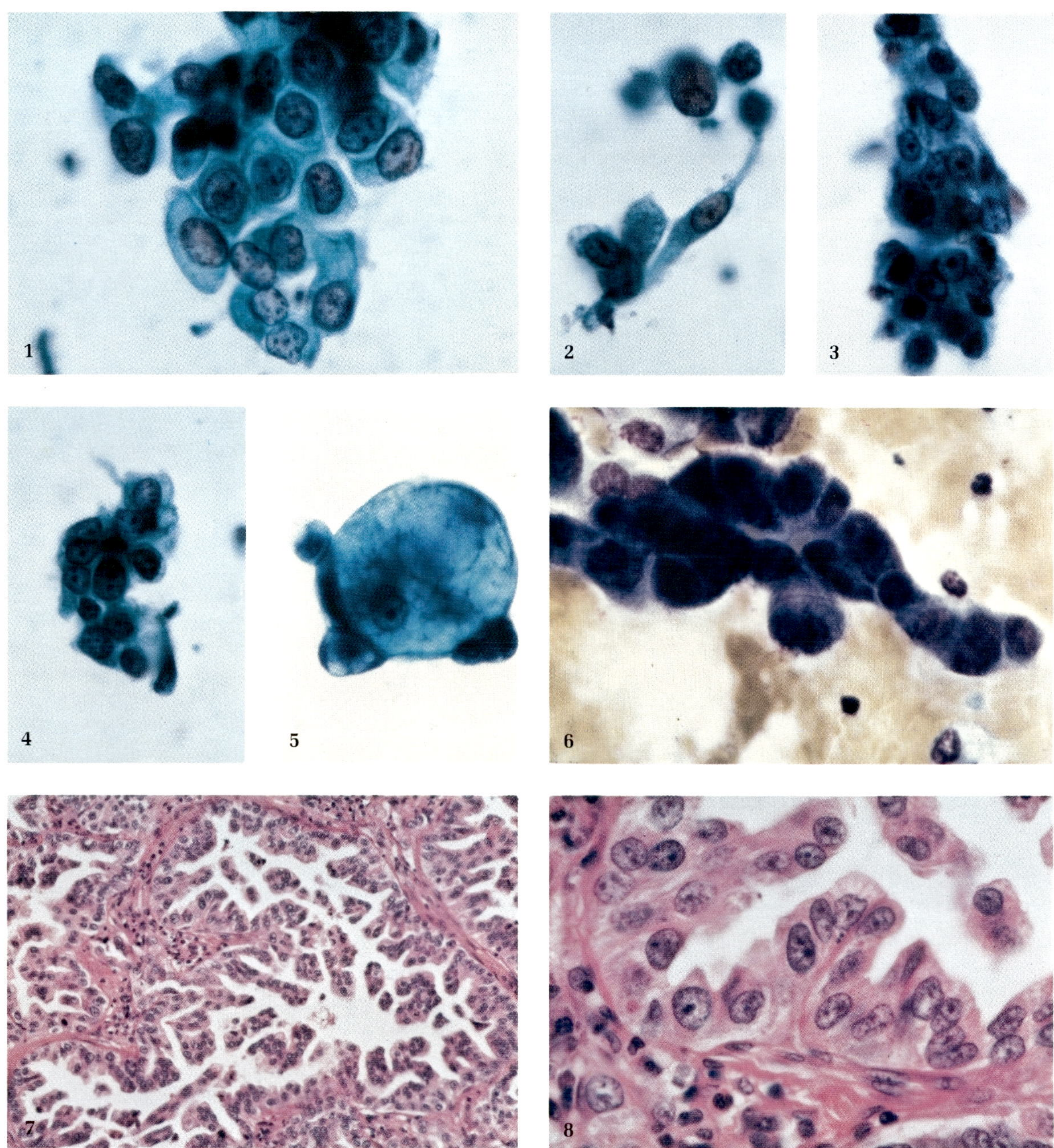

PLATE 39

Adenocarcinoma

Plate 39–1 to 39–5. Adenocarcinoma in filter preparation of needle washings of lung FNA (Papanicolaou stain, × 400).

Plate 39–6. Adenocarcinoma in lung FNA smear (modified Wright-Giemsa stain, × 400).

Plate 39–7, 39–8. Moderately differentiated to well-differentiated adenocarcinoma in microscopic sections of the lung (H & E; 39–7, × 100; 39–8, × 400).

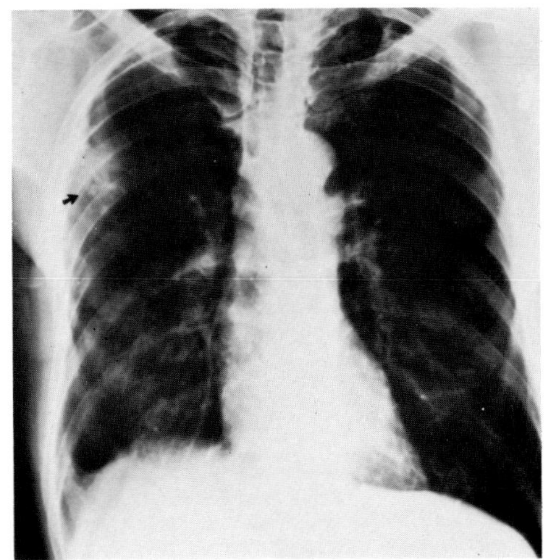

Figure A. Chest roentgenogram showing lesion in upper lobe of right lung *(see arrow).*

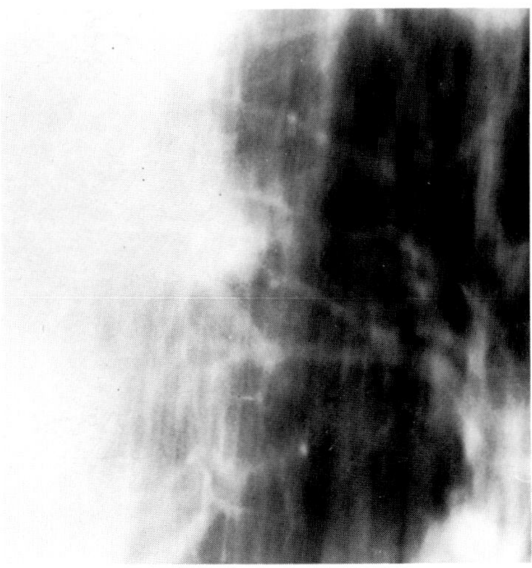

Figure B. Tomogram of same patient as seen in Figure A depicting mass in upper lobe of right lung at higher magnification.

PLATE 40

Adenocarcinoma

Clinical History. A 59-year-old man developed migratory thrombophlebitis three months before admission to another hosptial. Treatment with administration of heparin and crystalline warfarin sodium (Coumandin) was unsuccessful. During that time, the patient was experiencing pain in the right side of his chest and was coughing up blood-tinged sputum. A chest roentgenogram and tomogram taken at the time of admission revealed a right pleural effusion with a lesion in the upper lobe of the right lung (Figures A, B). He was then transferred to the University of Virginia Medical Center for further evaluation.

The physical examination showed that his chest was clear to percussion and auscultation. There was marked edema of the left lower extremity with erythema and a positive Homan's sign. The migratory thrombophlebitis was considered to be most consistent with the presence of a malignancy.

Cytologic Findings. A fluoroscopically directed FNA of the right lung mass revealed numerous malignant cells showing obvious nuclear pleomorphism (Plate 40–1 to 40–5). The round or oval, slightly hyperchromatic nuclei varied widely in size and contained single or multiple, sometimes irregular, prominent nucleoli (Plate 40–1). The nucleoli were sometimes surrounded by a clear halo (Plate 40–1, 40–2). The chromatin was finely granular and irregularly distributed (Plate 40–1). The cells were arranged singly with some syncytial arrangements. Some cells had vacuolated cytoplasm (Plate 40–4). Rare cell groups showed a suggestion of cellular molding (Plate 40–3). Although cell clustering was not observed, the presence of cytoplasmic vacuolization and rare molding suggested a malignant tumor of glandular origin. A diagnosis of adenocarcinoma was made.

Pathologic Findings. An upper lobectomy of the right lung was performed. The excised tissue contained a 5 × 6-cm, irregularly shaped, tan-grey peripheral mass adherent to the attached segment of parietal pleura. Microscopic section showed a moderately well-differentiated adenocarcinoma containing cells closely resembling those seen in the FNA (Plate 40–6 to 40–9). There was extensive invasion of lymphatics, blood vessels, parietal pleura, and hilar lymph nodes.

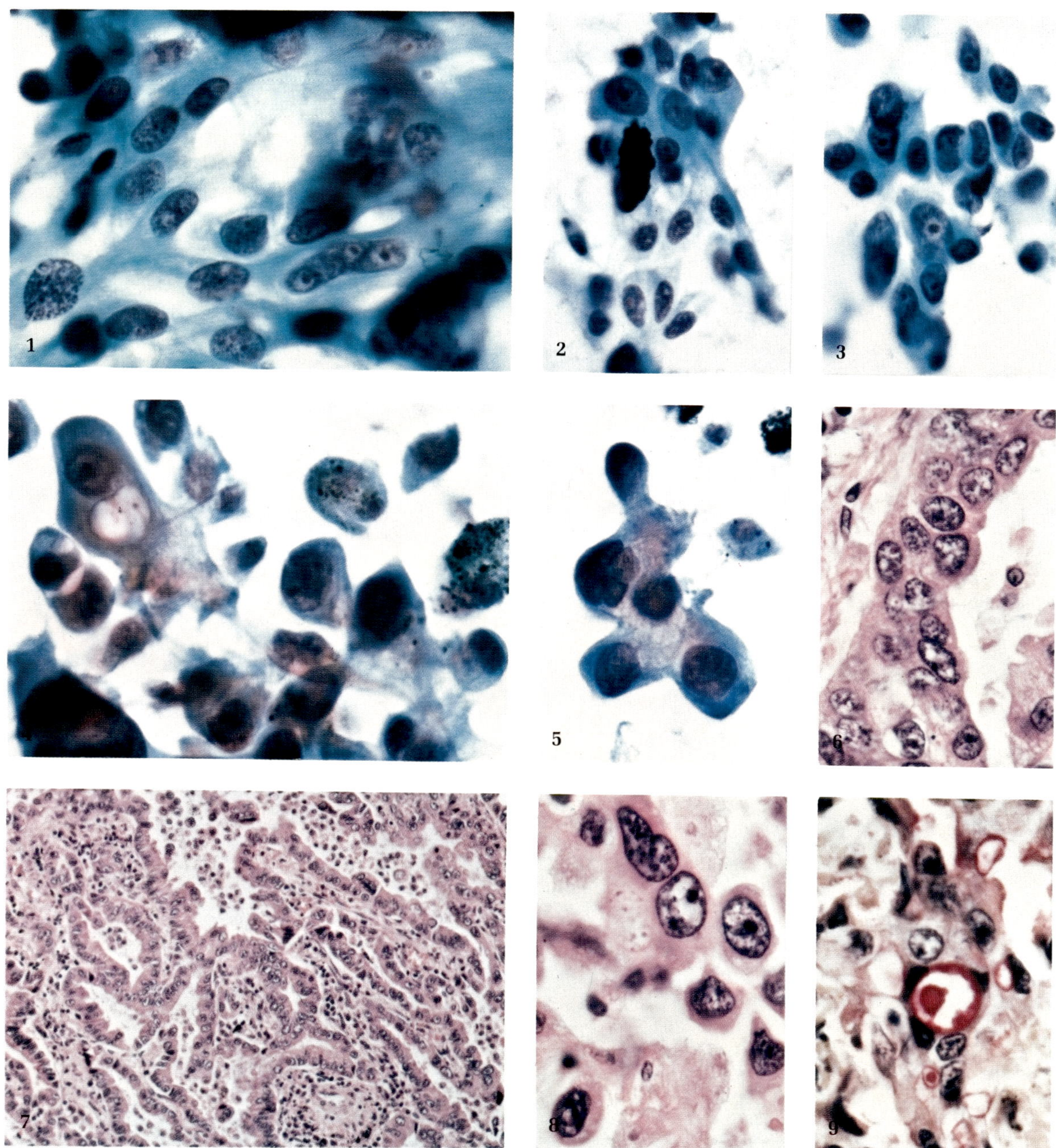

PLATE 40

Adenocarcinoma

Plate 40–1 to 40–5. Adenocarcinoma in lung FNA smear (Papanicolaou stain, × 400).

Plate 40–6 to 40–8. Lung sections showing moderately well-differentiated adenocarcinoma (H & E; 40–7, × 100; 40–6, 40–8, × 400).

Plate 40–9. Mucin-producing cell in microscopic section of adenocarcinoma of the lung (mucicarmine stain, × 400).

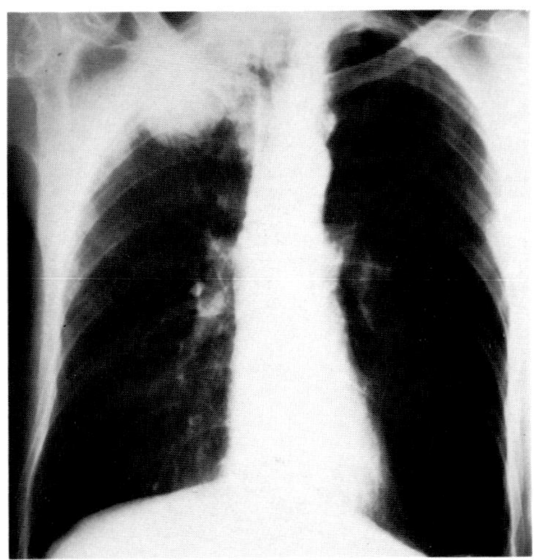

Figure A. Chest roentgenogram showing mass in upper lobe of right lung with destruction of right fourth and fifth ribs.

PLATE 41

Adenocarcinoma with Giant-Cell Component

Clinical History. A 57-year-old woman noticed the gradual onset of pain in her right scapula. A chest roentgenogram requested by her family physician demonstrated a large mass in the upper lobe of the right lung, and she was referred to the University of Virginia Medical Center.

Auscultation and percussion revealed that the lungs were normal. Examination of the back showed a mass medial to the right scapula. A chest roentgenogram showed a large mass in the upper lobe of the right lung with destruction of the right fourth and fifth ribs (Figure A).

Cytologic Findings. The FNA smears of the lung lesion contained numerous abnormal cells lying singly and in syncytial arrangements in a clean background (Plate 41–1 to 41–5). These cells varied widely in size and shape, and had moderate or abundant basophilic cytoplasm (Plate 41–1, 41–2). Frequent giant-cell forms were visible (Plate 41–4, 41–5). The large, pleomorphic, often multiple nuclei showed slight hyperchromatism and finely granular, irregularly distributed chromatin with parachromatin clearing (Plate 41–3). Irregularities in the nuclear membranes were also visible (Plate 41–2). The nucleoli were prominent, frequently multiple, and irregularly shaped (Plate 41–3). These cells were interpreted as a giant-cell variant of adenocarcinoma.

Pathologic Findings. A metastatic work-up showed no evidence of metastases. The patient received 4,500 rads of radiation to the right lung with no observed response. She underwent a palliative resection of the upper lobe of the right lung with an attached segment of the chest wall. The specimen submitted for pathologic interpretation consisted of hilar lymph nodes, the upper lobe of the right lung, and an attached segment of ribs and chest wall. Within the lung there was a 2 × 2-cm, mucoid, grey mass that extended to the adherent chest wall between the ribs to form a 5 × 4-cm tumor mass that was located just beneath the superficial surface of the chest wall. Microscopic sections showed an adenocarcinoma with a prominent giant-cell component (Plate 41–6 to 41–8). Sections of lymph nodes were free of carcinoma.

Refer to Slides 79 and 80 in Optional Slide Set.

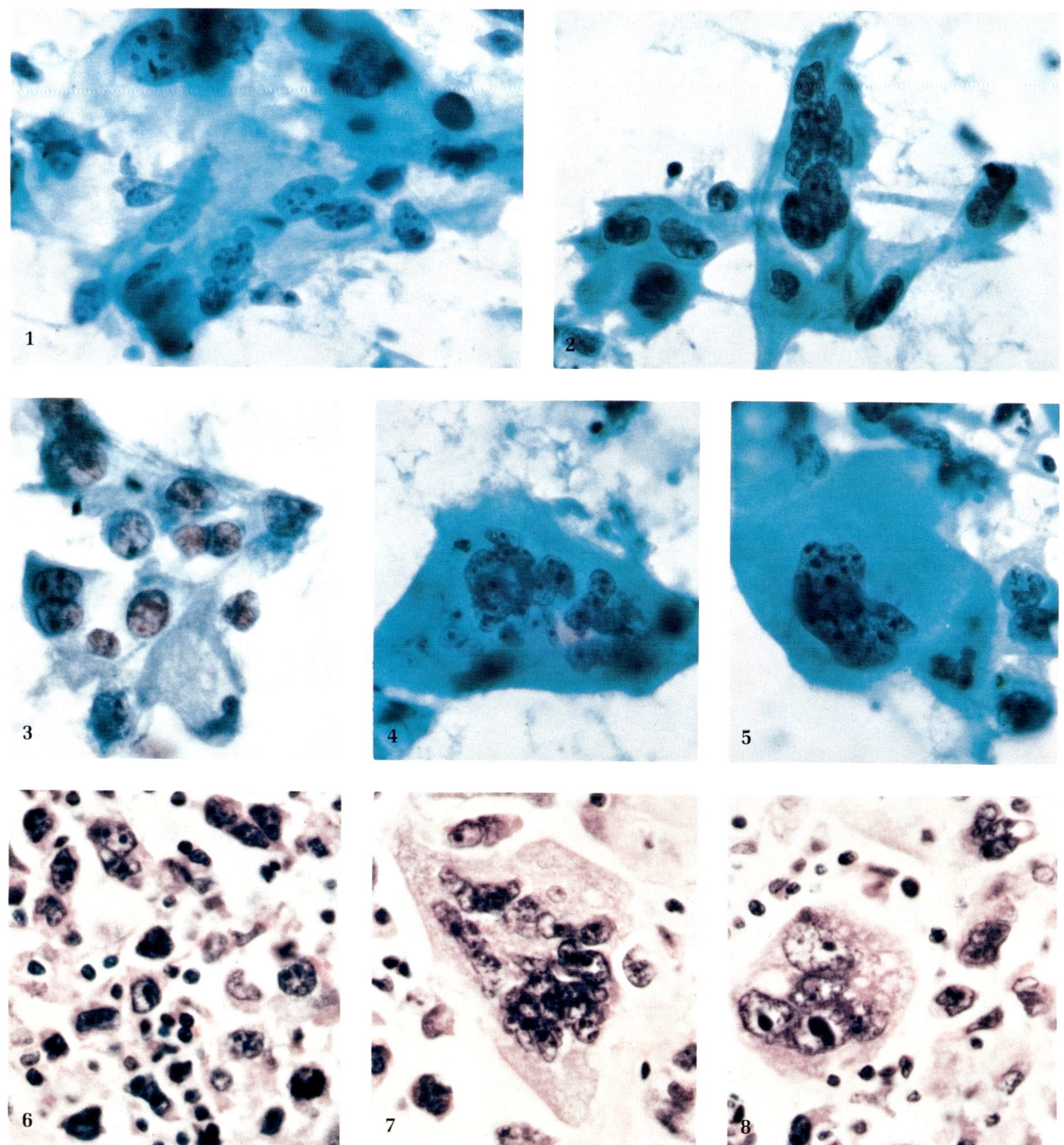

PLATE 41

Adenocarcinoma with Giant-Cell Component

Plate 41–1 to 41–5. Adenocarcinoma with giant-cell component in lung FNA smears (Papanicolaou stain, × 400).

Plate 41–6 to 41–8. Adenocarcinoma with giant-cell component in microscopic sections (H & E, × 400).

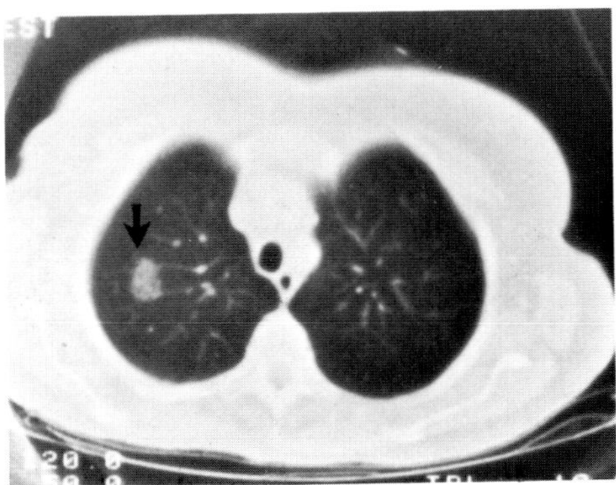

Figure A. Computerized tomography scan of chest revealing nodule in apex of right lung *(see arrow).*

PLATE 42

Bronchioloalveolar Carcinoma

Clinical History. A 56-year-old female smoker with myasthenia gravis had a six-week history of progressive weakness of her neck muscles. This weakness progressed to total neck drop the week before admission to the University of Virginia Medical Center. Nine years before, she had a laryngectomy and right radical neck dissection for squamous carcinoma of the larynx. The physical examination showed no evidence of recurrence in the head and neck area and no lymphadenopathy. Testing with edrophonium chloride solution (Tensilon) demonstrated diffuse weakness of the proximal muscles of all four extremities as well as diplopia in all directions. A computerized tomography scan of the chest revealed no thymoma but a 2.0 to 2.5-cm nodule in the apex of her right lung (Figure A). During thoracotomy, an FNA of the mass was performed.

Cytologic Findings. The FNA smears contained numerous round or oval abnormal cells arranged singly, in syncytial arrangements, and in papillary clusters (Plate 42–1 to 42–4). These clusters represented the cytologic counterpart of the tumor papillae seen in the histologic sections (Plate 42–5 to 42–7). The basophilic cytoplasm was scanty and finely granular. Cell borders were indistinct. The nuclei were generally round or oval, mildly hyperchromatic, and varied in size. Occasional indentations in the nuclear membranes were visible (Plate 42–2). Rare cytoplasmic invaginations into the nuclei forming a clear space were seen (Plate 42–1). The chromatin pattern was finely granular but irregularly distributed. One or more prominent nucleoli were found in every cell. A diagnosis of bronchioloalveolar carcinoma was made.

Pathologic Findings. An upper lobectomy of the right lung was performed, and the excised tissue contained a grey-tan, poorly defined 2-cm mass. Histologic sections showed an adenocarcinoma of bronchioloalveolar type that consisted of tall columnar epithelial cells lining the alveolar walls. The cancer cells often formed papillary projections within the alveolar spaces (Plate 42–5 to 42–7). The cells were frequently peg-shaped with nuclei situated near their points of attachment to the alveolar walls (Plate 42–6). Nuclei were quite variable in size and shape.

Refer to Slides 81 and 82 in Optional Slide Set.

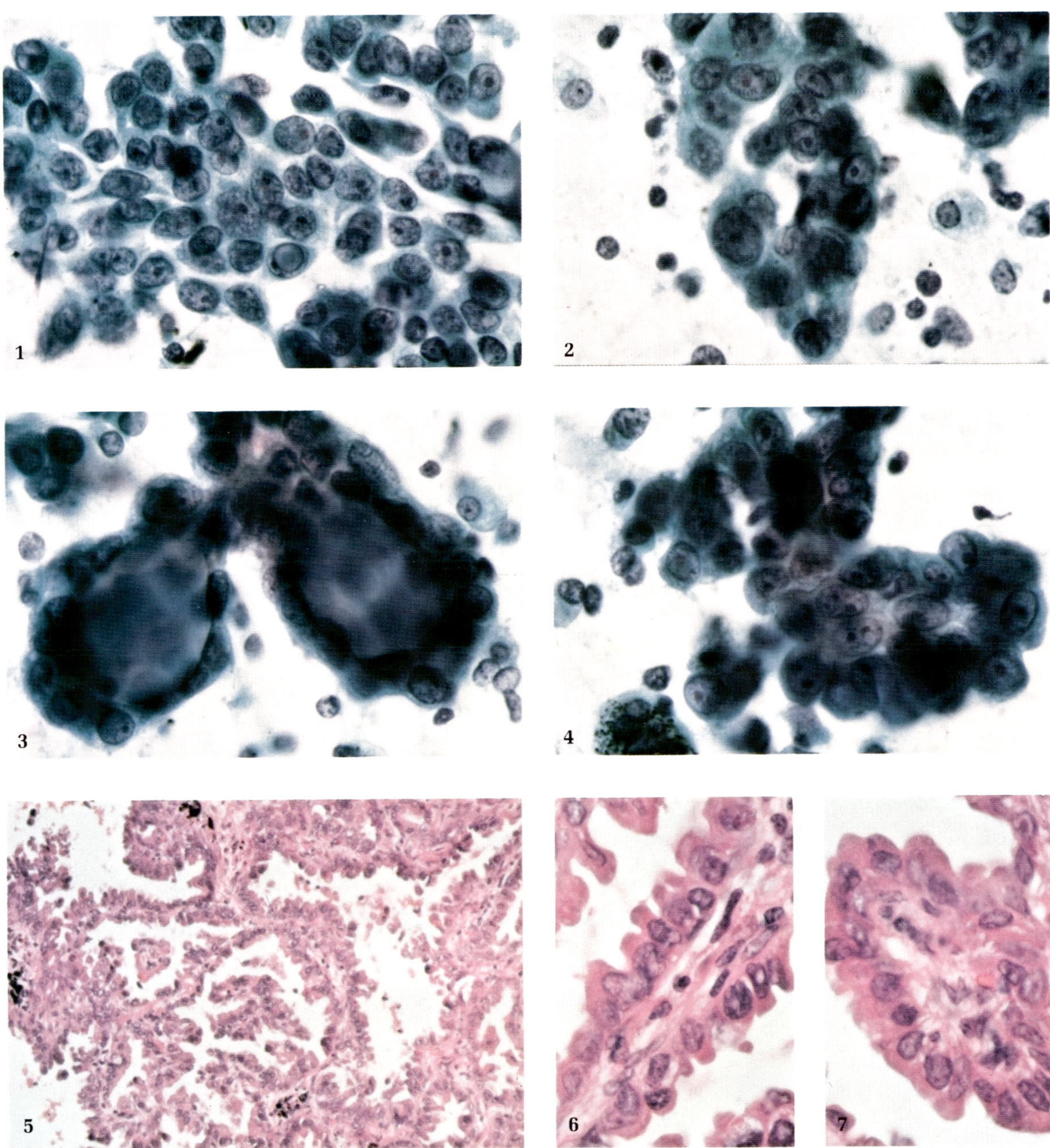

PLATE 42

Bronchioloalveolar Carcinoma

Plate 42–1 to 42–4. Bronchioloalveolar carcinoma in lung FNA smear (Papanicolaou stain, × 400).

Plate 42–5 to 42–7. Bronchioloalveolar-type adenocarcinoma in microscopic section of the lung (H & E; 42–5 × 100; 42–6, 42–7, × 400).

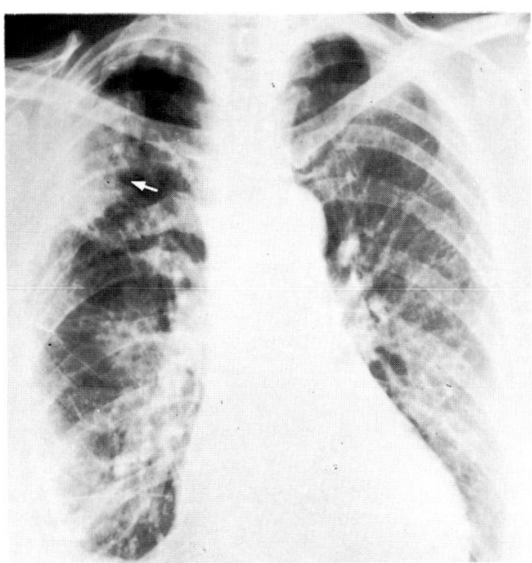

Figure A. Chest roentgenogram showing mass in upper lobe of right lung *(see arrow).*

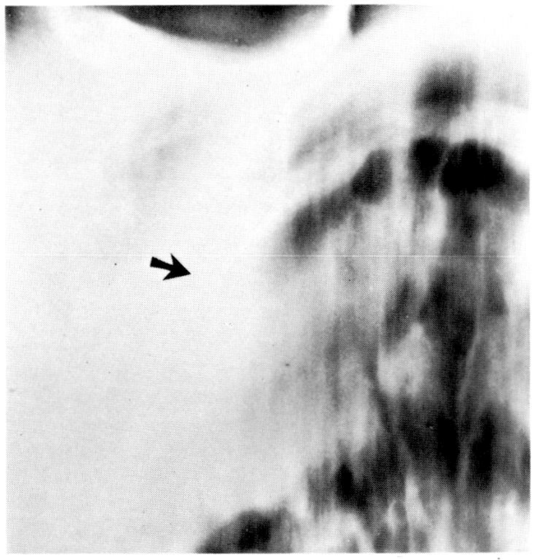

Figure B. Chest roentgenogram showing lateral view of patient shown in Figure A. A mass in upper lobe of right lung is visible *(see arrow).*

PLATE 43

Large-Cell Undifferentiated Carcinoma

Clinical History. A 65-year-old woman was referred to the University of Virginia Medical Center for evaluation of a mass in the upper lobe of the right lung. Two years before admission, she had an episode of hemoptysis. She again had hemoptysis three months before admission along with some pain over the right midthoracic area. The hemoptysis had persisted intermittently since then. She noticed a nonproductive cough but was unaware of fever, chills, or weight loss. Results of her physical examination were within normal limits. A chest roentgenogram and tomogram showed a mass in the upper lobe of the right lung (Figures A, B). Findings from bronchoscopy with biopsies and cell samplings were negative for malignancy. The patient then underwent an FNA of the mass under fluoroscopic guidance.

Cytologic Findings. The FNA smears contained a moderate number of large, irregular cells arranged singly and in aggregates (Plate 43–1). The variably sized nuclei were round or oval with some irregular forms (Plate 43–2). The chromatin pattern was finely granular but irregularly distributed. The nucleoli were large, round, and often multiple (Plate 43–2 to 43–5). The cytoplasm was moderate in amount, basophilic, and finely granular with occasional vacuoles. Rare mitotic figures were visible (Plate 43–4). Special stains for mucin were negative. Because none of the cells showed differentiation into glandular or squamous cells, a diagnosis of large-cell undifferentiated carcinoma was made.

Pathologic Findings. The patient received 4,500 rads of radiation preoperatively because the carcinoma had invaded the chest wall with destruction of portions of the second and third ribs. A composite resection of the second and third ribs with a large wedge resection of the upper lobe of the right lung was performed. Within the lung segment there was a firm, 3 × 2-cm tan-yellow mass that was adherent to the two attached ribs. Microscopic examination showed a large-cell undifferentiated carcinoma of the lung with direct extension into the adherent ribs (Plate 43–6 to 43–8). Mucicarmine stain was negative (Plate 43–8).

Refer to Slides 83 and 84 in Optional Slide Set.

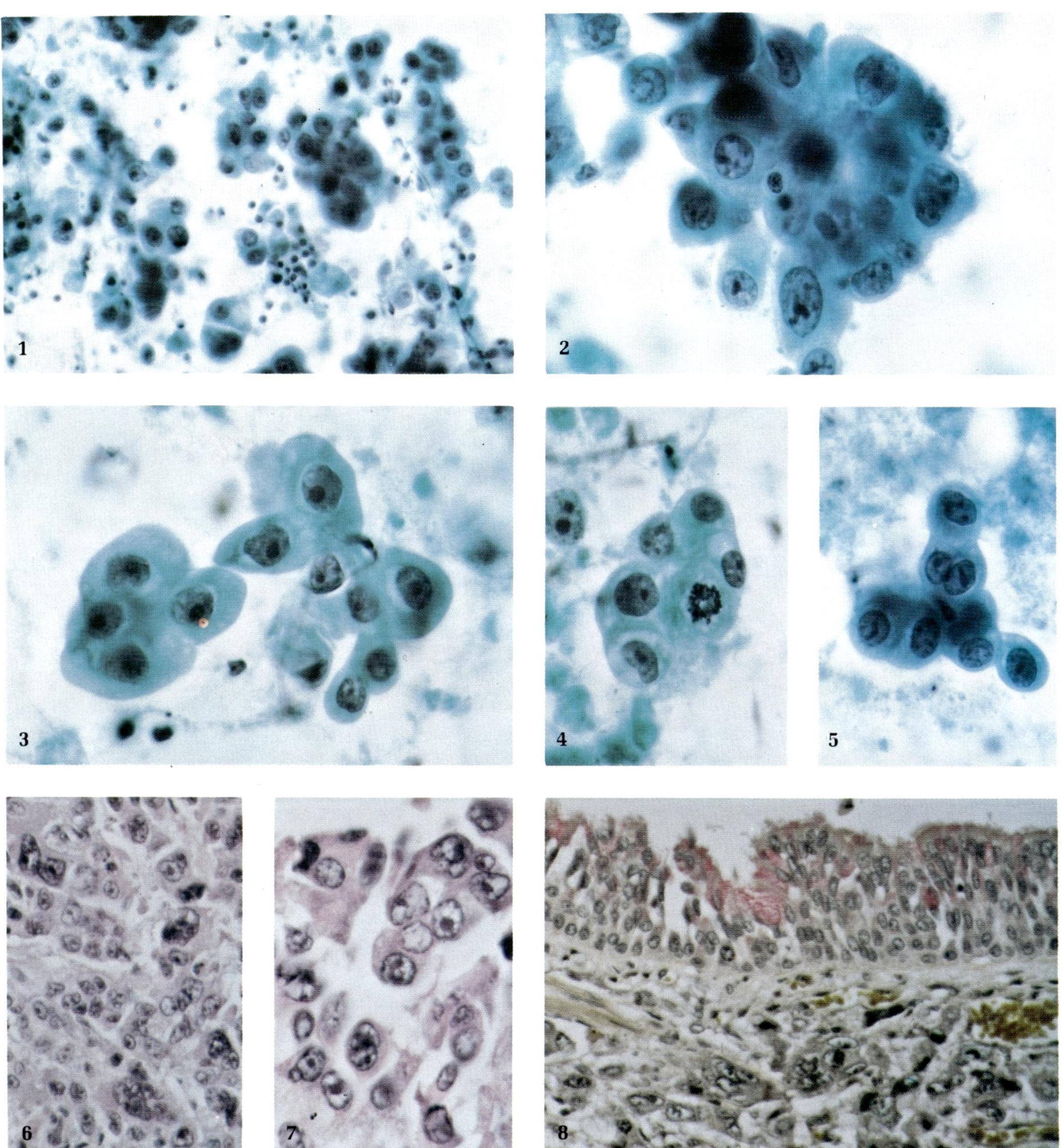

PLATE 43

Large-Cell Undifferentiated Carcinoma

Plate 43–1 to 43–5. Large-cell undifferentiated carcinoma in lung FNA smear (Papanicolaou stain; 43–1, × 200; 42–2 to 42–5, × 400).

Plate 43–6, 43–7. Microscopic sections of large-cell undifferentiated carcinoma of the lung (H & E; 42–6, × 200; 42–7, × 400).

Plate 43–8. Normal bronchial epithelium with underlying large-cell undifferentiated carcinoma in microscopic section of the lung (mucicarmine stain, × 200).

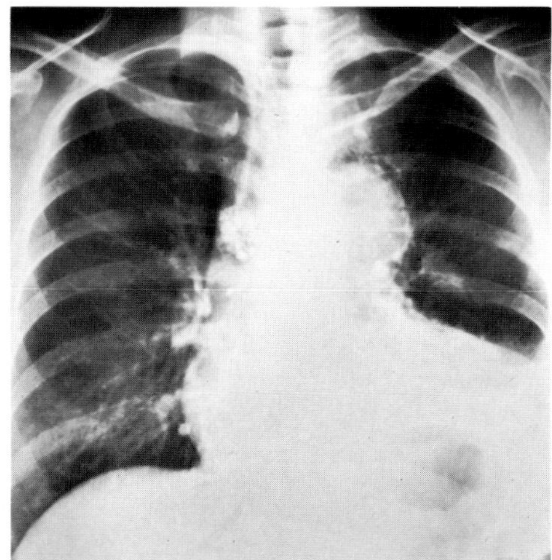

Figure A. Chest roentgenogram showing hilar mass in left lung with elevation of left hemidiaphragm and pleural effusion.

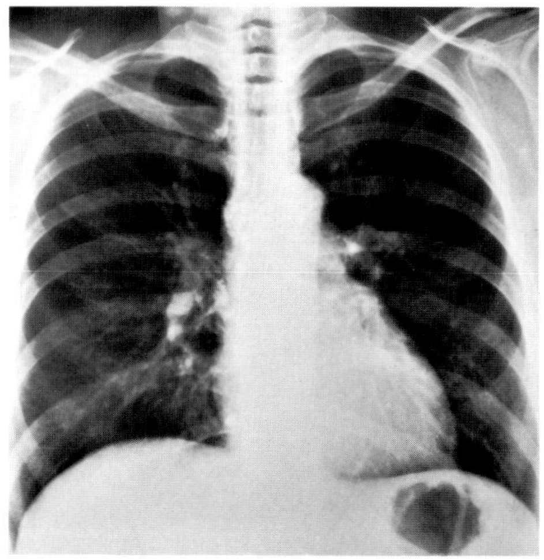

Figure B. Chest roentgenogram of same patient shown in Figure A six months before roentgenogram in Figure A was taken. No evidence of a mass is shown.

PLATE 44

Small-Cell Undifferentiated (Oat Cell) Carcinoma

Clinical History. A 57-year-old woman with a 30-pack year history of cigarette smoking developed a cough, hemoptysis, and hoarseness. A chest roentgenogram revealed a left hilar mass with elevation of the left hemidiaphragm and a left pleural effusion (Figure A). A chest roentgenogram done six months previously showed no evidence of a mass (Figure B). Bronchoscopy demonstrated paralysis of the left vocal cord and extrinsic narrowing of the bronchus in the upper lobe of the left lung with mucosal changes suggestive of carcinoma. Cells obtained from thoracentesis, bronchial washings and brushings showed no evidence of malignancy; but a biopsy was not performed because of an abnormal prothrombin time. The patient was referred to the University of Virginia Medical Center for further evaluation and treatment. Evaluation of cells obtained from sputum and a repetition of bronchial washing and brushing again revealed no evidence of malignancy. An FNA of the lung mass was performed under fluoroscopic guidance.

Cytologic Findings. The FNA smears contained numerous small but variably sized cells with scanty basophilic cytoplasm and indistinct cell borders (Plate 44–1 to 44–3). The cells were arranged singly and in aggregates with frequent nuclear molding (Plate 44–4). The enlarged nuclei varied in size and shape and were markedly hyperchromatic. The chromatin was granular and irregularly distributed. Some nuclei contained single, small nucleoli. Mitotic figures were frequent (Plate 44–1, 44–5). The smear background was composed of necrotic cellular debris. Because of the small size and prominent nuclear molding, these cells were obviously malignant and were diagnosed as small-cell undifferentiated (oat cell) carcinoma.

Pathologic Findings. Despite treatment with radiation and chemotherapy, the patient developed cerebral metastases and died eight months following the FNA diagnosis. Autopsy demonstrated a malignant tumor of the lung involving the brain, liver, and many lymph nodes. Microscopic sections of the lung showed a small-cell undifferentiated carcinoma characterized by small, hyperchromatic nuclei of varying size and shape, high nuclear:cytoplasmic ratio, and distinct nuclear molding, which were features identical to those seen in the FNA (Plate 44–6, 44–7).

Refer to Slides 85 and 86 in Optional Slide Set.

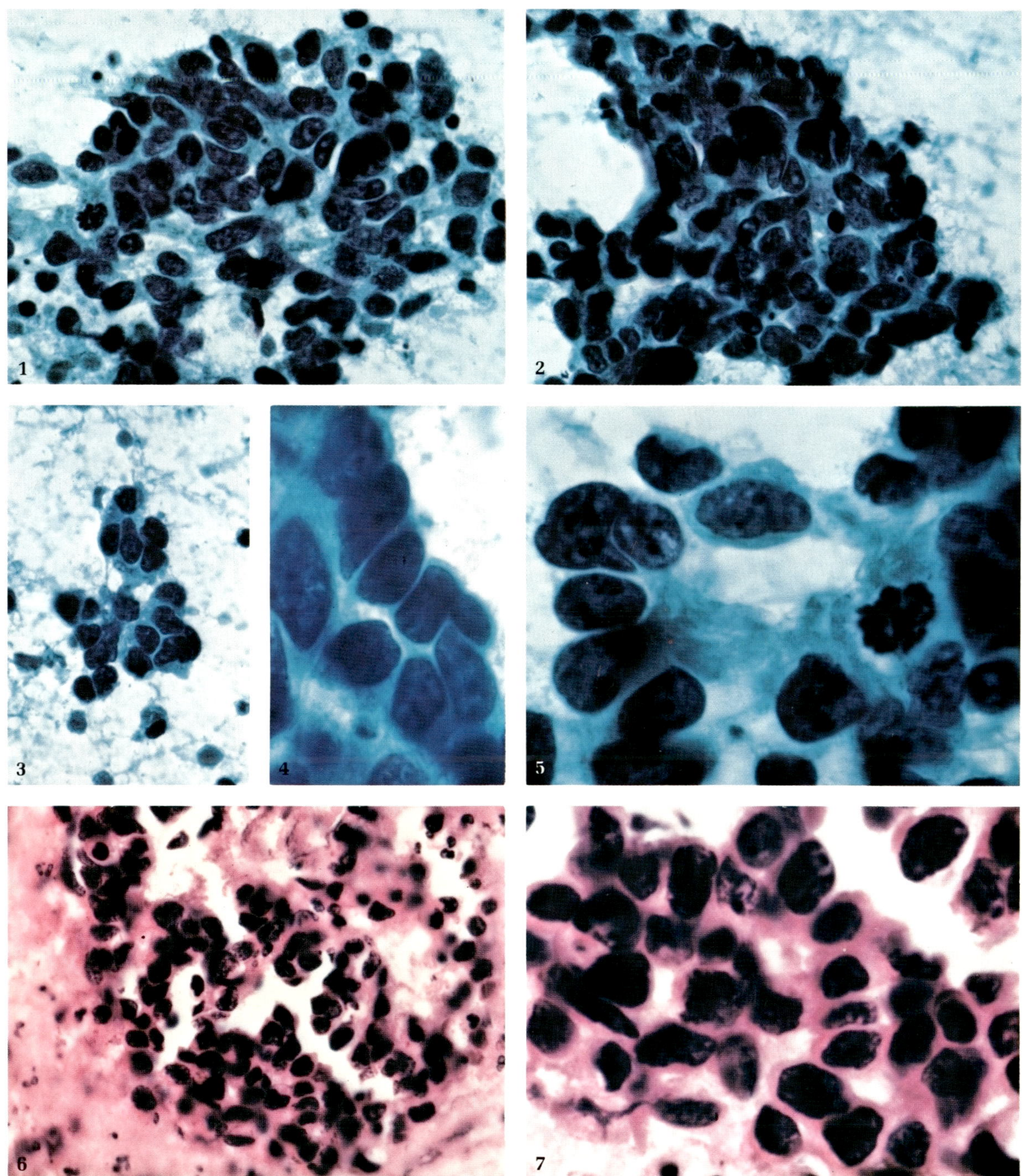

PLATE 44

Small-Cell Undifferentiated (Oat Cell) Carcinoma

Plate 44–1 to 44–3. Small-cell undifferentiated carcinoma in lung FNA smears (Papanicolaou stain, × 400).

Plate 44–4, 44–5. Prominent nuclear molding of small-cell undifferentiated carcinoma in FNA smear of the lung (Papanicolaou stain, × 1,000).

Plate 44–6 to 44–7. Microscopic sections of the lung at autopsy showing small-cell undifferentiated carcinoma (H & E; 44–6, × 400; 44–7, × 1,000).

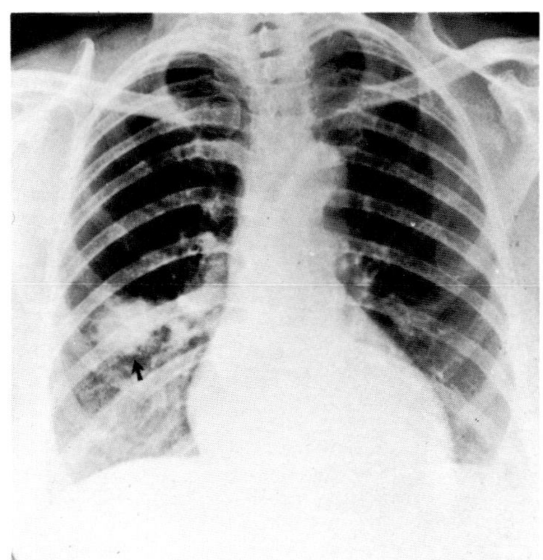

Figure A. Chest roentgenogram showing density in middle lobe of right lung.

PLATE 45

Carcinoid

Clinical History. A 69-year-old female nonsmoker was admitted to another hospital with a compression fracture of the first lumbar vertebra and resulting severe back pain after a fall. The physical examination showed no other abnormalities, although she had a history of abnormal chest roentgenograms, first noted two years before admission. After her back condition stabilized, the chest abnormality was evaluated. The chest roentgenogram taken at the time of admission showed a 4-cm density in the middle lobe of the right lung. The density appeared to be at the level of the minor fissure (Figure A). Cells from the sputum showed no evidence of malignancy.

The patient then underwent an FNA under fluoroscopic guidance. The FNA smears were interpreted as compatible with oat cell carcinoma. This diagnosis was inconsistent with the patient's lack of pulmonary symptoms. Additional evaluation for tumor staging yielded no further evidence of malignancy. Was this lesion truly an oat cell carcinoma of the lung? Perhaps it was a metastasis of another tumor that would be amenable to surgery. Bilateral bone marrow biopsies were performed and showed metastatic tumor that was most likely a carcinoid tumor. Because of the discrepancies in interpretation, the FNA and bone marrow slides were sent to the University of Virginia Pathology Department for evaluation.

Cytologic Findings. The FNA slides contained numerous syncytial masses of small cells with scant basophilic cytoplasm (Plate 45–1 to 45–3). The round or oval nuclei varied in size and often overlapped within the groups but did not show nuclear molding. The chromatin pattern was finely granular and evenly distributed with frequent chromocenters. The nuclear envelope was usually uniform and even. These cells lacked the pleomorphism and chromatin abnormalities of an oat cell carcinoma and were thought to represent a carcinoid tumor. Sheets of mesothelial cells easily recognized by their cuboidal shape, uniform vesicular nuclei, prominent nucleoli, distinct cell borders, and orderly arrangement were also present on the slides (Plate 45–4).

Pathologic Findings. Sections from the bone marrow biopsy showed a small-cell neoplasm, interpreted as a carcinoid (Plate 45–5, 45–6). Significantly absent in the tissue were the crush artifact and molding characteristics of oat cell carcinoma. Because of the presence of metastasis, no definitive therapy was recommended. Two years later, the patient was alive and without evidence of progressive disease.

Refer to Slides 87 and 88 in Optional Slide Set.

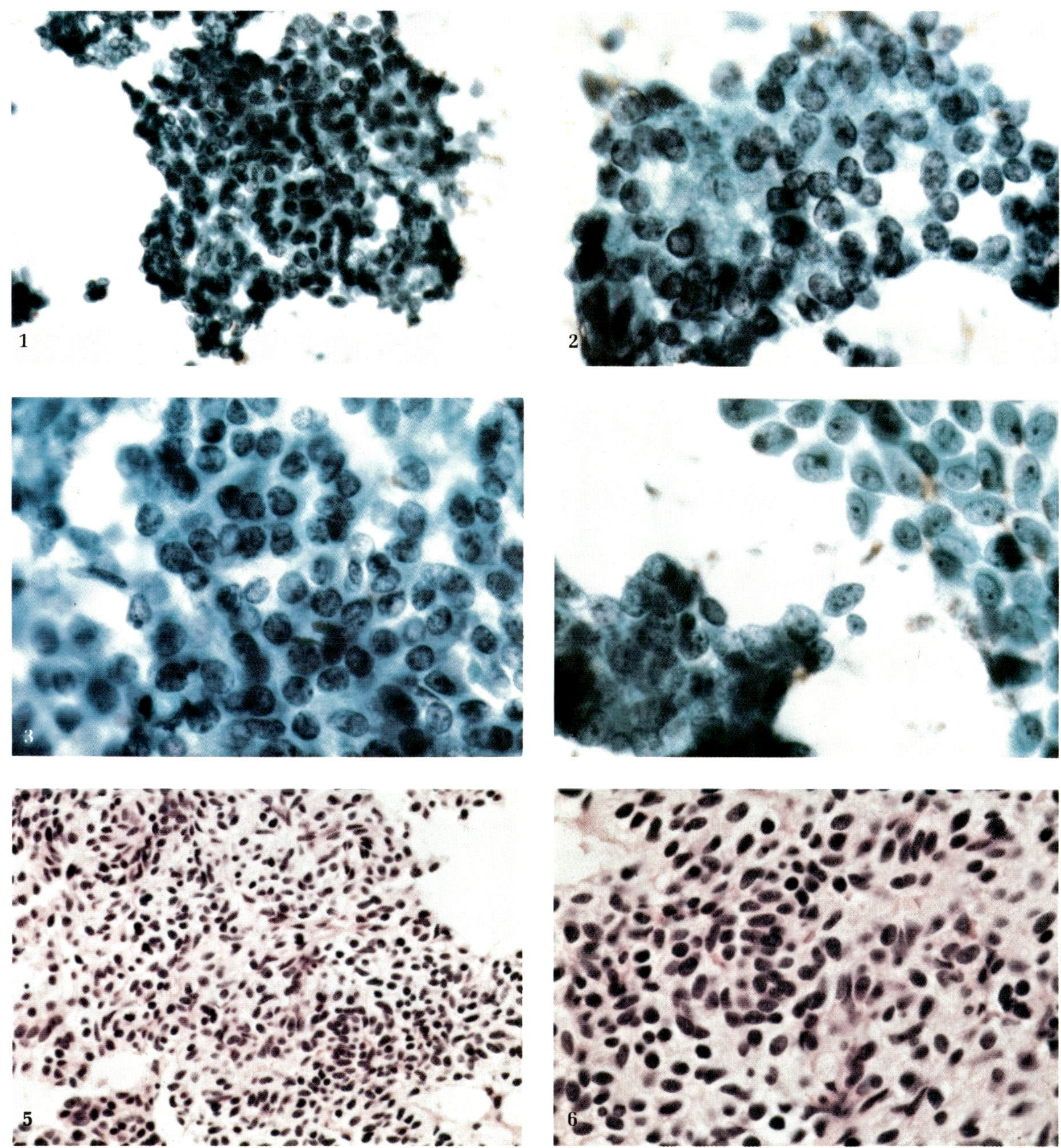

PLATE 45

Carcinoid

Plate 45–1 to 45–3. Carcinoid in lung FNA smear (Papanicolaou stain; 45–1, × 200; 45–2, 45–3, × 400).

Plate 45–4. Benign mesothelial cells and carcinoid cells in lung FNA smear (Papanicolaou stain, × 400).

Plate 45–5, 45–6. Microscopic section of metastatic carcinoid in bone marrow biopsy specimen (H & E; 45–5, × 200; 45–6, × 400).

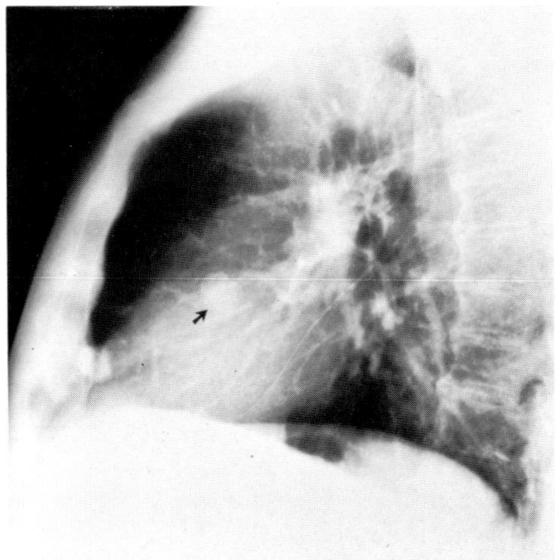

Figure A. Chest roentgenogram showing lateral view of mass in middle lobe of right lung *(see arrow)*.

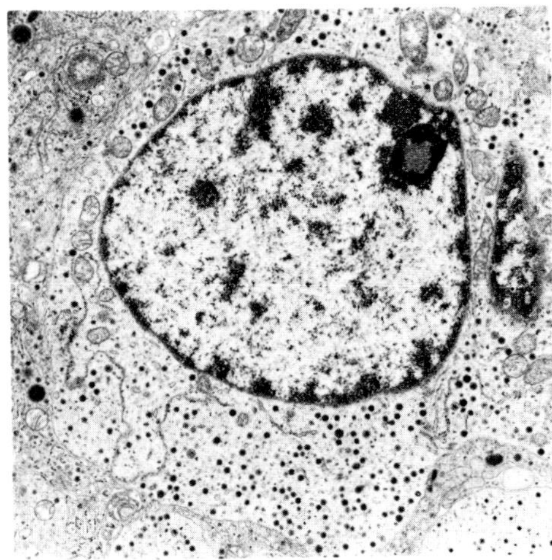

Figure B. Neurosecretory granules surrounding the nucleus of a tumor cell (× 7,800).

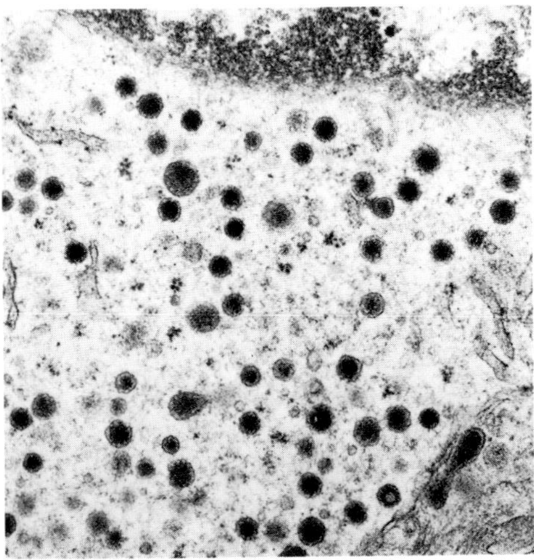

Figure C. High power magnification of neurosecretory granules seen in Figure B (× 20,000).

PLATE 46

Spindle Cell Carcinoid

Clinical History. A 64-year-old man with extensive coronary artery disease was admitted to the University of Virginia Hospital and prepared for a coronary bypass graft. His routine chest roentgenogram (Figure A) revealed a lung mass in the middle lobe of the right lung, which on tomography gave the impression of a primary lung carcinoma. An FNA of the mass was performed in the operating room during bypass surgery.

Cytologic Findings. The FNA smears contained numerous small cells with scanty, basophilic, delicate cytoplasm in a bloody background (Plate 46–1 to 46–4). The cell nuclei were variable in size, oval, elongated, or irregular in shape. The chromatin pattern was finely granular and evenly distributed. The nucleoli were small, occasionally irregular in shape, and frequently multiple. A diagnosis of carcinoid, spindle cell type, was made.

Pathologic Findings. A middle lobectomy of the right lung was performed at the time of the bypass surgery. In the excised tissue, there was a well-circumscribed, moderately soft, 1.7-cm mass that on cut section was solid and grey (Plate 46–5). Microscopic sections showed a tumor composed of nests of haphazardly arranged cells separated by a very vascular stroma (Plate 46–6, 46–7). These cells were characterized by variability in size and poorly defined cytoplasmic borders. Their nuclei were round-to-spindle-shaped with uniform, finely granular chromatin and micronucleoli. These features were thought to indicate a spindle cell carcinoid.

Electron microscopy demonstrated numerous membrane-bound, electron-dense neurosecretory granules measuring 90 to 150 nm in diameter. These granules confirmed the diagnosis of a carcinoid (Figures B, C).

Refer to Slides 89 and 90 in Optional Slide Set.

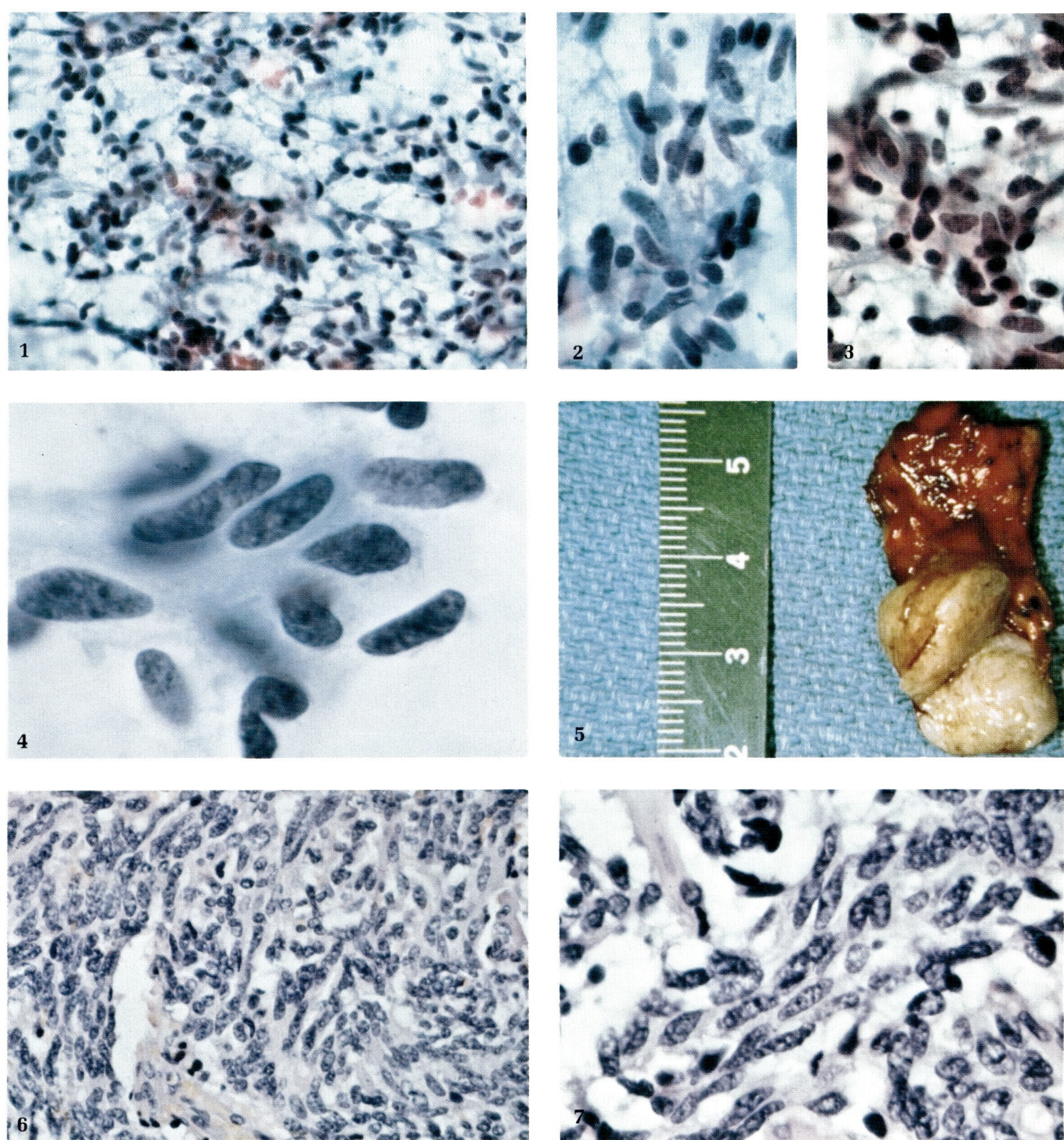

PLATE 46

Spindle Cell Carcinoid

Plate 46–1 to 46–4. Spindle cell carcinoid in lung FNA smear (Papanicolaou stain; 46–1, × 200; 46–2, 46–3, × 400; 46–4, × 1,000).

Plate 46–5. Gross lung specimen of spindle cell carcinoid. Scale is in centimeters.

Plate 46–6, 46–7. Microscopic section of spindle cell carcinoid of the lung (H & E; 46–6, × 200; 46–7, × 400).

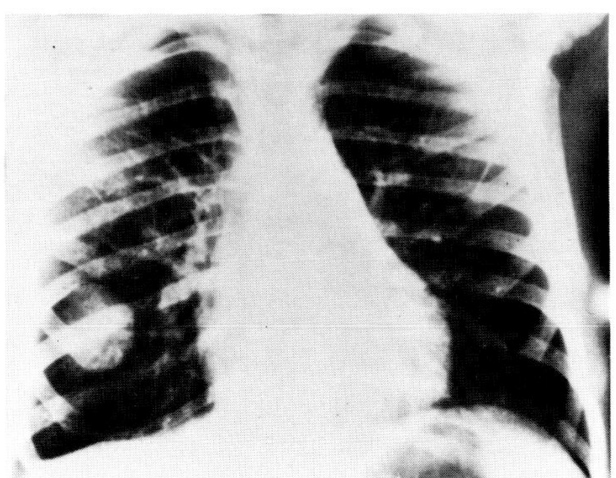

Figure A. Chest roentgenogram demonstrating spherical nodule in right lung.

PLATE 47

Pulmonary Blastoma

Clinical History. Three years previously, a 4-year-old girl had a resection of the middle and lower lobes of the right lung, which contained a multiloculated congenital cyst. A recent chest roentgenogram showed a spherical coin lesion in her right lung (Figure A). Fluoroscopically guided FNA of the lung lesion was performed.

Cytologic Findings. The FNA smears contained two distinct cell populations in a background of cellular debris (Plate 47–1 to 47–5). The first population consisted of numerous variably sized, round or oval cells lying singly and in aggregates (Plate 47–1, 47–2, 47–4). The cytoplasm was basophilic and scant. Cell borders were indistinct. The round or oval nuclei varied in size. The chromatin pattern was finely granular and occasionally clumped with parachromatin clearing (Plate 47–1). There was no significant hyperchromatism. Some nuclear molding was visible (Plate 47–4). Single, prominent nucleoli were seen in some cells. These cells were thought to be of glandular epithelial origin.

The second cell population consisted of syncytial arrangements of elongated, somewhat spindle-shaped cells with variably sized, oval or elongated nuclei (Plate 47–3, 47–5). The chromatin material was finely granular but irregularly distributed. Nuclear membrane indentations and irregularities were also visible (Plate 47–3). Occasional cells had prominent, single nucleoli. The cytoplasm was basophilic, and cell borders were indistinct. These cells were interpreted as mesenchymal in origin.

Because the cytologic pattern had both epithelial and stromal components, a diagnosis of pulmonary blastoma was made.

Pathologic Findings. A segment of the right lung contained a 4 × 5-cm, soft to rubbery, firm tumor. On cut surface, it was well circumscribed and tan to grey. Examination of microscopic sections showed a tumor having epithelial and mesenchymal components. Multilayered, columnar epithelium–lined tubules were surrounded by undifferentiated spindle- to round-shaped cells (Plate 47–6, 47–7). These histologic findings confirmed the diagnosis of pulmonary blastoma.

Refer to Slides 91 to 93 in Optional Slide Set.

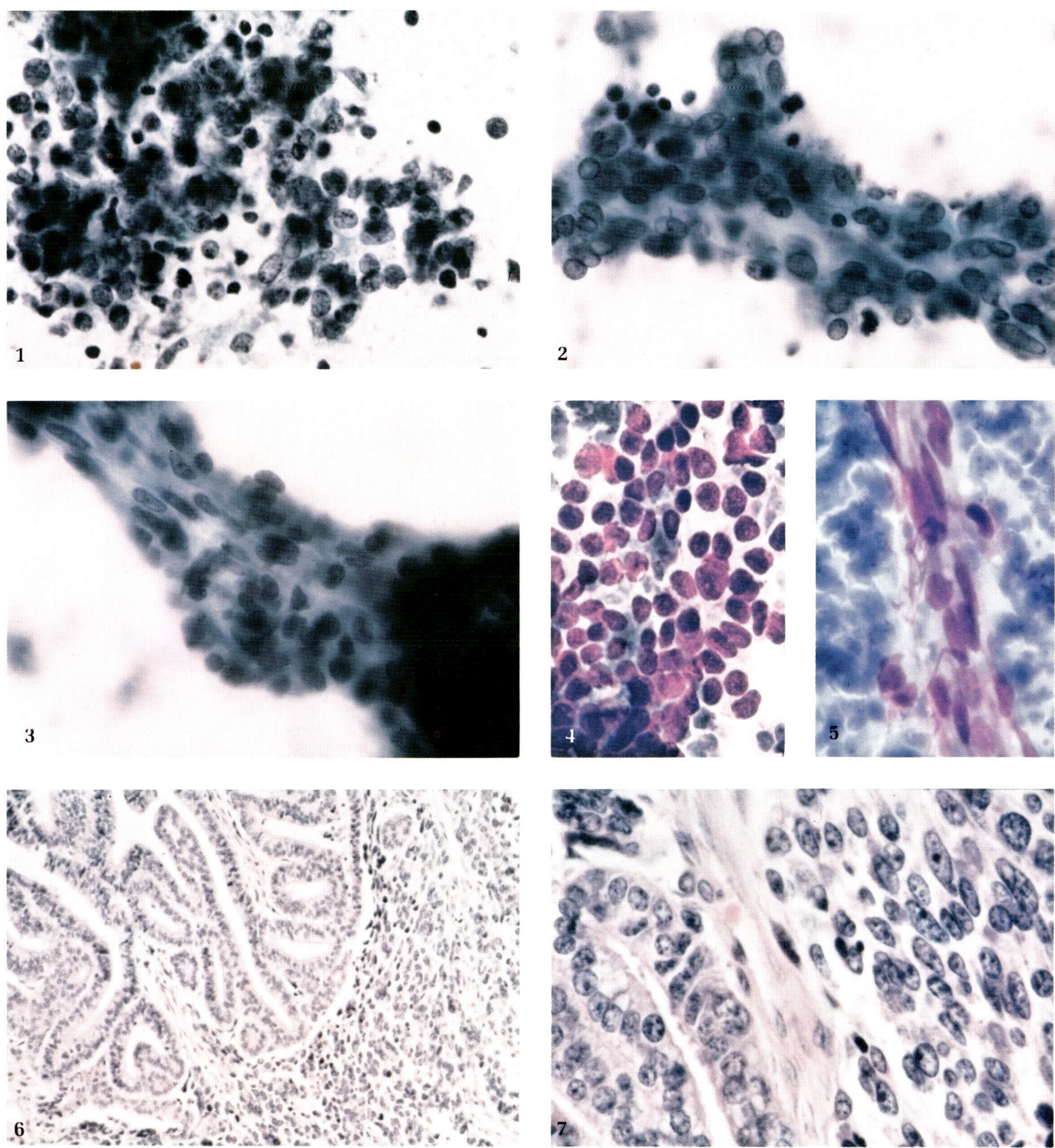

PLATE 47

Pulmonary Blastoma

Plate 47–1, 47–2. Epithelial glandular component of pulmonary blastoma in lung FNA smears (Papanicolaou stain, × 400).

Plate 47–3. Mesenchymal component of pulmonary blastoma in lung FNA smear (Papanicolaou stain, × 400).

Plate 47–4. Epithelial component of pulmonary blastoma in lung FNA smear (modified Wright-Giemsa stain, × 400).

Plate 47–5. Mesenchymal component of pulmonary blastoma in lung FNA smear (modified Wright-Giemsa stain, × 400).

Plate 47–6, 47–7. Microscopic sections of pulmonary blastoma in the lung (H & E; 47–6, × 100; 47–7, × 400).

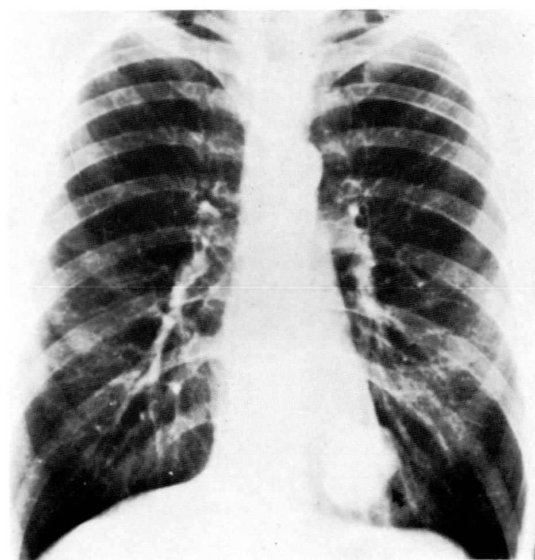

Figure A. Chest roentgenogram showing mass in lower lobe of left lung.

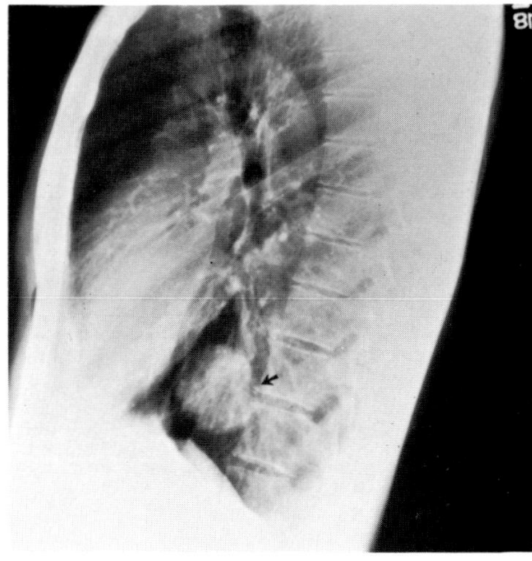

Figure B. Chest roentgenogram showing lateral view of mass in lower lobe of left lung *(see arrow).*

PLATE 48

Metastatic Malignant Melanoma

Clinical History. An asymptomatic 35-year-old man was admitted to the University of Virginia Hospital for evaluation of a mass in the lower lobe of the left lung. The mass was discovered on a routine chest roentgenogram (Figures A, B). Ten years ago, he had surgery for excision of a melanoma from the anterior right side of his chest. A right axillary lymph node dissection performed eight months after his surgery revealed metastatic melanoma. The physical examination on admission showed a well-healed scar on the anterior right side of the chest, but otherwise was within normal limits.

Cytologic Findings. Abundant tumor cells were observed in the FNA smears. These cells lay singly or in occasional aggregates (Plate 48–1 to 48–4). Cell clustering, sheets, and syncytia were not present. The nuclei were enlarged, varied in size and shape, and showed frequent irregularities in the nuclear membranes. The chromatin material was irregularly distributed with pronounced parachromatin clearing (Plate 48–4). The nucleoli were prominent. Eccentric nuclear placement and occasional binucleation were also seen (Plate 48–3, 48–4). Rare cells showed cytoplasmic invaginations into the nuclei, creating a clear space within the nuclei (Plate 48–3). The cytoplasm was basophilic and granular, without melanin pigment. Scattered mitotic figures were observed. These tumor cells were interpreted as being consistent with the amelanotic component of melanoma.

Pathologic Findings. The patient underwent a thoracotomy with lower lobectomy of the left lung. In the excised tissue near the base of the lobe, there was a well-circumscribed, multilobular, tan mass that was 4.5 cm at its greatest diameter (Plate 48–5). Histologic sections confirmed the diagnosis of melanoma (Plate 48–6 to 48–8). Hilar lymph nodes were free of tumor. Four years after the lobectomy, the patient was alive and well without symptoms.

Refer to Slide 94 in Optional Slide Set.

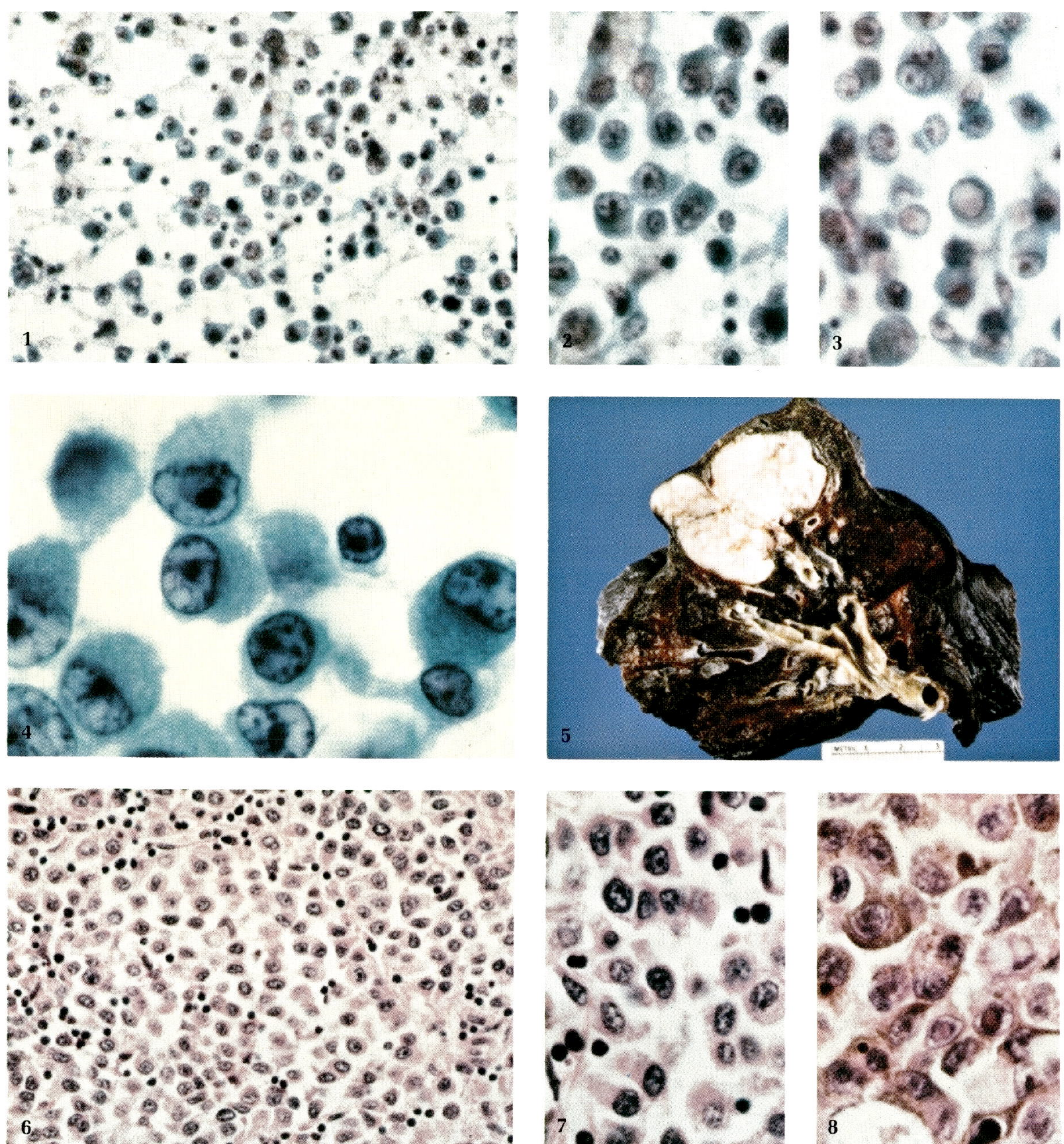

PLATE 48

Metastatic Malignant Melanoma

Plate 48–1 to 48–4. Metastatic malignant melanoma (amelanotic) in lung FNA smears (Papanicolaou stain; 48–1, × 200; 48–2, 48–3, 48–4, × 1,000).

Plate 48–5. Gross lobectomy specimen showing tumor mass.

Plate 48–6, 48–7. Metastatic malignant melanoma in microscopic section of the lung (H & E; 48–6, × 200; 48–7, × 400).

Plate 48–8. Microscopic section of pigmented portion of tumor mass (H & E, × 400).

PLATE 49
Metastatic Renal Cell Carcinoma

Clinical History. A 70-year-old man who had a nephrectomy for a renal cell carcinoma two years earlier was referred to the University of Virginia Medical Center for evaluation of an asymptomatic lung mass. His past medical history included chronic obstructive pulmonary disease and a smoking history of two packs per day for 15 years. The physical examination showed no abnormalities except for expiratory wheezes in the lungs. The results of pulmonary function tests were compatible with the presence of chronic obstructive pulmonary disease. A chest roentgenogram was obtained and showed areas suspicious for metastatic disease (Figure A). A percutaneous FNA of the lung was done under fluoroscopic guidance.

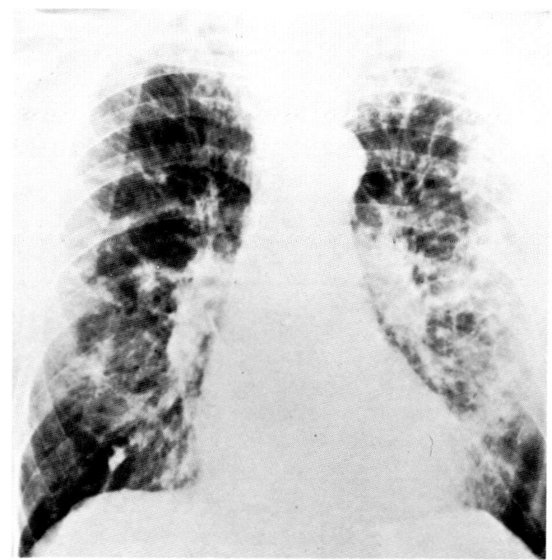

Figure A. Chest roentgenogram showing areas suspicious for metastases.

Cytologic Findings. The FNA smears contained numerous large, polygonally shaped cells with abundant, occasionally vacuolated, basophilic cytoplasm often containing pinkish-orange bodies (Plate 49–1, 49–2). The nature of these bodies was unclear. They possibly represented some form of storage vacuoles. The cell borders were indistinct. The nuclei were enlarged, round, and slightly hyperchromatic with finely granular, evenly distributed chromatin. The nucleoli were large, single, and rounded. These cells were similar to those seen in the previous nephrectomy specimen, and a diagnosis of metastatic renal cell carcinoma was made.

Pathologic Findings. A review of the slides from the patient's nephrectomy showed a renal cell carcinoma with nuclei of variable size, prominent nucleoli, and eosinophilic bodies within the cytoplasm (Plate 49–3). In other foci, the cytoplasm of the cancer cells was vacuolated (Plate 49–4).

Refer to Slide 95 in Optional Slide Set.

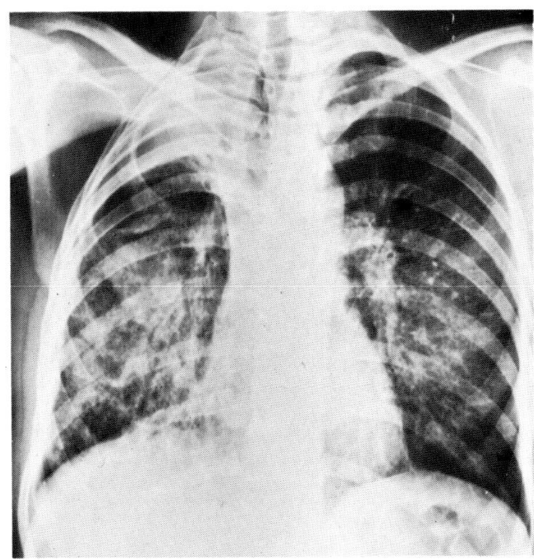

Figure B. Chest roentgenogram showing collapsed upper lobe of right lung with evidence of radiation fibrosis.

PLATE 49

Metastatic Breast Carcinoma

Clinical History. Five years before admission to the University of Virginia Medical Center, a 34-year-old woman had had a right radical mastectomy for an infiltrating duct carcinoma with two axillary lymph nodes containing metastatic carcinoma. She received radiation therapy and chemotherapy postoperatively. Despite this treatment, the carcinoma recurred in the wall of the right side of her chest and spread to her left breast.

She was admitted to the University of Virginia Medical Center because of shortness of breath. During the two weeks before admission, she had developed a cough with occasional hemoptysis. The physical examination showed many hard nodules over the right side of her chest in the region of the mastectomy scar. Similar nodules were palpable in her left breast. Examination of the lung revealed inspiratory wheezes and rhonchi. There was no evidence of consolidation. Chest roentgenograms showed a collapsed upper lobe of the right lung with evidence of radiation fibrosis. There were also changes suggestive of lymphangitic spread of the carcinoma (Figure B). Because the exact nature of the reticular infiltrates was uncertain, an FNA of the right lung was performed under fluoroscopic guidance.

Cytologic Findings. The FNA smears contained numerous abnormal cells with enlarged nuclei and abundant basophilic cytoplasm (Plate 49–5, 49–6). The mildly hyperchromatic nuclei were round or oval, but varied greatly in size. The chromatin pattern was finely granular and evenly distributed. Macronucleoli were present in many cells. Cell borders were often indistinct, creating syncytial cellular arrangements. These cells were interpreted as adenocarcinoma and were felt to be consistent with metastatic breast carcinoma.

Pathologic Findings. The original breast specimen slides were unavailable for review, but sections from the chest wall metastasis showed adenocarcinoma with cells similar to those seen in the lung FNA (Plate 49–7).

Refer to Slide 96 in Optional Slide Set.

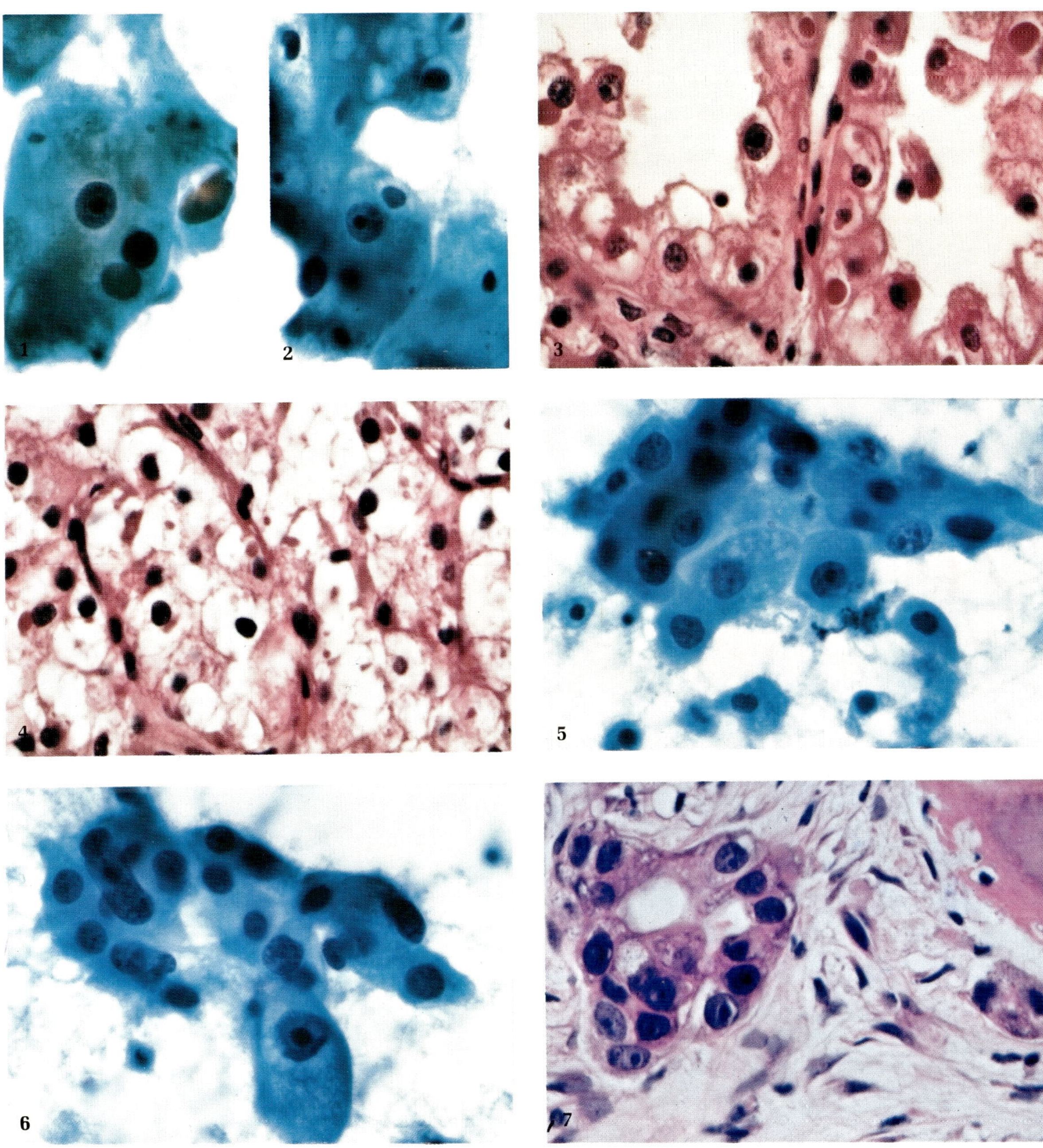

PLATE 49

Metastatic Renal Cell Carcinoma

Plate 49–1, 49–2. Metastatic renal cell carcinoma in lung FNA smears (Papanicolaou stain, × 400).

Plate 49–3, 49–4. Microscopic section of kidney tissue showing renal cell carcinoma (H & E, × 400).

Metastatic Breast Carcinoma

Plate 49–5, 49–6. Metastatic adenocarcinoma of the breast in lung FNA smears (Papanicolaou stain, × 400).

Plate 49–7. Microscopic section of metastatic breast carcinoma in bone biopsy specimen (H & E, × 400).

PLATE 50

Benign Metastasizing Leiomyoma

Clinical History. A 40-year-old woman, who five years previously had a hysterectomy for uterine leiomyomata, was admitted to another hospital for evaluation of an asymptomatic mass in her left lung. The mass was discovered on a routine chest roentgenogram (Figure A). Her physical examination on admission showed no abnormalities. A fluoroscopically guided FNA of the mass was performed.

Cytologic Findings. The FNA smears contained scattered, elongated, fiberlike cells either lying singly or in groups. The nuclei were thin and elongated (Plate 50–1 to 50–3), the chromatin pattern was finely granular and evenly distributed. Occasional small nucleoli were seen. The cytoplasm was basophilic and granular, and cell borders were often indistinct. Because obvious nuclear features of malignancy were absent and because the cells and nuclei had an elongated shape, these cells were interpreted as benign and consistent with leiomyoma.

Pathologic Findings. A biopsy of the lung mass was performed, and the excised tissue contained a 2 × 3-cm, well-circumscribed, tan-pink tumor (Plate 50–4). Microscopic sections demonstrated elongated, cigar-shaped nuclei with no mitoses (Plate 50–5). The cytoplasm was eosinophilic with the hematoxylin and eosin stain and red with the trichrome stain. These histologic features were interpreted as representative of a leiomyoma.

A review of the slides from her hysterectomy showed leiomyomata with an absence of mitoses. We favored the hypothesis that the lung tumor represented a metastasis from her uterus, a so-called benign metastasizing leiomyoma. Hendrickson and Kempson (see "Suggested Readings") refer to the possibility that some of these tumors may result from dissemination of benign uterine leiomyomata by surgical trauma. In this case, we have not excluded the possibility of a primary leiomyoma of the lung.

Refer to Slide 97 in Optional Slide Set.

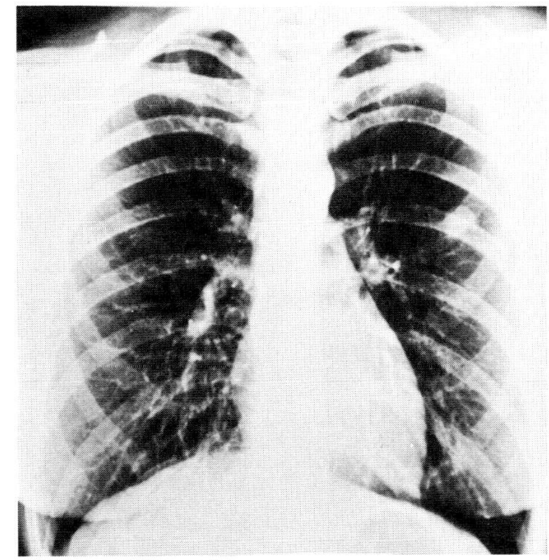

Figure A. Chest roentgenogram showing mass in left lung.

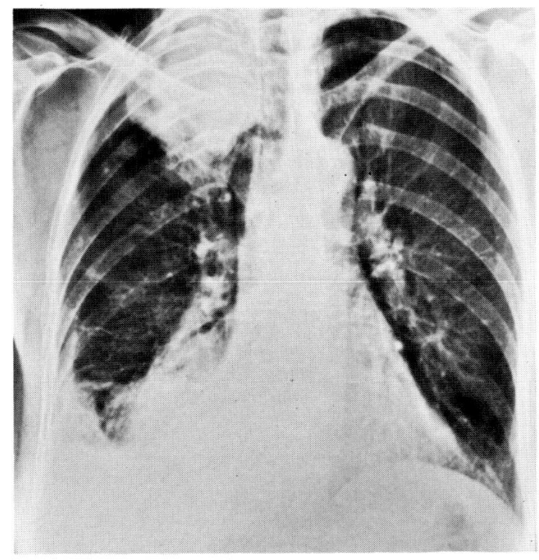

Figure B. Chest roentgenogram showing multiple lung masses.

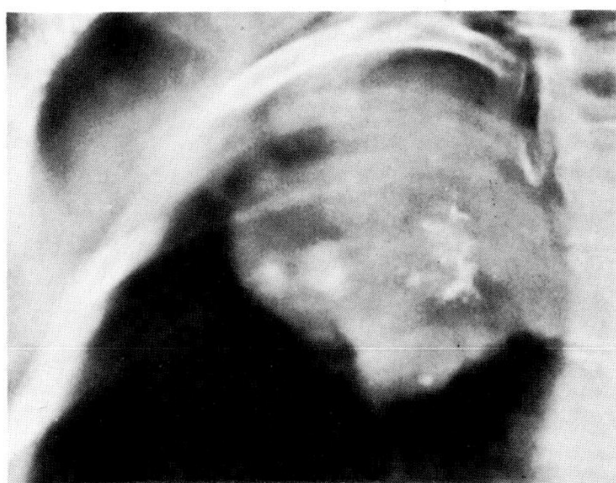

Figure C. Tomogram depicting mass in apical region of right lung at higher magnification.

PLATE 50

Extraskeletal Mesenchymal Chondrosarcoma

Clinical History. Ten years ago, a 53-year-old woman had an extraskeletal mesenchymal chondrosarcoma removed from her right thigh with a radical groin dissection. She had no further symptoms until three months before admission to the University of Virginia Hospital, when she noticed pain in her right scapula and shoulder and shortness of breath. Her chest roentgenogram and tomogram showed multiple lung masses (Figures B and C). Fine needle aspiration was performed under fluoroscopic guidance.

Cytologic Findings. The FNA smears contained scattered aggregates and sheets of abnormal, cuboidal-shaped cells in a clean background (Plate 50–6 to 50–8). Occasional overlapping of cells was visible within the groups (Plate 50–6). The cytoplasm of these cells was scant, finely granular, and basophilic-staining. Their nuclei varied in size and shape and showed moderate hyperchromatism (Plate 50–7, 50–8). The chromatin pattern was finely granular but irregularly distributed. Occasional nuclear membrane irregularities were seen (Plate 50–7). Prominent, rounded, and usually single nucleoli were identified in almost every cell (Plate 50–7, 50–8). These cells were interpreted as diagnostic of an undifferentiated malignant tumor.

Pathologic Findings. A review of tissue sections from the thigh mass revealed a sarcoma composed of undifferentiated mesenchymal cells that were round- to spindle-shaped and contained hyperchromatic nuclei and barely visible cytoplasm (Plate 50–9, 50–10). Islands of well-differentiated cartilage were scattered throughout the tumor (Plate 50–11). These features are characteristic of an extraskeletal mesenchymal chondrosarcoma, and the abnormal cells seen in the lung FNA were cytologically identical to those in the tissue sections from the thigh mass.

Refer to Slide 98 in Optional Slide Set.

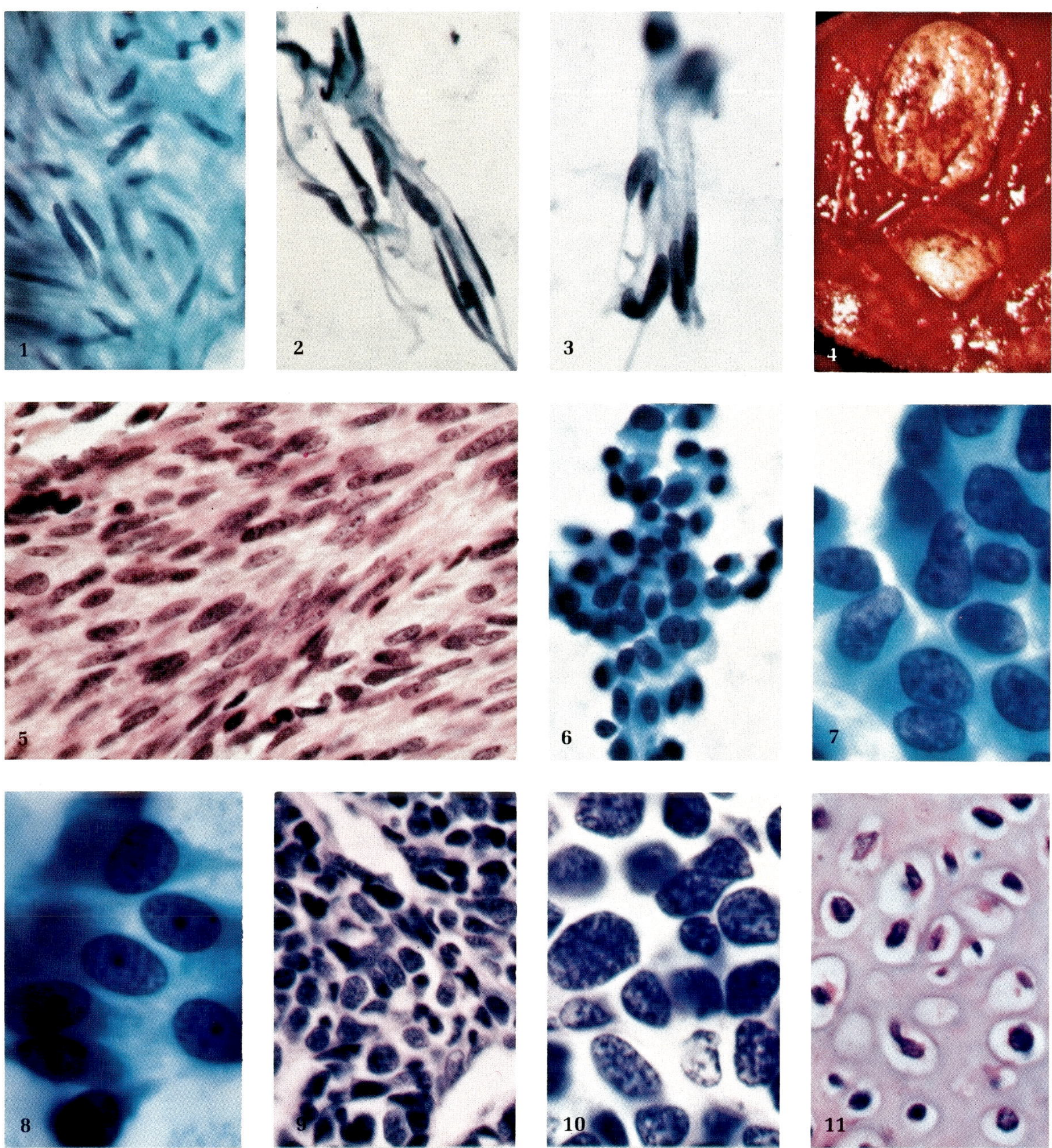

PLATE 50

Benign Metastasizing Leiomyoma

Plate 50–1 to 50–3. Benign metastasizing leiomyoma in lung FNA smears (Papanicolaou stain, × 400).

Plate 50–4. Gross appearance of tumor mass in the excisional biopsy specimen.

Plate 50–5. Microscopic section of leiomyoma in the lung (H & E, × 400).

Extraskeletal Mesenchymal Chondrosarcoma

Plate 50–6 to 50–8. Undifferentiated malignant cells consistent with sarcoma in lung FNA smears (Papanicolaou stain; 50–6, × 400; 50–7, 50–8, × 1,000).

Plate 50–9, 50–10. Microscopic sections of extraskeletal mesenchymal chondrosarcoma of thigh showing undifferentiated mesenchymal cells (H & E; 50–9, × 400; 50–10, × 1,000).

Plate 50–11. Well-differentiated cartilage seen in microscopic section of the tumor (H & E, × 400).

PLATE 51

Hodgkin's Disease

Clinical History. A 16-year-old boy came to the University of Virginia Hospital two years previously for evaluation of fatigue, weight loss, low-grade fever, and a mediastinal mass. A scalene lymph node biopsy revealed a nodular sclerosing type of Hodgkins's disease that was classified as Stage IIB after laparotomy. He received radiation therapy and chemotherapy. One year later, he suffered a relapse with mediastinal and pulmonary parenchymal disease.

Pulmonary biopsy of a persistent lingular infiltrate revealed Hodgkin's disease, and his condition was reclassified as a Stage IVB. He received additional chemotherapy. One month before his current admission he developed a temperature of 40 °C with neutropenia and a nonproductive cough.

He was readmitted to the University of Virginia Medical Center to rule out sepsis, and no evidence of sepsis was found. Oral candidiasis was diagnosed on admission, was treated, and resolved. The fever remained elevated with nightly spikes. His cough increased but was still nonproductive.

The physical examination showed that he had chills, a pulse rate of 100 beats per minute, temperature of 37.6 °C, and respirations of 24 per minute. He had markedly decreased breath sounds with decreased resonance over the left anterior midthoracic region. His chest roentgenogram showed a persistent lingular infiltrate (Figure A) that was unresponsive to a variety of strong antibiotics. The nature of the lung infiltrate was uncertain; possibilities included fungal and bacterial infection, *Pneumocystis carinii,* and neoplasm. A percutaneous FNA of the lung was performed under fluoroscopic guidance.

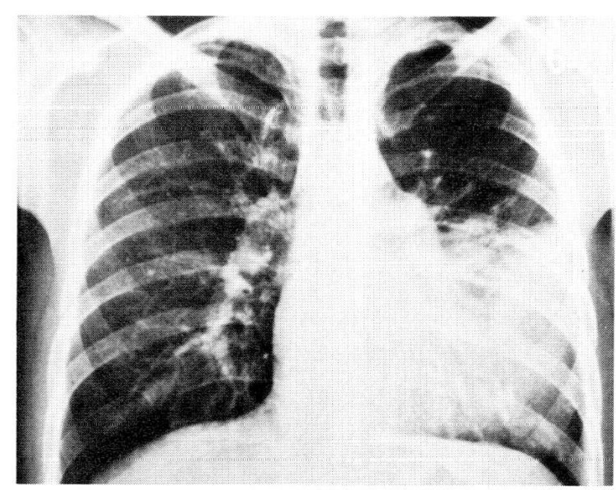

Figure A. Chest roentgenogram showing infiltrate in lingular region of left lung.

Cytologic Findings. The FNA smears contained enlarged mononucleated cells and giant cells with segmented or multiple nuclei (Plate 51–1 to 51–4). The nuclei were generally round or oval but varied widely in size. The chromatin was finely granular but irregularly distributed with obvious parachromatin clearing. Macronuleoli were often multiple and present in almost every cell. The cytoplasm was basophilic and moderate or scant in amount. The cells were arranged singly and in aggregates. True tissue formations were not observed. The cells were felt to represent malignant histiocytes (Plate 51–1 to 51–3) and Reed-Sternberg cells (Plate 51–4), and a diagnosis of Hodgkin's disease was made.

Pathologic Findings. The patient was treated with intensive chemotherapy and tolerated it well.

Six months later, the patient came to the emergency room in acute respiratory distress. He was treated, however, therapy was unsuccessful, and the patient died. The autopsy showed widespread Hodgkin's disease with extensive pulmonary involvement. Microscopic sections of the lungs confirmed the diagnosis of Hodgkin's disease. (Plate 51–5, 51–6).

Refer to Slide 99 in Optional Slide Set.

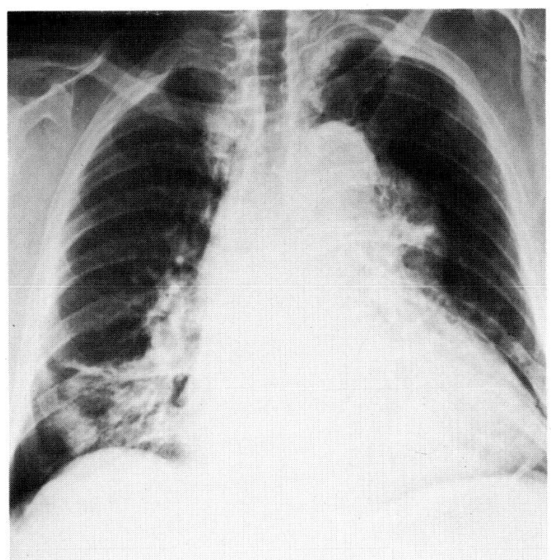

Figure B. Chest roentgenogram showing anterior mediastinal mass with hilar adenopathy and multiple lung lesions.

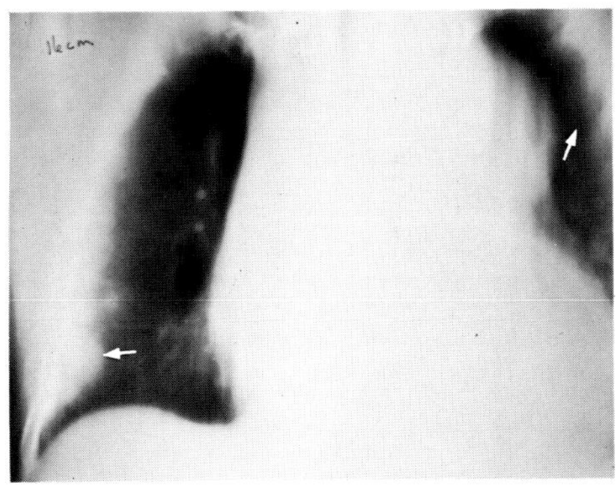

Figure C. Tomogram of chest showing multiple lung lesions *(see arrows).*

PLATE 51

Malignant Lymphoma

Clinical History. A 69-year-old man was in good health until he developed swollen testes and consulted his family physician who referred him to the University of Virginia Medical Center.

The physical examination on admission showed bilateral, swollen, nontender, firm testes and enlarged right inguinal lymph nodes. An FNA of his testes showed malignant lymphoma, and biopsy of an inguinal node showed malignant lymphoma, undifferentiated type. On the chest roentgenogram and tomogram, there was an anterior mediastinal mass with enlarged hilar lymph nodes and multiple lesions in his lungs (Figures B, C). An FNA of a peripheral lung mass was performed.

Cytologic Findings. The FNA smears contained numerous small, abnormal cells lying singly or occasionally in aggregates of three to five cells (Plate 51–7 to 51–9). Cell borders were poorly defined, and no true tissue formations were seen. The cytoplasm of these cells was scant and basophilic. Their nuclei varied in size and were usually round or oval with frequent nuclear membrane indentations or irregularities. The chromatin pattern was finely granular but irregularly distributed with chromocenters and parachromatin clearing. Mild or moderate hyperchromatism was visible. Prominent or macronucleoli were seen in almost every cell. The nucleoli were occasionally irregular in shape, multiple, or both. These cellular features were thought to represent a malignant lymphoma.

Pathologic Findings. A review of the FNA of his testes and the inguinal node biopsy (Plate 51–10, 51–11) showed cells identical to those seen in the lung aspiration. An abdominal computerized axial tomography scan showed tumor involvement of the kidneys and the para-aortic lymph nodes. He was treated with chemotherapy. Initially his testes decreased in size; however, the lymphoma progressed with central nervous system involvement. He died one year after his initial FNA diagnosis.

Refer to Slide 100 in Optional Slide Set.

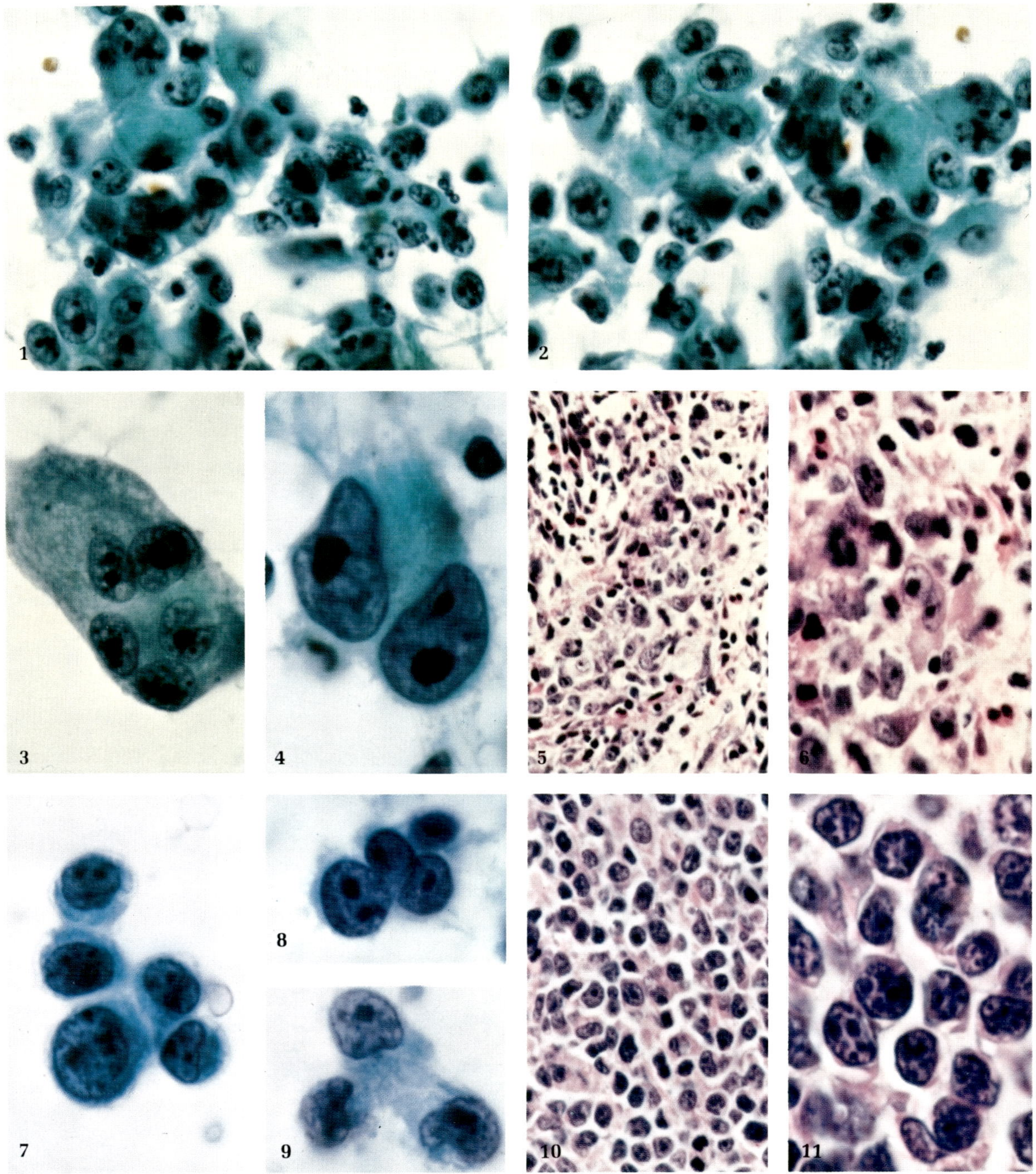

PLATE 51

Hodgkin's Disease

Plate 51–1 to 51–3. Malignant histiocytes of Hodgkin's disease in lung FNA smears (Papanicolaou stain, × 400).

Plate 51–4. Reed-Sternberg cell in lung FNA smear (Papanicolaou stain, × 1,000).

Plate 51–5, 51–6. Hodgkin's disease in microscopic sections of the lung at autopsy (H & E; 51–5, × 200; 51–6, × 400).

Malignant Lymphoma

Plate 51–7 to 51–9. Cells of malignant lymphoma in lung FNA smear (Papanicolaou stain, × 1,000).

Plate 51–10, 51–11. Microscopic sections of malignant lymphoma, undifferentiated type, in lymph node biopsy specimen (H & E; 51–10, × 400; 51–11, × 1,000).

Suggested Readings

Adenocarcinoma with Giant-Cell Component

Kallenberg F, Jaque J: Giant cell carcinoma of the lung. *Scand J Thorac Cardiovasc Surg* 1979;13:343–346.

Takenaga A, Matsuda M, Horai T, et al: Giant cell carcinoma of the lung. Comparative studies of the same cancer cells by light microscopy and scanning electron microscopy. *Acta Cytol* 1980;24:190–196.

Aspergillosis

Emmons C, Binford C, Utz J, et al: *Medical Mycology,* ed 3. Philadelphia, Lea & Febiger, 1977, pp 285–303.

Aspiration Pneumonia

Covell JL, Feldman PS: Fine needle aspiration diagnosis of aspiration pneumonia (phytopneumonitis). *Acta Cytol* 1984; 28:77–80.

Benign Metastasizing Leiomyoma

Hendrickson MR, Kempson RL: *Surgical Pathology of the Uterine Corpus.* Philadelphia, WB Saunders Co, 1980, pp 509-511.

Tench WD, Dail D, Gmelich JT, et al: Benign metastasizing leiomyomas: A review of twenty-one cases, abstract. *Lab Invest* 1978;38:37.

Blastomycosis

Emmons C, Binford C, Utz J, et al: *Medical Mycology,* ed 3. Philadelphia, Lea & Febiger, 1977, pp 342-363.

Johnston W, Amatulli J: The role of cytology in the primary diagnosis of North American blastomycosis. *Acta Cytol* 1970;14:200-204.

Bronchioloalveolar Carcinoma

Tao L, Delarue N, Sanders D, et al: Bronchiolo-alveolar carcinoma: A correlative clinical and cytologic study. *Cancer* 1978;42:2759-2767.

Carcinoid

Kyriakos M, Rockoff S: Brush biopsy of bronchial carcinoid—A source of cytologic error. *Acta Cytol* 1972;16:261–268.

Lozowski W, Hajdu S, Melamed M: Cytomorphology of carcinoid tumors. *Acta Cytol* 1979;23:360-365.

Coccidioidomycosis

Emmons C, Binford C, Utz J, et al: *Medical Mycology,* ed 3. Philadelphia, Lea & Febiger, 1977, pp 230-253.

Cryptococcosis

Emmons C, Binford C, Utz J, et al: *Medical Mycology,* ed 3. Philadelphia, Lea & Febiger, 1977, pp 206-229.

Gleason T, Hammar S, Barthas M, et al: Cytological diagnosis of pulmonary cryptococcus. *Arch Pathol Lab Med* 1980;104:384-387.

Extraskeletal Mesenchymal Chondrosarcoma

Guccion J, Font R, Enzinger F, et al: Extraskeletal mesenchymal chondrosarcoma. *Arch Path* 1973;95:336-340.

Histoplasmosis

Emmons C, Binford C, Utz J, et al: *Medical Mycology,* ed 3. Philadelphia, Lea & Febiger, 1977, pp 305-341.

Legionella micdadei Pneumonia

Hebert GA, Thomason BM, Harris PP, et al: "Pittsburgh Pneumonia Agent": A bacterium phenotypically similar to *Legionella pneumophila* and identical to the Tatlock bacterium. *Ann Intern Med* 1980;92:53-54.

Myerowitz RL, Pasculle AW, Dowling JN, et al: Opportunistic lung infection due to "Pittsburgh Pneumonia Agent." *N Engl J Med* 1979;301:953-958.

Rogers BH, Donowitz GR, Walker GK, et al: Opportunistic pneumonia. A clinicopathological study of five cases caused by an unidentified acid-fast bacterium. *N Engl J Med* 1979;301:959-961.

Walker AN, Walker GK, Feldman PS: Diagnosis of *Legionella micdadei* pneumonia from cytologic specimens. *Acta Cytol* 1983;27:252–254.

Mucormycosis

Emmons C, Binford C, Utz J, et al: *Medical Mycology,* ed 3. Philadelphia, Lea & Febiger, 1977, pp 254-284.

Nocardiosis

Emmons C, Binford C, Utz J, et al: *Medical Mycology,* ed 3. Philadelphia, Lea & Febiger, 1977, pp 103-115.

Pollack P, Valicenti J, Meyers D, et al: The use of fluorescent and special staining techniques in the aspiration of nocardiosis and actinomycosis. *Acta Cytol* 1978; 22:575–579.

Pulmonary Nodular Amyloidosis

Berclaz S: Amyloidose pulmonaire localisée multinodulaire. *Rev Med Suisse Romande* 1980;100:475-480.

Fénoglio C, Pascal R: Nodular amyloidosis of the lung. *Arch Pathol Lab Med* 1970;90:577-582.

Tomashefski J, Cramer S, Ambramowsky C, et al: Needle biopsy diagnosis of solitary amyloid nodule of the lung. *Acta Cytol* 1980;24:224-227.

Pneumocystis carinii Pneumonia

Demicco W, Stein A, Urbanetti J, et al: False negative biopsy in *Pneumocystis carinii* pneumonia. *Chest* 1979;75:389-390.

Dutz W, Burke B: Cytologic diagnosis of *Pneumocystis carinii. Natl Cancer Inst Monogr* 1976;43:157-161.

Kim H, Hughes W: Comparison of methods for identification of *Pneumocystis carinii* in pulmonary aspirates. *Am J Clin Pathol* 1973;60:462–466.

Pulmonary Blastoma

Anooshiravan N, Amir-Mokri E, Sarram A, et al: Pulmonary blastoma. *Chest* 1971;60:187-189.

Barnard W: Embryoma of the lung. *Thorax* 1952;7:299-301.

Francis D, Jacobsen M: Pulmonary blastoma—Preoperative cytologic and histologic findings. *Acta Cytol* 1979;23:437-442.

Karcioglu Z, Someren A: Pulmonary blastoma—A case report and review of the literature. *Am J Clin Pathol* 1974;61:287-295.

Spahr J, Draffin R, Johnston W: Cytopathologic findings in pulmonary blastoma. *Acta Cytol* 1979;23:454-459.

Spencer H: Pulmonary blastomas. *J Path Bact* 1961; 82:161-165.

Pulmonary Hamartoma

Dahlgren S: Needle biopsy of intrapulmonary hamartoma. *Scand J Resp Dis* 1966;47:187-194.

Ramzy I: Pulmonary hamartomas: Cytologic appearances of fine needle aspiration biopsy. *Acta Cytol* 1976; 20:15 19.

Spindle Cell Carcinoid

Craig I, Finley R: Spindle cell carcinoid tumor of lung. *Acta Cytol* 1982;26:495–498.

Ranchod M, Levine GD: Spindle-cell carcinoid tumors of the lung: A clinicopathologic study of 35 cases. *Am J Surg Path* 1980;4:315–331.

Squamous Carcinoma with Pancoast's Syndrome

Walls W, Thornbury J, Naylor B: Pulmonary needle aspiration in the diagnosis of Pancoast tumors. *Radiology* 1974;111:99-102.

Key to Optional Slide Set

Breast

Slide 1 **Abscess in Breast** Inflammatory cells, necrotic debris, and benign duct cells in FNA smear (Papanicolaou stain, × 400). *See Plate 1, Figures 1, 2.*

Slide 2 **Fat Necrosis of Breast** *Left:* Lipid laden macrophages in FNA smear (Papanicolaou stain, × 400). *Right:* Lipid material in FNA smear (Sudan IV stain, × 200). *See Plate 1, Figures 4, 8.*

Slide 3 **Gynecomastia** *Left:* Atypical ductal cells in FNA smear (Papanicolaou stain, × 400). *Right:* Microscopic section (H & E, × 400). *See Plate 1, Figures 11, 13.*

Slide 4 **Apocrine Metaplasia in Breast** *Left:* FNA smear (Papanicolaou stain, × 400). *Right:* Microscopic section (H & E, × 400). *See Plate 2, Figures 1, 5.*

Slide 5 **Fibrocystic Disease in Breast** Atypical cells in FNA smear, filter preparation of needle washings (Papanicolaou stain, × 400). *See Plate 3, Figures 1, 4.*

Slide 6 **Fibrocystic Disease in Breast** Atypical cells in cyst wall, microscopic section, (H & E, × 400). *See Plate 3, Figure 9.*

Slide 7 **Granular Cell Tumor in Breast** *Left:* FNA smear (Diff-Quik stain, × 400). *Right:* Section of breast tissue from excisional biopsy (H & E, × 400). *See Plate 4, Figures 1, 4.*

Slide 8 **Ductal Hyperplasia in Breast** *Left:* Mildly atypical ductal cells in FNA smear (Papanicolaou stain, × 400). *Right:* Microscopic section of breast tissue from biopsy (H & E, × 400). *See Plate 4, Figures 5, 9.*

Slide 9 **Atypical Ductal Hyperplasia in Breast** *Left:* Sheet of atypical ductal cells from FNA smear (Papanicolaou stain, × 400). *Right:* Microscopic section of breast tissue from excisional biopsy (H & E, × 100). *See Plate 5, Figures 3, 6.*

Slide 10 **Lactating Adenoma** *Top:* FNA smear (Papanicolaou stain, × 400). *Bottom:* Microscopic section of breast tissue from excisional biopsy (H & E, × 400). *See Plate 6, Figures 1, 5.*

Slide 11 **Tubular Adenoma in Breast** *Left:* FNA smear (Papanicolaou stain, × 400). *Right:* Microscopic section of breast tissue from excisional breast biopsy (H & E, × 400). *See Plate 6, Figures 7, 11.*

Slide 12 **Fibroadenoma in Breast** *Left:* Tissue fragment of benign ductal epithelium from FNA smear. *Right:* Fragment of stroma in FNA smear (Papanicolaou stain, × 200, left and right). *See Plate 7, Figures 1 (high power view), 7.*

Slide 13 **Fibroadenoma in Breast** *Left:* Fragment of benign ductal epithelium and numerous benign bare nuclei in FNA smear (Papanicolaou stain, × 200). *Right:* Benign ductal epithelium and stroma in FNA smear, (modified Wright-Giemsa stain, × 200). *See Plate 7, Figures 3, 8.*

Slide 14 **Papilloma in Breast** *Left:* Papillary cluster of benign ductal cells in FNA smear. *Right:* Connective tissue component from papilloma in FNA smear (Papanicolaou stain, × 200, left and right). *See Plate 8, Figures 1, 4.*

Slide 15 **Intraductal Papilloma in Breast** Microscopic section (H & E, × 40). *See Plate 8, Figure 8.*

Slide 16 **Infiltrating Duct Carcinoma in Breast** *Left:* FNA smear. *Right:* Benign ductal cells in FNA smear (Papanicolaou stain, × 400, left and right). *See Plate 9, Figures 3, 4.*

Slide 17 **Infiltrating Duct Carcinoma in Breast** Microscopic tissue sections from mastectomy specimen. (H & E, × 400). *See Plate 9, Figure 7.*

Slide 18 **Infiltrating Duct Carcinoma in Breast** *Left:* FNA smear (Papanicolaou stain, × 400). *Right:* Microscopic section (H & E, × 100). *See Plate 10, Figures 2, 3.*

Slide 19 **Infiltrating Duct Carcinoma in Breast** *Left:* FNA smear (Papanicolaou stain, × 400). *Right:* Microscopic section (H & E, × 400). *See Plate 10, Figures 6, 9.*

Slide 20 **Infiltrating Small-Cell Duct Carcinoma in Breast** Filter preparation of FNA needle washings. (Papanicolaou stain, × 400). *See Plate 11, Figures 3, 4.*

Slide 21 **Infiltrating Small-Cell Duct Carcinoma in Breast** Tissue section (H & E, × 400). *See Plate 11, Figure 9.*

Slide 22 **Comedocarcinoma in Breast** Papillary cluster of malignant cells in FNA smear (Papanicolaou stain, × 200, *left;* × 400, *right*). *See Plate 12, Figures 1, 2.*

Slide 23 **Infiltrating Comedocarcinoma in Breast** Microscopic section (H & E, × 100). *See Plate 12, Figure 9.*

Slide 24 **Tubular Carcinoma in Breast** Tubular structures in FNA smear (Papanicolaou stain, × 200). *See Plate 13, Figure 1.*

Slide 25 **Well-Differentiated Tubular Carcinoma in Breast** Mastectomy tissue section (H & E, × 200). *See Plate 13, Figure 6.*

Slide 26 **Inflammatory Carcinoma in Breast** *Left:* Malignant cells in filter preparations of FNA needle washings (Papanicolaou stain, × 400). *Right:* Tumor embolus present in dermal lymphatic (H & E, × 100). *See Plate 14, Figures 2, 4.*

Slide 27 **Male Breast Carcinoma** Infiltrating duct carcinoma in FNA smear (Papanicolaou stain, × 400). *See Plate 14, Figure 8.*

Slide 28 **Paget's Disease and Duct Carcinoma** Malignant cells in FNA smear (Papanicolaou stain, × 400). *See Plate 15, Figures 3, 6.*

Slide 29 **Paget's Disease** Infiltrating duct carcinoma in microscopic section (H & E, × 400). *See Plate 15, Figure 11.*

Slide 30 **Apocrine Cell Carcinoma in Breast** *Top:* FNA smear (Papanicolaou stain, × 200). *Bottom:* FNA smear (Diff-Quik stain, × 200). *See Plate 16, Figures 3, 5.*

Slide 31 **Infiltrating Carcinoma in Breast** Microscopic sections with apocrine features in mastectomy specimen (H & E, × 200). *See Plate 16, Figure 8.*

Slide 32 **Colloid Carcinoma in Breast** *Left:* Malignant cells in FNA smear (Papanicolaou stain, × 400). *Right:* Pool of mucin-containing tumor cells in FNA smear. (Papanicolaou stain, × 100). *See Plate 17, Figures 1, 2.*

Slide 33 **Colloid Carcinoma in Breast** Microscopic tissue section (H & E, × 400). *See Plate 17, Figure 7.*

Slide 34 **Signet-Ring Carcinoma in Breast** FNA smear (Papanicolaou stain, × 200). *See Plate 18, Figure 1.*

Slide 35 **Signet-Ring Carcinoma in Breast** Microscopic section of mastectomy specimen (H & E, × 400). *See Plate 18, Figure 8.*

Slide 36 **Papillary Carcinoma in Breast** FNA smear (Papanicolaou stain, × 400). *See Plate 19, Figure 2.*

Slide 37 **Papillary Carcinoma in Breast** Intraductal papillary carcinoma in microscopic section of breast tissue (H & E, × 100). *See Plate 19, Figure 3.*

Slide 38 **Medullary Carcinoma in Breast** Large tumor cells in FNA smear (Papanicolaou stain, × 400). *See Plate 20, Figure 4.*

Slide 39 **Medullary Carcinoma in Breast** Microscopic section (H & E, × 400). *See Plate 20, Figure 8 (high power view).*

Slide 40 **Lobular Carcinoma in Breast** FNA smear (Papanicolaou stain, × 400). *See Plate 21, Figure 1.*

Slide 41 **Lobular Carcinoma in Breast** Microscopic tissue section (H & E, × 200). *See Plate 21, Figure 8.*

Slide 42 **Lobular Carcinoma in Breast** *Left:* "Indian file" pattern in FNA smear (Papanicolaou stain, × 400). *Right:* Microscopic tissue section (H & E, × 400). *See Plate 22, Figures 1, 5.*

Slide 43 **Lobular Carcinoma in Breast** *Left:* Signet-ring forms in FNA smear (Papanicolaou stain, × 400). *Right:* Signet-ring pattern in microscopic section of infiltrating lobular carcinoma (H & E, × 400). *See Plate 22, Figures 6, 10, 12.*

Slide 44 **Malignant Cystosarcoma Phyllodes** Benign duct cells and sarcomatous cells in FNA smear (Papanicolaou stain, × 200). *See Plate 23, Figure 2.*

Slide 45 **Malignant Cystosarcoma Phyllodes** Microscopic section (H & E, × 400). *See Plate 23, Figure 10.*

Slide 46 **Angiosarcoma in Breast** Malignant cells in FNA smear (Papanicolaou stain, × 400). *See Plate 24, Figure 1.*

Slide 47 **Angiosarcoma in Breast** Microscopic section (H & E, × 400). *See Plate 24, Figure 7.*

Slide 48 **Osteosarcoma in Breast** *Left:* Benign osteoclast and malignant osteoblast in FNA smear. *Right:* Duct carcinoma component in FNA smear (Papanicolaou stain, × 400, left and right). *See Plate 25, Figures 4, 6.*

Slide 49 **Osteosarcoma in Breast** *Left:* Microscopic tissue section (H & E, × 200). *Right:* Duct carcinoma component in microscopic tissue section (H & E, × 400). *See Plate 25, Figures 7, 11.*

Slide 50 **Metastatic Carcinoma in Breast** *Left:* Metastatic small-cell undifferentiated carcinoma in FNA smear. *Right:* Metastatic ovarian carcinoma in FNA smear (Papanicolaou stain, × 400, left and right). *See Plate 26, Figures 1, 7.*

Lung

Slide 51 **Lipid Pneumonia** *Top:* Lipid-laden macrophages from lipid pneumonia in FNA smear (Papanicolaou stain, × 400). *Bottom:* Fat-positive material in macrophages (Sudan IV stain, × 400). *See Plate 27, Figures 1, 2.*

Slide 52 **Aspiration Pneumonia** Vegetable material in FNA smear (Papanicolaou stain, × 400). *See Plate 27, Figure 5.*

Slide 53 **Pulmonary Infarct** Benign histiocytes and atypical alveolar lining cells in FNA smear (H & E, × 400). *See Plate 28, Figure 1.*

Slide 54 **Pulmonary Infarct** *Left:* Atypical alveolar lining cells in FNA smear. *Right:* Atypical alveolar lining cells adjacent to pulmonary infarct in microscopic section of lung tissue (H & E, × 400, left and right). *See Plate 28, Figures 3, 8.*

Slide 55 **Chemotherapy and Irradiation Damage in Lung** *Left:* Highly atypical alveolar lining cells in FNA smear (Papanicolaou stain, × 400). *Right:* Diffuse alveolar damage in microscopic tissue section (H & E, × 400). *See Plate 29, Figures 1, 3.*

Slide 56 **Tuberculosis in Lung** *Left:* Multinucleated giant cell in FNA smear (Papanicolaou stain, × 400). *Right:* Acid-fast bacilli in FNA smear (acid-fast stain, × 1,000). *See Plate 29, Figures 4, 5.*

Slide 57 **Nocardiosis in Lung** *Left:* Marked, acute inflammation and necrotic debris in FNA smear (H & E, × 200). *Right:* Nocardia in FNA smear (Fite's acid-fast stain, × 1,000). *See Plate 29, Figures 8, 10.*

Slide 58 ***Legionella micdadei* Pneumonia in Lung** *Top:* Intracytoplasmic and extracellular acid-fast bacilli in FNA smear (Fite's acid-fast stain, × 1,000). *Bottom:* Direct fluorescent antibody stain for *L micdadei* in FNA smear (× 1,000). *See Plate 29, Figures 12, 14.*

Slide 59 **Histoplasmosis in Lung** *Left:* Macrophages containing *Histoplasma capsulatum* in FNA smear (Papanicolaou stain, × 400). *Right: H capsulatum* (Gomori methenamine silver stain, × 400). *See Plate 30, Figures 4, 5.*

Slide 60 **Cryptococcosis in Lung** Filter preparation of needle washings of FNA showing *Cryptococcus neoformans* (Papanicolaou stain, × 400). *See Plate 30, Figure 6.*

Slide 61 **Blastomycosis in Lung** *Left:* Epithelioid cells with *Blastomyces dermatitidis* in FNA smear (Papanicolaou stain, × 400). *Right:* Blastomyces organisms in FNA smear (Papanicolaou stain, × 1,000). *See Plate 31, Figures 3, 5.*

Slide 62 **Aspergillosis in Lung** *Left:* Hyphae of Aspergillus in filter preparation of FNA needle washings (Papanicolaou stain, × 400). *Right:* Hyphae of Aspergillus in FNA smear (Gomori methenamine silver stain, × 400). *See Plate 31, Figures 8, 10.*

Slide 63 **Coccidiomycosis in Lung** *Left:* Macrophage containing *Coccidioides immitis* in FNA smear (Papanicolaou stain, × 400). *Right:* Coccidioides spherule in FNA smear (Gomori methenamine silver stain, × 1,000). *See Plate 32, Figures 1, 4.*

Slide 64 **Mucormycosis in Lung** Fungal hyphae indicating presence of mucormycosis in FNA smear (Papanicolaou stain, × 400). *See Plate 32, Figure 6.*

Slide 65 **Cytomegalic Inclusion Disease in Lung** Viral changes in FNA smear (Papanicolaou stain, *left;* and H & E stain, *right,* × 1,000). *See Plate 33, Figures 2, 3.*

Slide 66 **Herpes Simplex Pneumonia Virus in Lung** Multinucleated giant cells showing the viral changes of herpes infection in FNA smear. (Papanicolaou stain, × 1,000). *See Plate 33, Figures 8, 9.*

Slide 67 ***Pneumocystis carinii* Pneumonia in Lung** *Left:* FNA smear (Gomori methenamine silver stain, × 1,000). *Right: Pneumocystis* wall with intracystic structures in FNA smear (modified

Wright-Giemsa stain, × 1,000). *See Plate 34, Figures 1, 2.*

Slide 68 ***Pneumocystis* Infection in Lung** Microscopic tissue section (H & E, × 400). *See Plate 34, Figure 4.*

Slide 69 **Pulmonary Nodular Amyloidosis** Amyloid *(left)* and normal bronchial epithelial cells *(right)* in FNA smear (Papanicolaou stain, × 400, *left;* × 1,000, *right*). *See Plate 35, Figures 2, 4.*

Slide 70 **Pulmonary Nodular Amyloidosis** *Left:* Microscopic tissue section (H & E, × 200). *Right:* Microscopic lung tissue section showing polarization of Congo red stain (× 100). *See Plate 35, Figures 6, 8.*

Slide 71 **Hamartoma in Lung** *Left:* Fragment of ciliated respiratory epithelium in FNA smear (Papanicolaou stain, × 400). *Right,* Cartilaginous matrix in FNA smear (H & E, × 200). *See Plate 36, Figures 1, 2.*

Slide 72 **Hamartoma in Lung** Benign cartilage admixed with cleft-like spaces lined by ciliated respiratory epithelium in microscopic tissue section (H & E, × 40). *See Plate 36, Figure 5.*

Slide 73 **Squamous Cell Carcinoma in Lung** "Cell in cell" arrangement of keratinized cells from well-differentiated squamous cell carcinoma in FNA smear (Papanicolaou stain, × 400). *See Plate 37, Figure 3.*

Slide 74 **Squamous Cell Carcinoma in Lung** Well-differentiated squamous cell carcinoma with focal necrosis (H & E, × 200). *See Plate 37, Figure 6.*

Slide 75 **Squamous Cell Carcinoma in Lung** Poorly differentiated squamous cell carcinoma in FNA smear (H & E, *left;* and Papanicolaou stain, *right,* × 400). *See Plate 38, Figures 2, 4.*

Slide 76 **Squamous Cell Carcinoma in Lung** Poorly differentiated squamous cell carcinoma in microscopic tissue section (H & E, × 400). *See Plate 38, Figure 7.*

Slide 77 **Adenocarcinoma in Lung** Filter preparation of FNA needle washings (Papanicolaou stain, × 400). *See Plate 39, Figures 1, 3.*

Slide 78 **Adenocarcinoma in Lung** Microscopic tissue section (H & E, × 400). *See Plate 39, Figure 8.*

Slide 79 **Adenocarcinoma in Lung** Giant cell component in FNA smear (Papanicolaou stain, × 400). *See Plate 41, Figures 2, 4.*

Slide 80 **Adenocarcinoma in Lung** Giant cell component in microscopic tissue section (H & E, × 400). *See Plate 41, Figure 7.*

Slide 81 **Bronchioloalveolar Carcinoma** FNA smear (Papanicolaou stain, × 400). *See Plate 42, Figures 2, 3.*

Slide 82 **Bronchioloalveolar Adenocarcinoma** Microscopic tissue section (H & E × 100). *See Plate 42, Figure 5.*

Slide 83 **Large-Cell Carcinoma in Lung** FNA smear (Papanicolaou stain, × 400). *See Plate 43, Figure 3.*

Slide 84 **Large-Cell Carcinoma in Lung** Normal bronchial epithelium in microscopic tissue section (mucicarmine stain, × 200). *See Plate 43, Figure 8.*

Slide 85 **Small-Cell Carcinoma in Lung** FNA smear (Papanicolaou stain, × 400). *See Plate 44, Figure 2.*

Slide 86 **Small-Cell Carcinoma in Lung** Microscopic section of lung tissue at autopsy showing small-cell undifferentiated carcinoma (H & E, × 400). *See Plate 44, Figure 6.*

Slide 87 **Carcinoid in Lung** FNA smear (Papanicolaou stain, × 400). *See Plate 45, Figure 3.*

Slide 88 **Carcinoid in Lung** Microscopic section of metastatic carcinoid in bone marrow biopsy specimen (H & E, × 400). *See Plate 45, Figure 6.*

Slide 89 **Carcinoid in Lung** Spindle cell carcinoid in FNA smear (Papanicolaou stain, × 400, *left;* × 1,000, *right*). *See Plate 46, Figures 2, 4.*

Slide 90 **Carcinoid in Lung** Microscopic section of spindle cell carcinoid (H & E, × 200). *See Plate 46, Figure 6.*

Slide 91 **Blastoma in Lung** Epithelial *(left)* and mesenchymal *(right)* components in FNA smear (Papanicolaou stain, × 400). *See Plate 47, Figures 1, 3.*

Slide 92 **Blastoma in Lung** Epithelial glandular *(left)* and mesenchymal *(right)* components in FNA smear (modified Wright-Giemsa stain, × 400). *See Plate 47, Figures 4, 5.*

Slide 93 **Blastoma in Lung** Microscopic section (H & E, × 400). *See Plate 47, Figure 7.*

Slide 94 **Melanoma in Lung** *Left:* Metastatic melanoma in FNA smear (Papanicolaou stain, × 400). *Right:* Metastatic melanoma in microscopic section (H & E, × 200). *See Plate 48, Figures 2, 6.*

Slide 95 **Carcinoma in Lung** *Left:* Metastatic renal cell carcinoma in lung FNA smear (Papanicolaou stain, × 400). *Right:* Microscopic section of the kidney showing renal cell carcinoma (H & E, × 400). *See Plate 49, Figures 1, 3.*

Slide 96 **Adenocarcinoma in Lung** *Left:* Metastatic adenocarcinoma of the breast in lung FNA smear (Papanicolaou stain, × 400). *Right:* Microscopic section of bone tissue biopsy specimen (H & E, × 400). *See Plate 49, Figures 6, 7.*

Slide 97 **Leiomyoma in Lung** *Left:* Benign metastasizing leiomyoma in FNA smear (Papanicolaou stain, × 400). *Right:* Microscopic tissue section (H & E, × 400). *See Plate 50, Figures 1, 5.*

Slide 98 **Sarcoma in Lung** *Left:* Undifferentiated malignant cells consistent with sarcoma in FNA smear (Papanicolaou stain, × 1,000). *Right:* Microscopic section of extraskeletal mesenchymal chondrosarcoma tissue from the thigh (H & E, × 400). *See Plate 50, Figures 7, 9.*

Slide 99 **Hodgkin's Disease in Lung** *Left:* Malignant histiocytes of Hodgkin's disease in FNA smear (Papanicolaou stain, × 400). *Right:* Microscopic tissue section (H & E, × 400). *See Plate 51, Figures 2, 6.*

Slide 100 **Lymphoma in Lung** *Top:* FNA smear (Papanicolaou stain, × 1,000). *Bottom:* Microscopic section of tissue specimen from lymph node biopsy (H & E, × 1,000). *See Plate 51, Figures 7, 11.*

Cross-Reference for Optional Slide Set

Breast

Plate 1	Slides 1, 2, 3
Plate 2	Slide 4
Plate 3	Slides 5, 6
Plate 4	Slides 7, 8
Plate 5	Slide 9
Plate 6	Slides 10, 11
Plate 7	Slides 12, 13
Plate 8	Slides 14, 15
Plate 9	Slides 16, 17
Plate 10	Slides 18, 19
Plate 11	Slides 20, 21
Plate 12	Slides 22, 23
Plate 13	Slides 24, 25
Plate 14	Slides 26, 27
Plate 15	Slides 28, 29
Plate 16	Slides 30, 31
Plate 17	Slides 32, 33
Plate 18	Slides 34, 35
Plate 19	Slides 36, 37
Plate 20	Slides 38, 39
Plate 21	Slides 40, 41
Plate 22	Slides 42, 43
Plate 23	Slides 44, 45
Plate 24	Slides 46, 47
Plate 25	Slides 48, 49
Plate 26	Slide 50

Lung

Plate 27	Slides 51, 52
Plate 28	Slides 53, 54
Plate 29	Slides 55, 56, 57, 58
Plate 30	Slides 59, 60
Plate 31	Slides 61, 62
Plate 32	Slides 63, 64
Plate 33	Slides 65, 66
Plate 34	Slides 67, 68
Plate 35	Slides 69, 70
Plate 36	Slides 71, 72
Plate 37	Slides 73, 74
Plate 38	Slides 75, 76
Plate 39	Slides 77, 78
Plate 40	None
Plate 41	Slides 79, 80
Plate 42	Slides 81, 82
Plate 43	Slides 83, 84
Plate 44	Slides 85, 86
Plate 45	Slides 87, 88
Plate 46	Slides 89, 90
Plate 47	Slides 91, 92, 93
Plate 48	Slide 94
Plate 49	Slides 95, 96
Plate 50	Slides 97, 98
Plate 51	Slides 99, 100

Index

Color figures are referred to by the plate numbers, and the page on which the plate appears is indicated in parentheses following the plate numbers. Slide numbers refer to the slides in the optional slide set. A list of the black and white figures in this book is found on page xi; a list of the tables, on page xiii. Black and white figures and tables are not distinguished from text in this index.

R

S

T

U-Z